Cholesterol, Children, and Heart Disease

An Analysis of Alternatives

DONALD M. BERWICK, M.D.
SHAN CRETIN, Ph.D.
EMMETT B. KEELER, Ph.D.

New York / Oxford
OXFORD UNIVERSITY PRESS
1980

Library of Congress Cataloging in Publication Data

Berwick, Donald M 1946–
Cholesterol, children, and heart disease.

Bibliography: p.
Includes index.
1. Hypercholesterolemia in children—United States—Diagnosis—Cost effectiveness. 2. Medical screening—United States—Cost effectiveness. 3. Cardiovascular system—Diseases—United States—Prevention.
4. Medical policy—United States. I. Cretin, Shan, joint author. II. Keeler, Emmett B., joint author.
III. Title. [DNLM: 1. Cholesterol, Dietary—Adverse effects. 2. Heart diseases—In infancy and childhood. 3. Heart diseases—In infancy and childhood. 4. Mass screening—In infancy and childhood.
5. Public policy—United States. WS290 B553c]
RJ399.H94B47 362.1'9612 80-12307
ISBN 0-19-502669-1

Printed in the United States of America

To Ann,
and to our children

Foreword

This fascinating volume deserves the attention of physicians, particularly pediatricians and cardiologists, as well as economists and health planners.

The interest for the physicians is based, on one level, on the excellent review of the voluminous cholesterol-atherosclerosis literature and the perceptive critique thereof. Through meticulous dissection, the book separates facts from inferences and from religious convictions. On a second level, this treatise deserves the attention of the physician of the last quarter of this century because its message extends beyond the cholesterol controversy. Specifically the authors, after examining the methods of dietary approaches to atherosclerosis control, turn their attention to the practicality and economic feasibility of three specific proposals: mass screening, screening of high-risk children, and mass propaganda as exemplified by Finland's North Karelia Project and Sweden's antismoking campaign. The importance of this analysis, the major portion of the book, obviously transcends cardiology. It presents a model applicable to almost all attempts at controlling disease on a national scale.

Up to perhaps the end of the 19th century, the ministrations of physicians were pretty ineffective, at least from the patients' points of view. In all fairness one has to recognize, however, that when no outright harm was done to the patient through bleeding, purging, or tooth extraction, or all the above, doctors may well have helped patients to feel better through moral support and kindness.

Although physicians have always lived relatively well and occupied a privileged position in society, there was no "Health Industry," up until quite recently, to drain the national economy. With the advent of modern medicine and technology, potent tools were given to the doctor to combat disease. At the same time, patients have come to bemoan the loss of personal attention from their family physicians. On careful consideration, patients probably would not want to give up the benefits of chemotherapy, modern surgery and anesthesiology, or radiology; but, obviously, the ideal is to have both: effective treatment delivered compassionately.

This luxurious goal is clearly very expensive. But, while the Health Industry claimed a larger and larger portion of the GNP, the conventional medical school curriculum did not face up to the problem of cost. Doctors, secure in their roles and incomes, did not worry directly about the cost of medical services, and even impoverished patients, by and large, received many of the benefits of modern medical services.

With the growth of the Health Industry, the development of expensive and effective diagnostic and treatment modalities, the emergence of propaganda as a tool to influence health practices, and the threatening control of third-party payers, economic considerations have today become central issues in the lives of every practicing doctor, public health physician, and investigator. Most of us had no training in economics and no interest in it; we wanted to track down disease and eradicate it. The cost did not matter. Now, with health consuming close to ten percent of the GNP, the finiteness of our resources becomes manifest. Governmental agencies, state and federal, are only too anxious to manage the financial limitations of health care. Many doctors are angry and frustrated, often finding solace in heady draughts of reactionary politics.

This book, over and beyond the trials and tribulations of cholesterol, teaches us an approach to analyzing health policy alternatives. It looks at dollars, atherosclerotic plaques, and epidemiology with equal expertise. It should inspire our young physicians to undertake this type of medico-economic research and to teach the economic facts of life to their colleagues. It is hoped that physicians with this type of training will enter the corridors of government and participate actively, with politicians, to forge an intelligent health policy for the nation.

Alexander S. Nadas, M.D.
Chief, Department of Cardiology
Children's Hospital Medical Center
Professor of Pediatrics
Harvard Medical School

Preface

This book is about strategies for fighting the greatest cause of mortality in the industrialized world, coronary heart disease, by attacking one of the most powerful risk factors for heart disease: elevated cholesterol levels in the bloodstream. Using cost-effectiveness analysis, we compare different programs which have been suggested for lowering cholesterol levels through childhood screening, through early dietary intervention, and through population-wide educational efforts. The programs we evaluate are in all cases hypothetical—extrapolations from pilot studies or from the recommendations of experts.

We are well aware that the evidence linking cholesterol and heart disease, though copious, does not prove unequivocally that cholesterol reduction will prevent heart disease. Indeed, we chose this problem partly *because* of that uncertainty, believing that in medicine, as in other fields, policies must often be formulated in the midst of controversy. The work in this book demonstrates a way to organize available information to aid in making decisions that cannot be delayed despite residual uncertainties.

We have intended from the outset that our readers, like the authors, should come from a variety of disciplines. For physicians, we offer a sound review of the relationship of cholesterol to coronary disease, a discussion of possible clinical approaches to the prevention of coronary disease, and an introduction to cost-effectiveness analysis. Physicians who specialize in cardiology, preventive medicine, genetics, or metabolic diseases may have special interest in our models and their conclusions. For public health professionals, we offer an example of a tool in policy analysis, using a case-study which demonstrates many of the strengths and weaknesses of applying cost-effectiveness analysis to questions of health policy. For professionals and researchers in public policy, economics, and statistics, we hope that our book can be a useful guide for undertaking similar studies of other issues. For students of these disciplines, we have tried to be clear enough and systematic enough to help the reader learn by example.

Finally, for all our readers, we have tried to offer a realistic view of how quantitiative analysis might best be used in policy making. Somewhere between blind faith in a new "science" that will generate perfectly rational policies and unalloyed cynicism about efforts to bring numbers into a purely political process lies a middle ground—a belief that systematic organization of what we know can improve our decision-making.

PLAN OF THE BOOK

The core of our book consists of seven chapters. Although our cost-effectiveness analysis employs a series of mathematical models, we have tried to make the body of our work as non-technical as possible, reserving the mathematics and theoretical work for a series of appendices which will be of interest primarily to methodologists in epidemiology, statistics, and economics. Our method, reasoning, and conclusions can be followed in the text without reference to the technical appendices.

Chapter 1 sets the stage, exploring the need for systematic methods for choosing among options in health care programs.

Chapter 2 reviews the voluminous literature on cholesterol and its relationship to coronary disease, and is designed primarily for those unfamiliar with that literature or with the vocabulary of lipids and heart disease. Knowledgeable readers may omit Chapter 2 without loss of continuity, or they may choose to refer to it for recapitulation of the literature.

Chapter 3 presents an overview of our methodology, and explores some of the major issues which arise when cost-effectiveness analysis is applied to a problem in health care.

Chapters 4, 5, and 6 contain the body of our analyses of, respectively, screening programs for all children, screening programs for high risk children, and community-wide efforts to control cholesterol levels without screening. In each category, we examine one typical program and one or more variations. We use sensitivity analysis extensively, testing the performance of these hypothetical strategies under varying assumptions about the biological, behavioral, and economic parameters affecting their cost-effectiveness.

At the end of Chapter 6 and throughout Chapter 7 we review and summarize the results of our analyses, and discuss the implications for heart disease prevention programs at both the community and national levels, for medical policy-making, and for biomedical and public health research priorities.

ACKNOWLEDGMENTS

This book began with the vision of Dr. Howard H. Hiatt, Dean of Harvard School of Public Health, who in 1974 established the Center for the Analysis of Health Practices as a laboratory for a new kind of interdisciplinary health-related research. In January 1975, under the umbrella of the Center, with support from the Robert Wood Johnson Foundation and the Commonwealth Fund, we three—a pediatrician, an operations researcher, and a mathematician—began looking at the question of the costs and benefits of screening for high cholesterol levels in children. Our immediate goal was to prepare a paper for presentation at a Conference on Genetic Counseling sponsored by the National Institute for Child Health and Human Development in Colorado Springs, Colorado. In two months, we uncovered hundreds of relevant, often conflicting articles and a dozen screening proposals worthy of consideration. Unable to represent the complexity of the issues fairly in a paper, we decided to follow up with a fuller treatment in what we then naively imagined would be a short monograph. Five years, two marriages, and four children later, we have finally produced this tome.

The path from paper to book was not always smooth. We received timely encouragement from Dr. Hiatt and from the Director of the Center, Dr. Howard Frazier, a man blessed with unusual patience, intelligence, and a sense of humor. The Center itself provided a supportive environment and resources, both physical and personal. Early in our work, we benefited from an exchange of ideas with Drs. William Stason and Milton Weinstein, who were then completing a similar analysis of hypertension screening programs. Other members of the Center, including Drs. Benjamin Barnes, Peter Braun, Harvey Fineberg, Don Shepard, Herb Sherman, and Mark Thompson, have critiqued our work at many stages. Patricia Hartge provided us with a thorough analysis of primary and secondary prevention studies. The Center's support staff, including Lind Fasciano, Penny Kefalas, Laurie Pearlman, Najla Salhaney, and Paula Zimlicki, patiently and efficiently plowed through many drafts to meet pressing deadlines. Eleanor Druckman allayed our administrative problems and our anxieties. Dawn Renear provided invaluable library services. Ms. Pearlman prepared our index.

We owe a particularly large debt to our Research Assistant, Christine Cann, who reviewed the extensive biomedical literature on cholesterol and kept us abreast of new developments. Her meticulous organization put this enormous body of information at our fingertips.

Our work has benefited, as well, from the criticism and suggestions of dozens of professionals outside of the Center. Professor John Farquhar and Ms. Nancy Ellsworth, of the Stanford Heart Disease Prevention Program, gave generously of their time to help us revise our analysis of cholesterol-lowering diets. Dr. Jan Breslow, of the Children's Hospital Medical Center, reviewed an early draft in detail and suggested many improvements in the organization and content. The Committee on Nutrition of the American Heart Association, chaired by Dr. Edwin Bierman, spent a number of hours exploring our work with us, as did the staff of the National Heart, Lung, and Blood Institute. The suggestions of these professional bodies have resulted in numerous adjustments and corrections. Other researchers who have contributed their time and ideas include Drs. Henry Blackburn, Michael Brown, Curt Ellison, Ralph Frerichs, Joseph Goldstein, Donald Lamphiear, Olli Miettinen, Arno Motulsky, Charles Phelps, Charles Sing, and Joan Slack. Not all of these investigators agree with our methods and conclusions—indeed, some have eloquently attacked them—but each has been generous in sharing his or her views with us.

Mr. Maurice Ford, of Harvard Law School, led a group of law students in exploring the legal implications of the programs we analyze in this book and helped us to modify our design accordingly. Mr. John Quelch, then of Harvard Business School, and Mr. Richard Manoff, of Manoff International, Inc., provided some of the background materials for Chapter 6. Ann Berwick spent many hours reading through several drafts, improving both style and substance.

We are grateful to the National Center for Health Services Research, whose small grants program, together with corporate funds from The Rand Corporation, funded the final year of work on this project. Computations were performed with the assistance of the Health Science Computing Facilities at UCLA, supported by NIH Special Research Resources Grant RR-3.

Finally, we wish to express particular gratitude to Mr. Jeffrey House, of Oxford University Press, who introduced us to the world of publishing. His support and encouragement have given us just the latitude we needed to bring this work to a close.

Without the help of these people, and many others unnamed, we could not have completed this book. The deficiencies that remain are solely our responsibility, but thanks to the interest and assistance of our colleagues, many errors have been caught and corrected. Thank you, one and all.

Boston D.M.B.
Los Angeles S.C.
Santa Monica E.B.K.
April 1980

Contents

Cholesterol, Children, and Heart Disease

1. Choosing policies in preventive medicine

INTRODUCTION: MEDICINE AND POSSIBILITY

The expansion of choice

The expansion of choice is both a boon and a burden for our times. From the modern near miracles of science and technology comes a constant stream of new opportunities to change the ways we live and work, opportunities that are nowhere more dramatic than they are in health and medical care. But with each new opportunity come new costs and hazards. If we refuse to use what science offers us, then we may forgo the chance to save lives and increase well-being, but if we too quickly adopt the newest device and the latest theory, we risk costly errors. When the early enthusiasm fades, the lifesaving miracle can prove to be an expensive disappointment that has drained our resources and disfigured our social systems without paying us back in proportion to our hopes.

This book is about making choices. We have chosen an example—the prevention of coronary artery disease by changing the diets of children—that is full of uncertainty. In the field of heart disease prevention, science has brought us to the brink of understanding, but we have not yet attained certainty. We can predict a person's risk of heart disease, we can describe the morphology and biochemistry of that disease with increasing precision, we can trace the course of disease in individuals from their early years, and we even know something about those special genes that render some of us unusually susceptible to premature heart disease. The evidence that we have leads us to suspicions and theories that, *if correct*, have strong implications for public policies in preventive medicine. Furthermore, with few exceptions, we have (or know how to find) the technologies that would make preventive programs feasible. The last link has not been forged, however; no irrefutable experimental proof exists that healthy diets reduce the risk of heart disease. The final choice remains difficult: We have clues about what we should do, and we know how to do it; but *should we act*?

In the chapters that follow, we will explore some of the current options in heart disease prevention, trying to describe in formal ways the dimensions of our uncertainty and to determine whether, within the boundaries of our knowledge, we may already be able to discover that some options are better than others. We will be studying cholesterol, a major risk factor for coronary artery disease, and we will evaluate primarily programs that are designed to prevent adult heart disease through childhood intervention. Before beginning that study, however, we will first, in this chapter, set our problem in perspective. We examine the use of a formal model to make choices in the field of preventive medicine. Why do we use a formal approach? Why must choices be made at all? And why do we focus here on prevention, instead of cure?

The explosion of cost

None of us gets a bill for "new medical possibilities," but we all pay. Our government supports new developments in medicine, as in other forms of technology, directly through its funding of medical research and indirectly through governmental health care programs like Medicare and Medicaid, through exemptions from income taxes for health care costs and insurance premiums, and through support for medical training. In 1977, the federal government financed over 60 percent of medical research expenses and almost half of our health care bill (Gibson and Fisher, 1978). As a result of these governmental contributions and the widespread use of private insurance, patients in 1977 paid out-of-pocket only 39 percent of their doctor's fees and only 6 percent of their hospital expenses. Even though universal national health insurance has not yet arrived, much of the burden of medical expenditures has already shifted from the sick to society as a whole.

With third parties paying so much of the bill, encounters between doctors and patients can have the freedom to be what most of us wish them to be: relationships of trust and personal advocacy. The physician in general need not ask about the costs of what he or she does, but only about how the patient can be best served. That is a property that we seem to want in our medical care, but it creates a serious problem; namely that while society has relieved many patients of the need for circumspection in incurring medical care costs, it has delegated to no one in particular the responsibility for making sure that the value of a service is, in fact, worth its cost. At a time when burgeoning technology is making available an expanding array of tests and treatments—the number of *types* of laboratory tests in general use, for example, doubles every 15 years—the resulting explosion of medical care expenditures is no surprise at all. If we multiply our rapidly expanding technology, with its new edifices, new machines, and new aggressiveness in diagnosis and treatment, times the rubric "money is no object"—the traditional guide of the physician and the patient—and add in the growing fear of "malpractice" suits because of too lax a diagnostic search or too limited a treatment, what we get is what we have—the exponentially increasing aggregate cost of medical care, shown in Figure 1-1.

Figure 1-1. National Health Care Expenditures.
(*Source.* Health: United States: 1976–77, DHEW pub. no. (HRA) 77-1232, 1977, p. 343.)

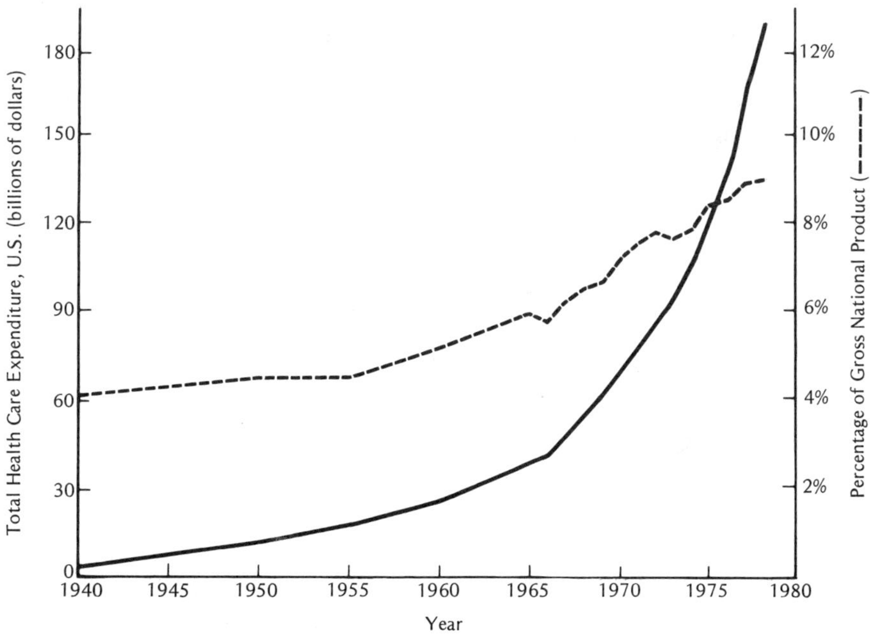

American political leaders are coming to realize that these costs must be contained and that only two broad strategies are available for containing them. On one hand, we can try to restore market incentives to patients by increasing their direct share of the costs or to providers by encouraging the formation of such provider groups as health maintenance organizations that can compete on the basis of price as well as quality of services (Enthoven, 1978). On the other hand, we can increase the legal and regulatory restrictions on resource use within which patients and physicians must operate. Either approach requires choices among the possible expenditures on health care. Some expenses will be accepted as reasonable, justified, and even necessary, but others will be rejected as ineffective or, even if effective, as beyond our capacity or willingness to pay.

The dilemma is uncomfortable. Either we must limit health care options, which forces us to make either tacit or explicit choices among possible technologies, or, in failing to limit options, we must pay a soaring bill that even today strains our willingness to pay.

What can we do? If we agree that we cannot afford to buy all technically feasible options, are there procedures short of political slugfests by which we can choose among them? Can we establish rational methods and guidelines for evaluation that will give us the chance to make reasonable and fair choices? In this book, we will work through in detail one type of health policy analysis that we believe should become part of decision making in the health field, a type of analysis that we believe can increase the odds for a rational and just decision.

With some readers, perhaps, we are already in trouble, for they may be offended by one of our central premises: that somebody must make choices. "Why," they ask, "can we not decide to buy all the options in health care that technology makes feasible? Health has the highest priority for individuals; why should that not be the case for our nation?" Indeed, almost any health care option does seem far more moral than many of the ways in which our government and industries spend billions of private and public dollars.

Yet the tethering of health care expenses is, in our opinion, an imperative, born not just of political pragmatism but also of reason. The currents of this argument will run through much of this book, but let us here make five points explicitly.

First, excellent health care can be purchased for much less than we spend now. The United States already devotes a larger portion of its gross national product to medical care than any other developed country except Sweden, including many nations with superb health care systems (Table 1-1).

Table 1-1. Private and governmental personal medical care expenditures per capita and percentage of gross national product spent on personal health care services, selected years

Country	*Year*	*Per capita gross domestic product (U.S. $)*	*Medical care share as % of gross domestic product*	*Per capita medical care expenditure (U.S. $)*
Australia	1972	3769	5.80	219
Austria	1971	2747	5.46	150
Canada	1971	4317	7.02	303
Finland	1972	2869	5.31	152
France	1970	2851	6.40	182
Germany, Federal Republic	1968	2246	6.07	136
Greece	1972	1374	2.51	34
Italy	1972	2164	6.12	132
Netherlands	1972	3437	6.78	233
Norway	1972	3889	5.18	201
Sweden	1971	4431	7.00	310
United Kingdom	1972	2742	4.45	122
United States	1972	5551	6.51	361

Source. J.P. Newhouse, Medical care expenditure: A cross-national survey. Rand Paper Series No. P-5608. Santa Monica, Rand Corporation, 1976.

Second, the contributions of the most expensive medical technologies to aggregate health (or even to individual health) often prove marginal or illusionary. Illich (1976) has argued at length that the overall impact of modern medical care is to *decrease* health. A more moderate view, with which we agree, was expressed by the participants in a recent conference on Technology and the Quality of Health Care (Egdahl and Gertman, 1978), where the problem addressed was more one of threshold: that is, ensuring that efficacious technologies survive, while ineffective ones are limited or made to wither. We believe that a significant portion of the most expensive technologies that come within our reach could disappear without much effect on our nation's health status.

Third, personal habits seem a far more potent determinant of health than does technology. Not only does this imply that behavioral changes, not better machines, promise a more satisfactory reduction of disease incidence, but it also tells us that people do not always value good health above all other goals. For many people, assuming that they are informed about what they do, the costs—either psychological or economic—of healthy behavior are too high to incur or the benefits of destructive behavior are too satisfying to reliquish.

Fourth, the constraints on medical dollars are imposed as much by politics as by laws of economics. Given the competing demands for public monies, the political pressures to control health expenditures eventually surface, as they have recently in congressional actions to control the costs of Medicare and Medicaid, two programs that uncontrolled, have wreaked havoc upon planned federal budget allocations for health care. In this political environment, the intelligent question to ask is no longer, "What is the best health care system available?" but rather, "What is the best system we can afford given alternative demands on our money?"

Fifth, as health care costs become increasingly the burden of society as a whole rather than of individual patients, a trend that is occurring even without formal national health insurance, the demand will increase for centralization of decisions about cost control and resource allocation. Recognizing this responsibility, both the U.S. Congress and the Department of Health, Education, and Welfare have added to their organizational charts in the past two years agencies whose primary responsibility is to evaluate and to encourage the evaluation of medical technologies. With the concentration of resource decisions in fewer hands, choices among alternatives will become increasingly explicit and will require comparably explicit criteria for choice. The search for such criteria is already under way, and our work is therefore as much a *description* of what is happening in medical decision making as a *prescription* for future decisions.

PREVENTION AND SCREENING

The rebirth of prevention

Although most of the recent attention to health resource allocation decisions has been directed at technologies, we have chosen a rather nontechnological public health issue to analyze. We have done so because we feel that the enterprise of disease prevention will become an increasingly important component in the health care of the future. We fear that in their fascination with scientific innovation, planners have tended to give the costs and benefits of prevention less serious scrutiny than they merit and that at least one important tool of prevention, screening for asymptomatic disease, is as susceptible as any modern miracle machine to misapplication and uncritical advocacy. Most of the costs and hazards in the road to modern acute-care medical technology lie equally in the path of modern disease prevention.

Traditionally, physicians and patients meet because the patient is ill. Without a complaint, there is no "patient," only an individual going about his or her daily work. The doctor, also, waits. In training, the physician learns to begin a case presentation with the "chief complaint"; "Using the patient's own words," begins the manual of medical reporting, "describe what is bothering him." The language of medicine preserves this passive attitude toward illness. It is no accident that the word "clinic"—the place where health care is delivered—derives from the Greek word for "bed."

That tradition is now changing. The growing awareness of both doctors and patients that their proper meeting ground extends far beyond the bedside has already fundamentally altered American health care. We are learning that the respondent attitude toward disease may not be the best. By waiting for illness to announce its presence, the patient and the doctor often lose time, money, the opportunity to relieve suffering, and sometimes even the chance to cure. Many diseases have asymptomatic stages, long periods during which a pathologic condition takes hold and during which the process may most easily be interrupted; the onset of symptoms may mark, not the beginning of the need to treat, but rather the end of the opportunity to treat effectively.

The challenge of disease in its asymptomatic stages creates a new problem: detection. Discovering disease without a patient-initiated complaint requires activists for whom health care is a process of reaching out, not merely responding. The search for hidden illness—screening—has had many meanings in the medical literature; for our purposes, screening is defined satisfactorily as *the testing of an individual for a personal attribute with the intent to intervene (if the test is positive) so as to prevent or mitigate the effects of a symptomatically silent disease process.*

This book is an effort to evaluate screening for high cholesterol levels, a risk factor for cardiovascular disease. We chose this particular topic in part because we believe that the years ahead will witness major expansion of preventive efforts in heart disease, and we would like that expansion to be less chaotic and costly than the explosion of high-technology, hospital-based medicine has been in the mid-twentieth century.

Why now?

The interest we see today in the early detection and prevention of disease is no whim; it is the product of several crucial trends in the way we Americans have come to think about disease and medical care.

Four of these trends have been particularly important: the limitations of therapeutic medicine, the changing nature of disease, the concept of a risk factor, and technological advances.

Therapeutic medicine, alone, holds little hope of dramatic improvements in morbidity and mortality in the next few decades. Despite impressive advances in some fields, such as the treatment of hyaline membrane disease and childhood leukemias, we have witnessed *a steadily decreasing return in health benefits for an exponentially increasing investment of dollars in health care.* The gains in life expectancy in the past two decades—amounting to one or two years for the American adult—though not negligible, are small, and the steady increase in the prevalence of chronic disease in our nation suggests that although we are living slightly longer, thanks in part to our medical care, the extra years may be ones burdened by pain and disability. In the absence of revolutionary breakthroughs in the treatment of established disease, improving the health of Americans is coming to require that we prevent disease before it expresses itself in symptoms.

An interest in prevention draws energy, as well, from *the changing nature of our burden of disease.* Instead of diseases of invasion from foreign organisms, the major threats of a century ago, we suffer today from the illness of cumulative damage to our bodies that results from our behaviors: what we eat, what we breathe, and how we spend our leisure. As Table 1-2 shows, seven of the ten major killers today are illnesses that are, in large part, the consequences of chosen behaviors. It seems a far better strategy to prevent these problems by changing how we live than to try to improve health by treating the morbid consequences of our choices.

A third development that increases our stock in prevention is the emerging of the concept of risk factors, the notion that people differ in their risks of developing particular diseases and that preventive efforts therefore need not always be distributed evenly across a population.

Without the idea of risk, we face enormous barriers to the management of asymptomatic disease. Everyone appears the same in the absence of a symptom; efforts to prevent a disease must be applied to *all* people, not just to the few who would eventually succumb. Only a few preventive measures—such as mass immunization or population-wide sanitation efforts—can be practicable if everyone merits treatment equally.

The concept of varying risk helps make prevention practical. The ability to distinguish among individuals in their chances of develop-

Table 1-2. Ten leading causes of death (United States, 1976) all ages

Male	*Female*
Heart diseases 400,536	Heart diseases 323,193
Cancer 205,406	Cancer 171,906
Cerebrovascular disease 80,597	Cerebrovascular disease 108,026
Accidents 70,277	Accidents 30,484
Pneumonia, influenza 32,513	Pneumonia, influenza 29,353
Cirrhosis of the liver 20,668	Diabetes 20,483
Suicide 19,493	Arteriosclerosis 17,553
Homicide 15,142	Cirrhosis of the liver 10,785
Diseases of infancy 14,198	Diseases of infancy 10,611
Diabetes 14,025	Suicide 7,339

Source. Vital Statistics of the United States, 1976.

ing symptomatic illness permits a concentration of effort on individuals at high risk and allows us to make a rational allocation of limited resources in preventive efforts. If a risk factor is causally connected to the disease process, then it may offer a specific lever for preventive intervention. If a risk indicator has no such causal connection but merely labels someone as highly liable to develop the disease, it may nonetheless be useful in allowing us to focus our nonspecific preventive resources on those individuals who will reap the most benefit.

Preventive medicine, finally, has benefited from some of the same *technological advances* that have altered the face of acute medical care. Most important among these advances have been the automation, miniaturization, and computerization of laboratory methods. A battery of tests that would have cost a patient $100 or more barely a decade ago can be performed today on multichannel autoanalyzers for less than one-tenth as much.

Because of innovations like this, what was a dream for the preventive medicine enthusiast of the past, the testing of large populations for biochemical abnormalities, has become a possibility. Technology has made mass screening practical.

In preventive medicine, however, no less than in acute care, the *ability* to act does not necessarily correlate with the *wisdom* of acting. It is highly unlikely that we should do all that we can do, even in prevention of disease. We have many reasons, only some of which have been mentioned here, to turn the attention of our health care industry toward prevention, but that attention must be tempered and must be informed by reasonable methods for sorting from our capabilities those enterprises that merit action.

The limitations of screening

The checkoff list: desirable criteria for screening

We err if we assume that when treatment of a disease falters or fails, detection and prevention will work. Despite the appeal of the idea that preventive medicine might solve problems before they overwhelm therapeutic medicine, prevention and screening have important limitations all their own. These limitations derive primarily from the following circumstances: prevention of a disease must involve many more people than will actually fall victim to that disease, while attempts to cure can be focused on only those few who are actually ill. Screening programs attempt to avoid wasting effort by testing a population to find those who would later be afflicted with disease, but unless the test used is extremely accurate, indentifying those people and *only* those people who would later acquire the disease, screening can be prohibitively wasteful.

In the pediatric literature of the last ten years alone, we can count nearly 100 conditions for which authors have shown screening to be possible, if not desirable. How can we possibly choose, aware as we are that some screening programs might cost far more in resources than they would return in added health?

The most frequent approach to the evaluation of screening proposals is a "checkoff list," a filtering device to detect faulty proposals. One such reasonable list of criteria to be met is presented in Table 1-3 and is similar to those published by Wilson and Jungner (1968), the World Health Organization (1971), and McKeown (1968)

For mass screening to be worthwhile, the disease for which we search must be socially significant and amenable to advantageous detection and treatment in presymptomatic stages, stages prior to those in which the patient would spontaneously seek out care. The screen-

Table 1-3. Screening is more advantageous if:

The disease

1. is an important cause of morbidity, mortality, or medical expense;
2. has asymptomatic stages;
3. is treatable, or progression is preventable during asymptomatic stages, or there is advantage to others in early detection.

The treatment

1. is more effective or efficient in early stages;
2. costs are low;
3. is acceptable to the people treated.

The screening process

1. is inexpensive;
2. is reliable, with few false-positive or false-negative results;
3. is acceptable to the subject population.

The population

1. suffers from the disease;
2. is accessible to the screening test;
3. is compliant with presymptomatic treatment.

The health care system

1. can offer diagnostic confirmation;
2. can offer therapeutic intervention;
3. shows consensus about diagnostic and therapeutic policies.

Note. The more fully each of the listed criteria is met in the conditions under which screening is conducted, the more cost-effective will be the related screening program. Such a list of criteria, however, is of little use in selecting from among alternative programs, each of which offers a different set of advantages.

ing test must be inexpensive, reliable, and acceptable to the screenees. The presymptomatic treatment must be relatively inexpensive and acceptable, as well, and must offer advantages over postsymptomatic treatment. The subject population must be afflicted to some degree with the disease, accessible to screening, and compliant with treatment. Finally, the local health care system must be or become able to offer diagnostic confirmation, effective treatment and follow-up, and some consensus about diagnostic and therapeutic policies.

Such lists of criteria are useful to filter out proposals that have severe deficiencies, but they are not panaceas for policymakers. There are inherent limitations to "checkoff" approaches. The criteria label important dimensions but do not specify where along those dimensions the margins of acceptability fall. Treatment, for example, must not be too costly, but how much is too much?

Furthermore, filters are not mechanisms for choice. The number of programs that successfully run the gauntlet of criteria may be beyond our ability to mount all at once, and we therefore need ways to choose among good programs, not merely to discard the bad.

The need to choose is not really new. Individual physicians have always chosen among available therapies for individual patients; institutions have elected to offer some services but not others; governments and private systems have adopted some public programs and voted down alternatives. A look at past social decisions may help us understand how choices like these have been made. In particular, we can enrich our understanding of the circumstances that tend to increase or decrease the value of screening by drawing on the growing number of evaluative accounts of screening programs. With this intent, we will review three short case histories: one of a conspicuous success (screening for phenylketonuria), one of a definite failure (screening for congenital heart disease), and one of a program that is difficult to categorize but that is rich in lessons for those who propose screening programs in the future (the use of mammography to screen for breast cancer).

Three case studies

Screening for phenylketonuria—a successful gamble. Phenylketonuria (PKU) is an inborn error of metabolism of amino acids leading, in the young infant, to the accumulation of a substance, phenylalanine, which is toxic to the brain. Untreated, PKU produces irreversible brain damage within the first several months of life, rendering the child retarded and often in need of institutionalization. Treatment consists of altering the diet in infancy and childhood to decrease the intake of phenylalanine and thus prevent the accumulation of this amino acid to toxic levels in the blood. The therapeutic diet must be adjusted so that amino acid levels are high enough to permit adequate growth and nutrition but low enough to prevent brain damage.

In 1961, Guthrie described a method of measuring phenylalanine in the blood so quickly and inexpensively that large numbers of infants could be screened for their phenylalanine levels—an immense technological breakthrough permitting the early detection of PKU and requiring only that all neonates be screened. Those with high levels, presumed to have PKU, could be placed on therapeutic diets *before* severe brain damage had occurred.

The rate of spread of this metabolic screening program has been dizzying. Barely a decade after Guthrie's test for PKU was introduced,

Levy (1973) reviewed the results of screening 13 million infants worldwide for PKU (with 1199 cases found). This rapid dissemination occurred despite persisting uncertainty about PKU intervention. In 1961, the following questions about PKU were unanswered.

1. What percentage of newborns with high phenylalanine would become retarded from PKU if untreated?
2. At what age (days? weeks?) did PKU produce measurably high phenylalanine levels?
3. Would diets that lowered phenylalanine intake reduce retardation, and to what degree?
4. Were "therapeutic" diets potentially harmful to normal children and/or to children with PKU?

With the Guthrie test available, a few well-controlled studies of these questions began to emerge, but the spread of the social policy of mandatory PKU screenings far outpaced the certainty of the evidence that dietary treatment would be efficacious in preventing retardation.

Bessman and Swazey (1971) reviewed the gaps between legislative initiatives in PKU detection and proof of the scientific assumptions underlying mass screening. Throughout the 1960s, our knowledge of PKU was insufficient to support at least two of these assumptions—that high phenylalanine *means* that symptomatic PKU will develop in the untreated infant and that treatment prevents retardation. As late as 1973, Nitowsky noted that our knowledge of the natural history of PKU was incomplete, that the degree of effectiveness of treatment was unmeasured, and that guidelines for treatment (age, phenylalanine levels, length of treatment) could not be set owing to a lack of information. At the time Nitowsky wrote, 43 out of 50 states had mandatory PKU screening programs.

Bessman and Swazey document the political steps that led from proposal to law in PKU screening and show clearly that the process was not one of orderly analysis and prediction but of impassioned advocacy swaying legislatures and executives. Suspicion became conviction, aspiration became intent, and tentative exploration became fervent advocacy—all in the absence of firm, scientifically valid evidence that the benefits of PKU screening would be anything near the costs. The advocacy for PKU programs in the mid-1960s was well intentioned, but it could not have been well informed; the evidence simply did not exist then.

Good fortune prevailed. The programs were adopted widely and, in retrospect, wisely. Some uncertainties remain about the absolute efficacy of PKU dietary treatment, but that treatment has proved safe in competent hands, and the rates of admission of PKU victims to institutions for the retarded have fallen far enough that we must rate the programs as very successful. Still, the history of this movement must leave us pleased, not with our wisdom, but with our luck. As Bessman and Swazey conclude: "What we have done so far with PKU should give us no cause for pride or self-satisfaction. If we examine the situation in which we find ourselves, we may be able to construct a more intelligent and effective approach to the application of science to social questions." It is such an approach that we seek to develop in this book.

Phonocardiographic screening for childhood heart disease: the components of a failure. In the mid-1960s, a computerized machine became available to record heart sounds, thereby permitting the examination of large groups of people for variations in heart sounds that are associated with congenital malformations and rheumatic fever. To test the value of this new technology in routine screening of asymptomatic children, a program was organized in Baltimore that screened almost 19,000 elementary school children over a two-year period (Matanoski et al., 1977).

The results were disappointing. From the entire group of 19,000, only one child was discovered to have a previously unknown condition (rheumatic heart disease) that required treatment (prophylactic antibiotics). Furthermore, the three hospital centers that participated in this project reported widely different rates of positivity on both initial and follow-up screens, and the overall detection rate for previously known and previously unknown congenital heart disease was far less than would have been predicted on the basis of the epidemiology of these conditions.

The elements of failure in this program are several. First, the conditions found tended to be known already to the participants' families. Screening can be of little value if the health care system without screening has a high detection rate. Second, the sensitivity and specificity of the screening test were not high enough for use in screening for extremely rare diseases. The program wasted effort in referring well children to cardiologists because of suspicious screening results, and the epidemiologic calculations suggest that a high proportion of the children who did have congenital heart disease may have been missed by the screening test. In general, when a "positive" screening result initiates an expensive process of confirmation or treatment, the screening test must perform exceptionally well (especially in its specificity) in order to be efficient. If, for example, a test with a sensitivity of 100 percent and a specificity of 99 percent—an excellent test by most standards—is used to screen for a disease with a prevalence of 1 in 1000, the test will falsely label ten screenees as positive for every one truly diseased person found.

Third, the performance of the screening test in the Baltimore study varied greatly among the participating centers, indicating that the abilities and thresholds of the people using the machine were as important as the characteristics of the machine itself in determining the program's efficiency. We must characterize, not the *screening test*, but rather the *screening test in actual use* in order to know how much cost and benefit will derive from a screening program. Programs with spectacular laboratory results may founder on the shoals of real-world application.

The Baltimore study thus suggests at least three questions to be asked before attempting mass screening. Are the conditions that are worth discovering truly unknown to the potential positive screenees? Are the specificity and sensitivity of the test sufficiently high to avoid an expensive rate of false-positive errors (a question that can be answered only with reference to the prevalence of the disease to be detected)? And, will the test "in the field" actually perform as well as it can in theory? A negative answer to any of these questions casts doubt on the usefulness of a proposed screening program.

Mammography in breast cancer screening—some complex lessons. In 1963, the Health Insurance Plan of Greater New York (HIP) began a large, long-term, randomized trial to study the usefulness of screening and early detection of breast cancer. Over 20,000 women aged 40 to 64 years underwent a series of screening procedures, including the taking of a medical history, a physical examination, and mammography. In all, almost 65,000 mammographic studies were performed on these women. The screening program detected a total of 132 cancers of the breast in the study group, and an additional 167 cases appeared in the same group but outside of the study examinations. Of those breast cancers detected through the screening program, 44 (15 percent) were diagnosed first because of mammographic findings alone (Shapiro et al., 1973).

Bailar (1976) has published a detailed analysis of the implications of the results of the HIP study for the widespread use of mammograms in screening. As he shows, the simple calculation that mammograms can detect 44 cases of breast cancer in 20,000 women (or 1 case in about 450) is a misleading and incomplete statement of the worth of the screening procedure. (We should note that the HIP study was designed with great sophistication and carefully avoided such a simplistic statement as this of its results.)

The results of a screening program for breast cancer fall victim to several important statistical biases. First, the "lead time bias," which results from the confusion of *early detection* with *prolonged survival*, can make screening appear more effective than it is in truth. If we are able to detect an untreatable, inevitably fatal disease two years before it would otherwise become manifest, then the "beneficiaries" of our screening program would have an apparent survival time two years longer than those who are not detected early. The benefit, however, would be an illusion.

Second, those cases of asymptomatic disease that have the most indolent and benign courses would be overrepresented in a cross-sectional screening study, and therefore positive screenees would, for this reason alone, have more favorable outcomes than average. Imagine, for example, that some forms of breast cancer were so aggressive as to be, for practical purposes, instantly fatal, while other forms grew slowly and caused death only after many years. A screening program at one point in time would detect far more cancers of the second type than of the first type, and it would appear that those cases "detected early" benefited from that detection, even though the effect was again a statistical illusion.

Third, symptomatic people might use a screening program as a source of diagnosis, whereas they would go elsewhere if no screening program existed. We overestimate the yield of screening if we assume, without question, that *all* cases detected would have been missed without the screening program.

Fourth, "early detection" may uncover and result in the treatment of diseases that, left alone, would run benign courses and never need to be treated. If, for example, some forms of breast pathology *look* cancerous but do not behave so in the long run, then early detection is a disservice to those women who would *never* become symptomatic.

Bailar argues that, for these and other reasons, it is an error to equate the *success* rate of a screening program with its *discovery* rate. Of the 44 women discovered to have breast cancer through mammography for example, some will die despite early detection, some would have gotten better (either spontaneously or with later treatment) without early detection, and some of those who do benefit from detection may have been symptomatic already and would have gone elsewhere promptly for diagnosis. Before undertaking any new screening program, we would be well advised to ask how strongly considerations such as these apply to the disease for which we intend to screen.

Another potential problem with screening becomes evident upon further scrutiny of the example of mammography; namely hazards in the screening procedure itself. X-ray exposure in large doses is known to be carcinogenic, and even the low-dose exposure involved in mammography may not be entirely safe. Bailar calculates, based upon extrapolations from high exposure levels, that the irradiation of routine mammography may well *cause* as many new cases of breast cancer as it detects. The lesson is that when screening tests are used to detect rare conditions in large populations, even tiny hazards associated with the test may become important in comparison to the benefits of early detection.

The breast cancer screener is fortunate in having several screening devices available, including, in the HIP study, medical history and physical examination in addition to mammography. When alternatives exist, it is useful to study the incremental value of one test as a supplement to another. This view helps to expose the limited value of mammography, since a number of cancers were detected in the HIP study by both mammography and history or physical examination. Bailar need ask not only what the value of mammography would be if used alone but also what the marginal value of the procedure is when added to more benign forms of screening. On this basis, he concludes that mammograms add little or no extra benefit, at least for younger women, when appended to a simple history and physical examination. A preventive medicine policymaker who is considering implementing a particular screening program should ask if simpler screening devices, perhaps with less associated hazard, are available.

The breast cancer example teaches one final lesson about evaluating a screening program; namely, it may not be obvious at first who can truly benefit from the program. Bailar concludes, for example, that the risk of cancers induced by mammographic x-ray exposure is considerably less for older women than for younger ones, since the latency period between exposure and induced disease is probably many years. In addition, women of advanced age are at especially high risk for cancer of the breast. The conclusion is that, although mammograms are probably not beneficial to all adult women, they may nonetheless be of significant benefit to women over the age of 60 or 65. Thus the simple question "Is screening worthwhile?" may not have a clear answer until we also ask, and think hard about, for whom we intend to use it.

THE VALUE OF ANALYSIS

How can we predict what will work? The proponents of each of these screening devices—PKU testing, phonocardiograms, and mammography—doubtless both hoped and believed that they possessed tools for improving the health of the population. Could they have known in advance whether they did, in fact, have such a tool or which subgroups of the population really stood to gain from their efforts?

Failures, or at least limitations on success, are unavoidable. We believe, however, that the formal techniques of quantitative analysis can greatly improve our ability to spot success or failure from a distance. Nothing can really replace the hard-earned lessons of experience in knowing how a proposed program will perform, but experience is not the only teacher. The methods we will demonstrate in this book can help us go a long way toward understanding where our future efforts may bear the most fruit and where, however attractive an idea may seem at first, disappointment lurks.

We are advocates of analysis. We propose to demonstrate the worth of our approach to evaluating proposed health programs through a case study in one area—the possible prevention of heart disease by alteration of diet.

Lowering the cholesterol levels of Americans, beginning with children, may prevent heart disease. The level of cholesterol in the individual's bloodstream correlates with the risk of subsequent heart disease, and many people now believe that lowering cholesterol levels through diet or drugs can reduce risk. Conceivably, all Americans could be screened for their cholesterol levels, apprised of their associated risks, and advised and guided to change their diets to achieve cholesterol reductions. Such a program is within our technical reach and already has strong advocates. Sooner than the wary may wish, choices may be made—to screen or not, to encourage dietary changes or not, to deal with subgroups of the population or with the entire population. Should we—physicians, health departments, legislators, private agencies, individuals—use what we now know about cholesterol and heart disease to mount preventive programs? Or, should we wait?

We could wait. The temptation is strong to delay until the data are clearer and the evidence more secure. Cautious writers underline the uncertainty: lowering cholesterol *may* reduce risk, but proof is lacking; public programs *may* persuade people to alter their diets, but we can only guess at the likely costs and magnitude of the effects. With such uncertainties, postponing a decision would seem a responsible plan.

In public health policy, however, social action has not always awaited the resolution of scientific uncertainty. Programs are often adopted, not when the data are conclusive, but rather when the data are suggestive and the political pressures are conclusive. Interest groups in our medical past have forced the enactment of health-related programs well in advance of sound information about costs, benefits, hazards, and efficacy. History suggests that to wait for certainty may be to yield the field to pressure groups less interested in analysis than in advocacy.

Once enacted, public health policies can become resistant to retrospective, impartial analysis. The programs generate in their own employees and clients alert groups whose interests are more in perpetuating the programs than in rating them. "Advocates" can be relabeled "experts," who monopolize access to information about the programs and claim unique competence to judge the propriety and efficacy of what they do.

Because enacted programs generate their own momentum and become relatively impervious to effective evaluation, systematic analysis of costs and benefits, if it is to be useful, must begin *before* programs are adopted, not after. It is therefore appropriate that the public health issue that we will explore is nascent; it concerns programs not yet in place and proposals still in their formative stages. In being early, we must use ambiguous information, but to wait may be to permit the issue to move out of reach of analysis—to allow rhetoric to replace reason and programmatic momentum to replace more impartial scrutiny.

In our analyses, we will address these questions: when to decide, how to decide, and which of several possible choices to select. However, athough we will address these issues, we will not produce a single, conclusive "right answer" to any of them. The tentative and even conflicting data on which we rely make predictions of policy outcomes uncertain. Even if this were not the case, even if the results of different policies could be perfectly foreseen, choices among those policies depend on the value systems of the decision makers and ultimately on the values of the people they represent. Under such conditions, the realistic demand to be made of quantitative analysis is not that it solve problems but that it illuminate and refine our understanding of them. The measure of our success at the end of this book should be, not whether we know for sure which choice to make, but rather whether our choice has been made a more enlightened one.

2. Cholesterol, heart disease, and policy

Cardiovascular risk factors in general, and cholesterol in particular, have been the objects of intensive medical study for decades, and a body of literature has accumulated whose review is well beyond the scope of this book. Excellent summaries already exist reviewing cholesterol* and its relationship to heart disease (Keys et al., 1966; Inter-Society Commission for Heart Disease Resources, 1972; National Heart and Lung Institute, 1972; Stamler, 1978; Blackburn, 1974; Kannel, 1974). This chapter will provide a brief overview for the newcomer and focus most intensively on the crucial parameters for our subsequent analysis. We will lay the groundwork for making the best guesses we can about the unknown and the partially known properties of cholesterol. We will touch first on the burden of cardiovascular disease in the United States; second, on the biochemical properties of cholesterol and its distribution in the population; third, on the circumstantial evidence linking cholesterol with cardiovascular disease; fourth, on the limited information we have about controlling human cholesterol levels through diet; and fifth, on the possible consequent effect on risk. Finally, we will consider some of the current recommendations for public programs to control cholesterol.

In the final analysis, though we can martial an impressive volume of circumstantial evidence linking cholesterol with heart disease, we

*For the sake of brevity, we will frequently use the term "cholesterol" in place of the more precise designation "plasma cholesterol."

have no conclusive scientific experiments demonstrating once and for all that the reduction of cholesterol through diet reduces the morbidity and mortality of cardiovascular disease. These residual uncertainties have been used to support attacks against the thesis that dietary change can be a lever on heart disease (Mann, 1977). We hope, nonetheless, to show that diet-changing programs, if not of proven worth, are at least promising and plausible public health measures, worthy of the analysis we give them.†

THE BURDEN OF CARDIOVASCULAR DISEASE

The distribution of disease

Of the burdens on our American health and life span, none weigh more heavily than the diseases of the heart and circulation. Among these diseases, the most significant causes of death and disability are those in which the central pathological process is atherosclerosis: the gradual narrowing of arteries as a result of the collection of fatty substances within the blood vessel walls. As an artery becomes narrower, the blood supply to the tissue fed by that artery is decreased, with a resulting compromise of the function of that tissue. If the blood supply is limited severely enough, the tissue dies. More than one-half of all deaths in the United States are attributable to diseases of the heart and blood vessels, the vast majority caused by the narrowing of arteries and the consequent damage to the tissues thus deprived of blood.‡

†Readers who have substantial familiarity with the biomedical and epidemiologic evidence on cholesterol may skip over this chapter and proceed directly to Chapter 3.

‡We name the clinical syndromes that result from narrowed arteries according to the location of the tissue *affected* by the narrowing and according to the type of damage or disability manifested by that tissue. For example:

(a) *Angina pectoris* (or *angina*) is the syndrome of pain in or near the chest caused by a compromise of the blood supply to the heart, usually as a result of the narrowing of one of the major arteries that supply blood to the heart muscle (called *coronary* arteries). Angina occurs when the blood supply to an area of heart muscle is too small for the muscle's metabolic needs but not so small that the muscle dies.

(b) *Myocardial infarction* (MI, or heart attack) occurs when an area of the heart muscle receives so little blood that the tissue is irreversibly damaged. If the patient survives the MI, the damaged tissue will undergo a process of inflammatory change eventually leading to the formation of a scar of fibrous tissue, replacing muscle in the area of tissue death.

(c) *Stroke* (or cerebral vascular accident, CVA) refers to the death of brain tissue usually as a result of a loss of local blood supply. Depending on the region of the brain damaged, the patient will exhibit a variety of combinations of loss of function—paralysis of a limb, perhaps, or loss of speech. A stroke may result from the gradual occlusion of a blood vessel supplying the brain, or the sudden lodging of a small blood clot in an artery, or, more rarely, leakage of blood from a torn or damaged blood vessel into an area of brain tissue which is thereby injured. The brain is not capable of regen-

Figure 2-1 shows the percentage of total mortality by age in the United States for each major cardiovascular condition. As can be seen, stroke tends to cause death later in life than does myocardial infarction, angina, or sudden death. In males especially, myocardial infarction is largely a disease of occupationally productive years, causing nearly 30 percent of all male deaths between the ages of 55 and 65. The risk of heart attack before age 60 in American males is approximately one in five, and the risk of death from heart attack before age 60 is one in ten (Stamler et al., 1972; Inter-Society Commission for Heart Disease Resources, 1972). Overall, 39 percent of deaths in 1973 were attributable to some form of ischemic heart disease. In the same year, diseases of the heart and circulation accounted for 13 percent of all short-stay hospital discharges and 19 percent of all hospital days (Table 2-1), ranking above all other causes of short-stay hospitalizations (National Center for Health Statistics, 1975). As causes of chronic limitation of physical activity, heart conditions also ranked first for all adult age groups, including those under age 45. Between the ages of 45 and 74 years, heart conditions limited the activity of 25 percent more people than did arthritis and rheumatism and nearly four times as many people as all recorded mental and nervous conditions in the household survey summarized in Table 2-2.

An assessment by Braun et al. (1976) of years of productive life lost places ischemic heart disease at the top of the list of the American

---

eration once damaged, and therefore, if the patient survives a stroke, the recovery of function depends on the degree to which other areas of the brain are capable of taking over the function of the damaged area. This capability is highly variable, and the disability from a nonfatal stroke is frequently permanent.

(d) *Sudden death* can result from a variety of disease processes but is frequently attributable to events that follow the obstruction of blood flow through a coronary artery. Those events can include the sudden disarrangement of the normally orderly cyclical flow of electrical impulses through the heart muscle. In the healthy heart, these impulses result in highly organized contraction of the heart muscle and an effective pumping activity; in the heart receiving insufficient blood supply, these electrical impulses can become suddenly disorganized, turning the heart as a whole into an ineffectively quivering mass of anarchical muscle (a phenomenon called ventricular fibrillation) or causing electrical activity suddenly to cease entirely (cardiac standstill). Even a small area of heart muscle damage can be a focus for this electrical anarchy or cessation of function to begin, and with the pumping activity of the heart interrupted, death will follow within minutes.

(e) *Peripheral vascular disease* is the damaging and occluding of arteries in the body other than those that supply the heart or brain. The effects of blockage of blood flow to a foot or leg may be less catastrophic than a heart attack or a stroke but may nonetheless be disabling, causing, for example, ulceration of the skin, muscle pain upon exercise, or susceptibility to local infection. The most common and troublesome form of severe peripheral vascular disease occurs in the abdominal portion of the aorta, the main artery leading away from the heart, and can cause leg trouble, pain, impotence, and, in the most serious circumstances, rupture of the aorta and death from internal bleeding.

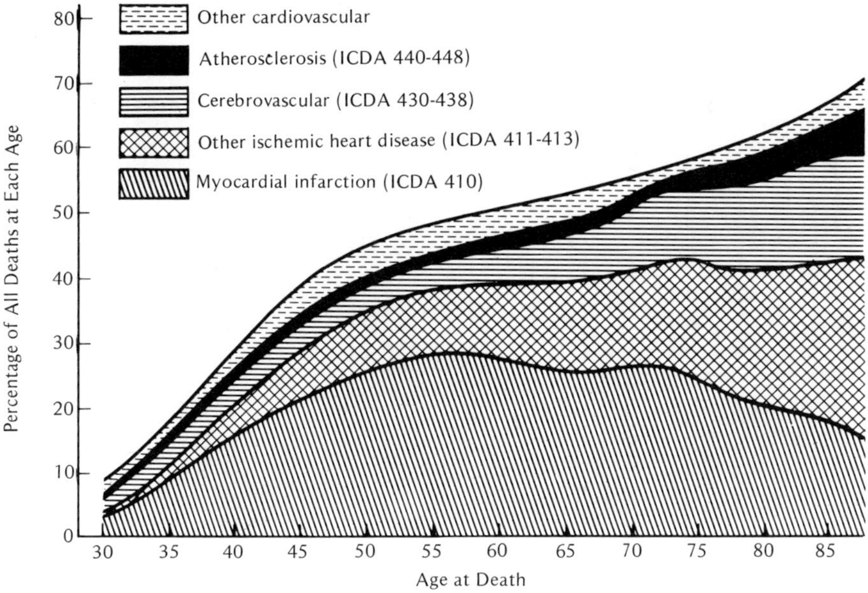

Figure 2-1A. Percentage of Deaths from Cardiovascular Disease vs. Age (Men, 1973, United States), by Disease. Myocardial infarction causes a higher proportion of deaths in men in middle age (45 to 65 years) than in the oldest age groups.

Figure 2-1B. Percentage of Deaths from Cardiovascular Disease vs. Age (Women, 1973, United States), by Disease. Ischemic heart disease and myocardial infarctions cause death in women somewhat later than in men.

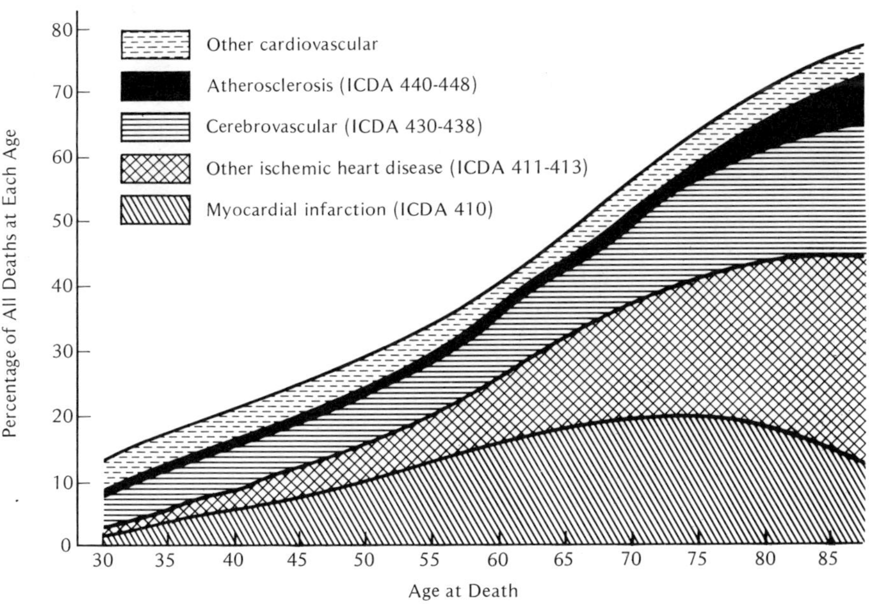

Table 2-1. Number of inpatients discharged from short-stay hospitals: class of first-listed diagnosis and selected diagnostic categories

All conditions	*Discharges (000's)*	*Hospital days (000's)*	*Average length of stay (days)*	*Rank order hospital days*	*% of hospital days*	*% of discharges*
Total	32,125	244,666	7.8			
1. Diseases of the circulatory system	4,110	46,854	11.4	1	19.1	12.8
Acute myocardial infarction	354	5,552	15.6			
Other ischemic heart disease	1,353	14,612	10.8			
All other heart and hypertensive disease	897	8,970	10.0			
Cardiovascular disease	602	8,187	13.6			
2. Diseases of the digestive system	3,999	31,592	7.9	2	12.9	12.4
3. Complications of pregnancy, childbirth, and the puerperium	3,971	14,692	3.7	8	6.0	12.3
4. Diseases of the respiratory system	3,427	20,562	6.0	6	8.4	10.6
5. Diseases of the genitourinary system	3,390	21,357	6.3	5	8.7	10.6

Source. National Center for Health Statistics, Utilization of short-stay hospitals, by diagnosis: United States, 1973. Monthly Vital Statistics Report, 24(3) Suppl. 2 (DHEW Publication No. (HRA) 75-1120). Washington, D.C.: Government Printing Office, 1975.

Note. Diseases of the heart and blood vessels account for more hospitalizations and more hospital days in the United States than any other disease category.

Table 2-2. Chronic conditions ranked by numbers of persons with limitation of activity*

Chronic conditions	*Persons with limitation of activity/year all ages*	*Percentage of total*
Heart conditions	3,609,000	15.5
Arthritis, rheumatism	3,265,000	14.1
Impairments of back and spine (except paralysis)	1,613,000	6.9
Impairments of lower extremities and hips (except paralysis and absence)	1,551,000	6.7
Hypertension without heart involvement	1,059,000	4.6
Mental and nervous conditions	1,033,000	4.4
Asthma, with or without hay fever	1,010,000	4.3
Other musculoskeletal disorders	914,000	3.9
Diabetes	865,000	3.7
Paralysis, complete or partial	817,000	3.5
All other causes	7,501,000	32.3
Total persons with limitation of activity	23,237,000	100

Source. National Center for Health Statistics, Limitation of activity due to chronic conditions, U.S., 1969 and 1970. Vital and Health Statistics, Series 10, No. 80, Table 16 (DHEW Publication No. (HSM) 73-1506). Washington, D.C.: Government Printing Office, 1973.

Note. Heart diseases rank first among causes of restricted activity. They predominate especially in the age group from 45 to 74 years.

*Data are based on household interviews of the civilian, noninstitutionalized population. Limitation of activity is defined as inability or reduction in ability to carry on a major activity such as working, keeping house, or attending school.

burden of illness according to this measure and further underlines the enormous indirect economic impact of this disease category (Table 2-3). By comparison, motor vehicle accidents result in only one-fourth as many lost years of life as do diseases of the heart and circulation.

Alterability of the burden

At least three lines of evidence suggest strongly that our burden of atherosclerosis is not inevitable but rather that it is largely a culturally determined phenomenon, the product of our choices and behaviors. The first clue comes from studies of other cultures, showing enormous variability of cardiovascular disease rates. Table 2-4 shows a sample of the countries for which data are available.

Coronary disease kills 40 percent of Finnish men who die between the ages of 55 and 64 years; it is only half as common a mode of death in Switzerland, Belgium, and Italy and only one-fourth as common in Japan. In absolute rates, Taiwanese men aged 55 to 64 have only

Table 2-3. Leading causes of potential years of life lost due to death, United States, 1970

Cause	*Potential years lost**
Diseases of the circulatory system	11,927,887
Ischemic heart disease	7,824,626
Cerebrovascular disease	2,201,229
Accidents, poisoning, and violence	8,587,741
Neoplasms	5,415,546
Mortality—early infancy	3,023,285
Diseases of the respiratory system	2,076,496
Diseases of the digestive system	1,414,220
Congenital anomalies	1,042,002

Source. P. Braun, M. Weinstein, and M. Farber. An inventory for health care research. (Discussion paper), Boston: Center for the Analysis of Health Practices, Harvard School of Public Health, 1974.

Note. More years of life are lost to circulatory diseases than to any others.

*The number of deaths resulting from each of the listed causes of death in 1970 (1) for 5-year age groups (under 5, 5–9, 10–14, 15–19, 20–24. 25–29, 30–34, 35–39, 40–44, 45–49, 50–54, 55–59, 60–64, 65–69. 70–74, 75–79, 80–84, 85 and over) was multiplied by the remaining life expectancy at the midpoint of each interval (2) and summed to estimate potential years of life lost.
Sources. National Center for Health Statistics. Vital Statistics of the U.S. 1970, Vol. II, Mortality, Part A. Table 1-26. Deaths from 281 selected causes by age, race and sex: United States, 1970 (DHEW Publication No. (HRA) 75-1101). Washington, D.C.: Government Printing Office, 1974; and National Center for Health Statistics. Vital Statistics of U.S. 1971, Vol. II, Section 5. Life tables (DHEW Publication No. (HRA) 74-1147). Washington, D.C.: Government Printing Office, 1974.

one-eighth the risk of dying of coronary disease as do Finnish men. In many less developed countries, among African Pygmies, some Nigerian tribesmen, and natives of St. Kitts, for example, ischemic heart disease as a clinical entity is practically nonexistent (Keys, 1975).

Cross-cultural differences in morbidity may result in part from uncontrollable genetic variation, but a second clue indicates that environmental variation may be more critical; namely the changes over time in the coronary disease burden within our own society.

Trends over time must be measured not by the crude death rates, which are heavily influenced by the aging of our population, but rather by age-adjusted death rates, which reflect mortality patterns independently of trends in age distribution. From 1940 to 1960, the age-adjusted death rate from coronary disease rose 26 percent in white males (Gordon and Thom, 1975). From the peak in 1963 to 1976, rates fell by 20 percent in men and 28 percent in women (Walker, 1977).

These variations in morbidity occurred in too short a period to allow for major changes in our genetic pool, and so environmental factors must explain both the increase and the subsequent decrease in disease rates. Stamler (1978) believes that improvements in our smoking

Table 2-4. Death rates for men aged 55–64 reported by the World Health Organization (1970)

	Coronary heart disease	
Country	*Deaths due to CHD (%)*	*Death rate per 100,000*
Australia	44	945
Belgium	23	498
Ceylon	10	160
Columbia	11	243
Czechoslovakia	23	483
England and Wales	34	695
Finland	40	1,045
France	10	199
Germany (West)	28	658
Greece	14	197
Italy	20	363
Japan	9	162
Mexico	6	129
Spain	10	174
Switzerland	24	416
Taiwan	3	64
United States	40	929
Yugoslavia	24	277

Source. A. Keys, Coronary heart disease. The global picture. Atherosclerosis 22:149–192, 1975.

Note. Wide variations in coronary heart disease rates exist from nation to nation.

habits, diets, and blood pressure control are responsible for the recent decline in cardiovascular disease. Whereas genetic factors can explain differences among individuals in their susceptibility to an improved environment, genes cannot explain the observed short-term variations in morbidity. What we do, what we breathe, what we eat—these are the more likely culprits.

The third clue comes from studies of migrating populations, and this evidence also undermines a purely genetic theory of heart disease. If cardiovascular disease were determined only by genetic endowment, then we might expect a first- or second-generation immigrant population's morbidity pattern to resemble more closely the pattern of its ancestral group than that of its adoptive neighbors. Such is not the case with cardiovascular disease. Study after study shows that foreign-born inhabitants of a nation resemble their adoptive countrymen more than their ancestors in their pattern of heart disease (Krueger and Moriyama, 1967).

The hope that we could reduce our burden of cardiovascular disease depends on the discovery of control levers on risk, behaviors or biological variables that are subject to intentional manipulation and through which risk itself can be manipulated. Decades of effort have been devoted to the search for such levers, and there are several promising leads, among them, blood pressure, body weight, dietary fat content, cigarette smoking habits, stress of living and working, personality type, amount of physical exercise, and the mineral content of drinking water. Each of these has been found, with some confidence, to be predictive of risk of cardiovascular disease and, with less confidence, to be a possible control lever on future risk. Cigarette smoking and hypertension are the most thoroughly explored and currently the most intensively studied, but cholesterol has not lagged far behind. We will soon explore the specific evidence, but first let us introduce our enemy and get to know its several names.

CHOLESTEROL

Biochemistry

We will be discussing assumptions and conclusions about connections between the levels of cholesterol in human blood and the development of common sorts of cardiovascular disease. Even a brief dip into the relevant literature, however, seems to the newcomer like a cold bath in technical terms, neologisms, and acronyms. To ease the shock, we will provide a brief summary of the ways in which the body makes and uses cholesterol and of the terms biochemists and lipid researchers have come to use to describe cholesterol and its relatives. Excellent summaries exist of terminologies and pathways in human lipid metabolism (Fredrickson et al., 1967; Bortz, 1974; Fredrickson et al., 1978), and the confused reader can refer to these if the words used here are entirely unfamiliar.

Cholesterol is a lipid or, in common terms, a fat, one of the basic components of biochemical systems. (Other categories include proteins, carbohydrates, and free ions such as sodium and potassium.) Lipids are defined by the general chemical formulas that they share—carbon, hydrogen, and oxygen in particular proportions—and by their behavior in solutions. In the human bloodstream, two main sorts of lipid are transported: fatty acids, which are long strings of carbon atoms with accompanying hydrogen and oxygen atoms, and cholesterol, a molecule of complex structure that is the way station relative of an enormous number of very active biochemical compounds and an important constituent of biological membranes.

Lipids come from one of two sources. *Endogenous* lipids are produced by the body from basic building blocks that are assembled in, for example, the liver, the intestinal wall, or fat cells. *Exogenous* lipids are those taken into the body in food and utilized directly without being broken down and resynthesized. Since exogenous lipids make up only a small fraction of circulating lipids, diets to reduce cholesterol are concerned not only with cholesterol in food but also with the ingested fats that the body uses to produce endogenous cholesterol.

Cholesterol, whether directly absorbed or synthesized, circulates in the human bloodstream primarily not as free molecules but rather bound to protein in complexes called *lipoproteins*. It is in the classification of these lipoproteins and in the description of their interrelationships and constituents that most of the terminologic headaches in lipidology lie.

Terminology

For purposes of classification, the lipoprotein packages in which most lipids are carried in the bloodstream have now been grouped into four basic categories, the components of each category sharing similar size, similar proportions of lipids and protein, similar migratory behavior when placed in a special medium in a strong electrical field, and usually similar biological roles. Table 2-5 displays these four categories and some of their important properties and synonyms.

Chylomicrons are the largest and lightest lipoproteins, consisting mostly of triglycerides. They are synthesized in intestinal cells during fat digestion and serve to transport lipids from there to the rest of the body. *Very low density lipoproteins* (VLDL) are synthesized both in

Table 2-5. Major forms of lipoproteins in human plasma

Ultracentrifugical characteristics	*Electrophoretic characteristics*	*Contents*		
		Cholesterol	*Triglyceride*	*Phospholipids*
Chylomicrons	(at origin)	~2%	~95%	~3%
Very low density lipoproteins (VLDL)	Pre-beta	20–30%	50%	30%
Low-density lipoproteins (LDL)	Beta lipoproteins	50–60%	15%	35%
High-density lipoproteins (HDL)	Alpha lipoproteins	18–25%	3%	67%

the liver and in the intestines and, in humans, are mainly converted to the third lipoprotein class, *low-density lipoproteins* (LDL), where the majority of circulating cholesterol is found. LDL appears to play an active role in cells of many different types and is the lipoprotein fraction most closely associated with heart disease. The fourth class of lipoprotein, *high-density lipoproteins* (HDL), are synthesized in both the liver and the intestine. HDL may play a role in controlling the uptake of LDL by some tissues, but neither its metabolism nor its biologic function is yet clearly understood. With the discovery of an apparent protective effect of HDL against heart disease, this class of lipoprotein has recently become the object of intense interest and investigation (Miller and Miller, 1975; Miller et al., 1977). Unfortunately, the HDL story has emerged too recently to have a central role in our discussion, and we will not deal with it further in this book.

Cholesterol in the bloodstream is partitioned among these different lipoprotein families. It accounts for 50 to 60 percent by weight of low-density lipoprotein, 20 to 30 percent of very low density lipoprotein, and 18 to 25 percent of high-density lipoprotein. Of all the cholesterol circulating in the bloodstream, 50 to 75 percent is bound to LDL, and it is this LDL cholesterol that is usually regarded with most suspicion by those who are interested in the effects of cholesterol levels on coronary artery disease risk. In general, however, when we refer to "cholesterol" here, we will mean *total* plasma cholesterol; that is, all the circulating cholesterol, no matter how packaged in lipoprotein. When we mean LDL cholesterol, we will so specify.

In the population as a whole, lipid levels exhibit a "log normal" statistical distribution,* with a mean level characteristic of the particular group involved. Within large groups, however, scientists now distinguish discrete subpopulations of "hyperlipidemics," people with atypically high lipoprotein levels in patterns that at least suggest an underlying genetic or biochemical defect. The mode of inheritance of some of these hyperlipidemic states is a subject of current debate, a debate that we will enter in Chapter 5.

For the present, clarity demands a brief discussion of the labels applied to the hyperlipoprotein phenotypes. In the original classification, proposed by Fredrickson, Levy, and Lees (1967), five types of hyperlipidemia were designated, with a subsequent further division

*The graph of the frequency distribution of a "log normal" variable is skewed to the right, with a long "tail" at the upper end. The logarithm of such a variable is normally distributed, and its graph exhibits the familiar symmetrical shape of the "bell-shaped curve."

of type II into IIa and IIb as shown below. A simplified terminology for the most common variants has gained common usage in the past several years, with three of the major classifications designating conditions with single-gene inheritance: familial hypercholesterolemia, familial hypertriglyceridemia, and familial combined hyperlipidemia. Table 2-6, modified from Motulsky (1976), relates the Fredrickson typology to the newer version. We will make use of both terminologies in subsequent discussion.

Since cholesterol and triglyceride levels assume a continuous distribution in the population, criteria for "abnormality," and thus criteria for assignment of a diagnosis of hyperlipoproteinemia, are somewhat arbitrary. Investigators have not achieved widespread consensus on thresholds for abnormality. The 95th percentile is often used to define normality, but the distribution of cholesterol levels differs from one population to another, and the issue is further complicated by the tendency of lipid levels to rise with age, requiring different diagnostic criteria at different ages. Underlying biochemical disorders remain incompletely understood and cannot generally be used for diagnosis of most borderline cases. Thus, although the classification systems for hyperlipidemia are in common use, one cannot assume strict criteria for membership or reliable interobserver agreement on labeling of borderline cases.

Cholesterol and risk: five clues

The definitive study demonstrating beyond reasonable doubt that lowering an individual's serum cholesterol by diet or drugs reliably reduces the risk of morbidity from atherosclerosis has not been done. Instead, we have a web of evidence connecting cholesterol and cardiovascular disease. Though no strand by itself can support a firm conclusion, the web as a whole is consistent and strong.

Five categories of circumstantial evidence exist:

1. Observations of the nature of the obstructive lesion of atherosclerosis
2. Experiments with animal models
3. The results of longitudinal epidemiological observation studies
4. Cross-cultural investigations, including studies of primitive cultures, comparisons among industrialized cultures, and observations of migrating populations
5. Investigations of unusual populations, including especially victims of early myocardial infarction and genetic hyperlipidemics.

Table 2-6. Classification and characteristics of genetic hyperlipidemias

Name of condition	*Fredrickson lipoprotein type*	*Cholesterol*	*Triglycerides*	*Most common electrophoretic pattern*	*Premature coronary heart disease*	*Approximate frequency in adult population*
Familial hypercholesterolemia (FHC)	IIa (rarely IIb)	Elevated	Normal	LDL increased	4+	0.1–0.5%
Polygenic hypercholesterolemia	IIa or IIb	Elevated	Normal	LDL increased	2+	5%
Familial hypertriglyceridemia (FHT)	IV (rarely V)	Normal	Elevated	VLDL increased	1+	1%
Familial combined hyperlipidemia (FCH)	IIa, IIb, IV (rarely V)	Elevated in 2/3 of cases	Elevated in 2/3 of cases	LDL and VLDL increased	3+	1.5%
Broad beta disease	III	Elevated	Elevated	Abnormal beta band	4+	Rare
Familial lipoprotein lipase deficiency	I	Slightly elevated	Very high	Chylomicrons increased	0	Very rare

Source. Adapted with permission from A. Motulsky, The genetic hyperlipidemias, N Engl J Med 294: 823–827, 1976.

Coronary pathology and cholesterol: guilt by association

Even if no other evidence existed, knowing the morphology and constituents of the occlusive lesion of atherosclerosis would at least raise our suspicions about cholesterol. Both free cholesterol and LDL are at least present at the scene of the crime, the atherosclerotic plaque, and have no visibly useful function there.

The *fibrous plaque* of the mature atherosclerotic lesion is a firm, thick deposit of fibrous tissue cells and fats, most prominently cholesterol, occupying the innermost layer of the arterial wall—the *intima*. The oldest plaques contain rock-hard deposits of calcium and their consistency is more like that of an old clay pot than the rubbery, elastic feel of the normal arterial wall. Such plaques are the site of tiny hemorrhages and breaks in the smooth inner surface of the artery, breaks that can result from the pulsatile pressure of the arterial blood against this noncompliant surface.

At sites of such disruption, the artery may burst and bleed, or more commonly, a clot may form on the inner surface of the artery, accelerating occlusion of blood flow. Successive clots may form and become incorporated into the arterial wall, further distorting its architecture and occluding the vessel still more. Figure 2-2 shows a photomicrograph of an occlusive atherosclerotic lesion in a coronary artery, with the distortion of normal architecture, the layers of fat, fibrous tissue, old clot, and the fresh new hemorrhage that may finally have blocked the last pinpoint channel through which blood had been squeezing to the needy tissue beyond. The artery shown here is from a human heart, but it may as easily have been from a major artery supplying the brain. In the latter case, the occlusion would cause a stroke, resulting perhaps in paralysis or loss of speech or, ultimately, even death.

The occlusive lesion of the mature atherosclerotic plaque does not spring de novo in an arterial wall. It is an end-stage lesion, whose history is long, beginning perhaps in the individual's infancy and progressing silently through the stages. At every stage, cholesterol is involved.

"Fatty streaks" probably mark the earliest stages of plaque formation. In the aortas of many infants and of all children by the age of 3 years, autopsies reveal light yellow streaks of lipid embedded in the intima. By the second decade of life, similar streaks appear in the coronary arteries, with cholesterol by far the predominant lipid. These fatty streaks, and their natural history, have been the object of much research. From these efforts, a few conclusions now seem clear.

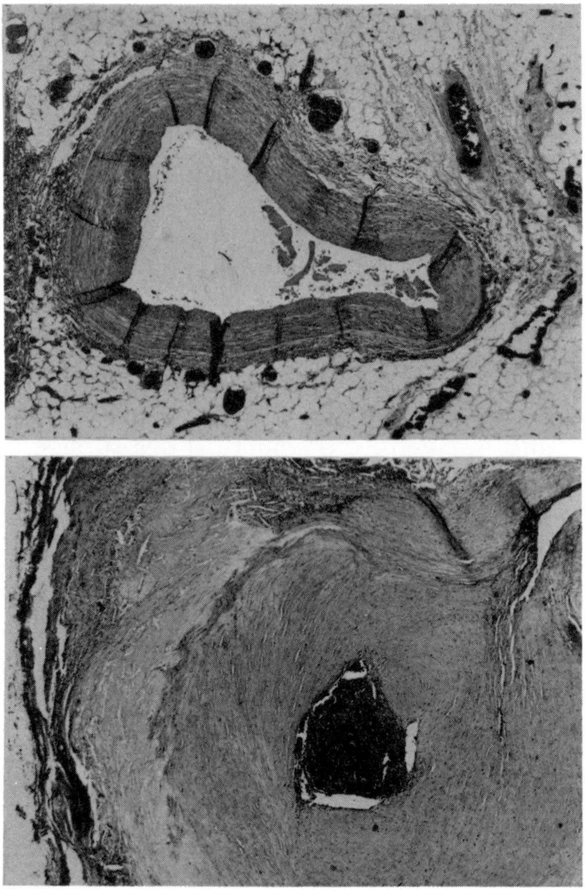

Figure 2-2. Normal and Diseased Coronary Arteries. The photograph at top is of a normal human coronary artery. The artery shown below is partially occluded by severe atherosclerosis, with a plaque containing cholesterol crystals and fibrous tissue. The cholesterol crystals appear as thin, elongated slits in this preparation. A more recent thrombus, or blood clot, in the arterial channel has completed the obstruction to blood flow. The thrombus is adherent to the wall of the channel. Both arteries have been photographed at a magnification of 40×. Notice how much smaller the channel for blood flow is in the diseased artery (ignoring the thrombus) than in the normal artery. (Photomicrographs courtesy of Dr. Leonard Berwick, University of Pennsylvania School of Medicine.)

First, not all fatty streaks become atherosclerotic plaques. Virtually no human culture, no matter how low the incidence of atherosclerosis, is spared fatty streaks at some age. They develop independent of diet, weight, geography, or concurrent disease (McGill et al., 1968). Even malnourished people show fatty streaks at autopsy in both aortas and coronary arteries (Sackett and Winkelstein, 1965). Findings of the International Atherosclerosis Project suggest that fatty streaks in coronary arteries may have more predictive value for ischemic heart disease than do aortic fatty streaks (McGill et al., 1968), but it is equally clear that the occurrence of fatty streaks is not a sufficient condition for atherosclerosis to proceed.

Second, some fatty streaks do progress to fibrous plaques (McMillan, 1973). All transitional stages between the two have been observed (McGill et al., 1968), and plaques rarely, if ever, are found unaccompanied by fatty streaks (Pomeranze, 1961). The International Study of Atherosclerosis concluded on the basis of over 23,000 autopsies from 19 population groups that there is a sequential relationship between fatty streaks, fibrous plaques, and prevalence of coronary heart disease.

The burden of evidence is that fatty streaks are probably necessary though not sufficient precursors of occlusive atherosclerosis. Some other factor is needed—behavioral, dietary, anatomical (Kannel, 1974), or genetic (Neufeld, 1974)—to convert these soft irregularities of arterial walls into hard, occlusive deposits; they are but the seeds of destruction.

Although cholesterol is a major constituent of the fatty streak, it has not been shown that dietary content influences the formation of the lesions. Few people argue that the prevention of fatty streaks through dietary intervention would be a rational or achievable goal. Instead, interventionists argue, we should attempt to interrupt the transition from fatty streak to fibrous plaque, a transition that begins in late childhood, that has progressed substantially in American men by the second decade of life (Rigal et al., 1960; McNamara et al., 1971; Enos et al., 1953), and that includes the further laying down of lipid in an already existing lesion. In this process, cholesterol is implicated by the company it keeps. It is there throughout—in the seedling fatty streak, in the developing plaque, and in the occlusive mass.

Animal models

The investigation of disease processes often requires intervention designs that cannot ethically or practically be applied to human beings. Experiments in humans are limited furthermore by the length of our lives. Lifelong pathological processes in humans take, of course, lifetimes to observe, and we tend to ask for answers more quickly, in months or years, not generations.

We turn therefore to animal models, which are more susceptible to manipulation and in which the pace of disease is often faster. Scientists consider it a breakthrough when a human disease can be reproduced convincingly in an animal, thereby rendering the disease susceptible to experimental control.

Atherosclerosis was first produced experimentally in animals early in this century (Anitschkow, 1913), and models now exist in rats (Hartroft and Thomas, 1959), chickens (Katz and Stamler, 1953), rabbits (Vesselinovitch et al., 1974), swine (Reiser, 1971), dogs (Malmros, 1969), and a variety of other creatures including primates (Mann and Andrus, 1956; Taylor et al., 1962; Wissler, 1968; Younger et al., 1969). Wissler et al., (1965) produced lesions in monkeys fed the constituents of the usual American table diet, and primates can now be shown to develop occlusive atheromata with moderate cholesterol increases comparable to that found in many human populations (Armstrong et al., 1974).

Among the most exciting results from animal models are those that show a *regression* of atherosclerotic lesions in animals on cholesterol-lowering diets. Decreases in plaque size with dietary changes under some conditions have been reported in chicks (Horlick and Katz, 1949), dogs (Bevans et al., 1951), pigeons (St. Clair et al., 1972), and rabbits (Lisovskii and Mikushkin, 1962; Bortz, 1968), although some investigators report only minimal changes without adjunctive drug or high-oxygen treatment (Vesselinovitch et al., 1974). Armstrong and collaborators (1970) have demonstrated regression of lesions in male rhesus monkeys, among which narrowing of coronary arteries by atherosclerosis decreased from 50 to 60 percent narrowing to 15 to 25 percent narrowing when diets were switched from high fat, high cholesterol (for 17 months) to low fat, low cholesterol (for 40 months). A polyunsaturated fat or a low-fat, low-calorie diet in rhesus monkeys studied by Chakravarti et al., (1977) similarly led to regression of atherosclerosis. Wagner et al. (1976) have demonstrated regression of lesions in monkeys whose cholesterol levels were lowered by either drug or diet.

Extrapolation from the results of these animal studies (even primate studies) is risky. We must first have evidence that animal models of atherosclerotic disease are indeed comparable in mechanism to disease processes in humans. Moreover, even if the progress of atherosclerotic lesions can be manipulated in humans as in animals, we must ask whether the change in morphology leads to a decrease in cardiovascular morbidity or mortality, for, as we will see, although atherosclerosis is associated with diseases such as stroke and myocardial infarction, it is not the sole cause. These diseases can occur in the absence of atherosclerosis, and conversely, many people with severe atherosclerosis live symptom-free into old age. For further confirmation of our suspicions about cholesterol, we must look to human populations.

Epidemiologic observation

Numerous studies in the past three decades have measured cholesterol levels in large populations of adults free of cardiovascular disease and subsequently observed whether the subgroup that developed disease differed in lipid profile from those who escaped disease.

In its overall significance, the Framingham Study of Cardiovascular Disease looms above the others. It was the first major longitudinal study, among the largest ever done, and it has never been superseded in sophistication of design, comprehensiveness of data collection, or inventiveness of statistical analysis.

The Framingham study began in 1948 with an initial enrollment of 2336 men and 2873 women between the ages of 30 and 62 years who were free of cardiovascular disease at entry. At two-year intervals since the study began, subjects have been restudied with note being taken of the presence or absence of 14 types of cardiovascular disease "events" and a large variety of individual characteristics, among them the serum cholesterol level.

Over the years, the Framingham study has demonstrated serum cholesterol level at entry to be among the most powerful predictive variables in separating subjects who later developed coronary artery disease from those who did not (Kannel, 1974; Kannel et al., 1971a; Gordon and Kannel, 1972 a). In predicting myocardial infarction, only blood pressure among all the variables studied was a match for the serum cholesterol level. Specifically, the Framingham study has produced the following conclusions about cholesterol as a predictor of heart disease:

Total serum cholesterol is a better predictor than any other lipid fraction studied, including casual triglycerides, LDL, and VLDL.

Cholesterol is a good predictor of risk in men until the age of 65 and in younger women (Kannel and Castelli, 1972).

Even in the mid-range, near the mean cholesterol level, risk varies with level; that is, subjects whose cholesterol levels are below the mean have lower risk than do subjects whose cholesterol levels are at the mean.

Cholesterol contributes to risk independently of other useful predictors such as blood pressure, smoking history, and family history.

The effect of cholesterol as a risk factor is not merely additive with other risk factors but is multiplicative.

For example, as shown in Table 2-7, a 45-year-old Framingham man who does not smoke and whose electrocardiogram (ECG) does not show left ventricular hypertrophy (LVH) has about 2.5 times the chance of developing coronary heart disease if his systolic blood pressure is 180 mm Hg as if it is 105 mm Hg. The same man has a risk about three times as high with a cholesterol level of 310 mg/dl as he does with a cholesterol of 185 mg/dl. The risks are multiplicative: if both factors are elevated (cholesterol over 310 mg/dl and systolic blood pressure over 180 mm Hg), then the risk is over seven times greater than if both factors are low (cholesterol under 180 mg/dl and systolic blood pressure under 105 mm Hg) (American Heart Association, 1973b).

As a mathematical model of the contribution of cholesterol level to cardiovascular risk, the Framingham analysts chose the so-called logistic function, in which risk varies as an exponential function of the risk factor. Cornfield (1962) has discussed the derivation of this mathematical risk model, which leads to the following expression of

Table 2-7. Probability* of developing coronary heart disease in eight years (for a 45-year-old man, with no LVH on ECG, no glucose intolerance, and no cigarette smoking)

	Systolic blood pressure (mm Hg)		
Serum cholesterol (mg/dl)	105	135	180
185	20	29	51
235	31	45	79
310	60	87	146

Source. William B. Kannel, The role of cholesterol in coronary atherogenesis, Med Clin North Am 58:376, 1974.

Note. Coronary disease risk factors, such as cholesterol and hypertension, interact multiplicatively with each other.

*Probability in thousandths.

the relationship between P, the probability of developing coronary heart disease, and X, the log of serum cholesterol level:

$$P = \frac{1}{1 + e^{-(\alpha + \beta X)}}$$

The analysis leads to empirical estimations of α and β such that the data fit this S-shaped logistic risk curve as closely as possible (Gordon, 1974). Within the range of cholesterol levels observed in the Framingham study, the relationship between risk of myocardial infarction in men and cholesterol level is depicted in Figure 2-3.

Several features of this risk curve deserve our attention, for reasons that will become more apparent later. First, at any point, lower cholesterol levels are preferable to higher levels; there is no discontinuity above which an individual is clearly ill or below which he is as well as he could be. Second, the risk function is not straight but curves up-

Figure 2-3. The Framingham Logistic Curve: Cholesterol Level vs. Risk of Infarction. For any age group, the logistic function shows risk to be a steadily increasing function of cholesterol level. Similar curves could be shown for other cardiovascular events associated with cholesterol level.

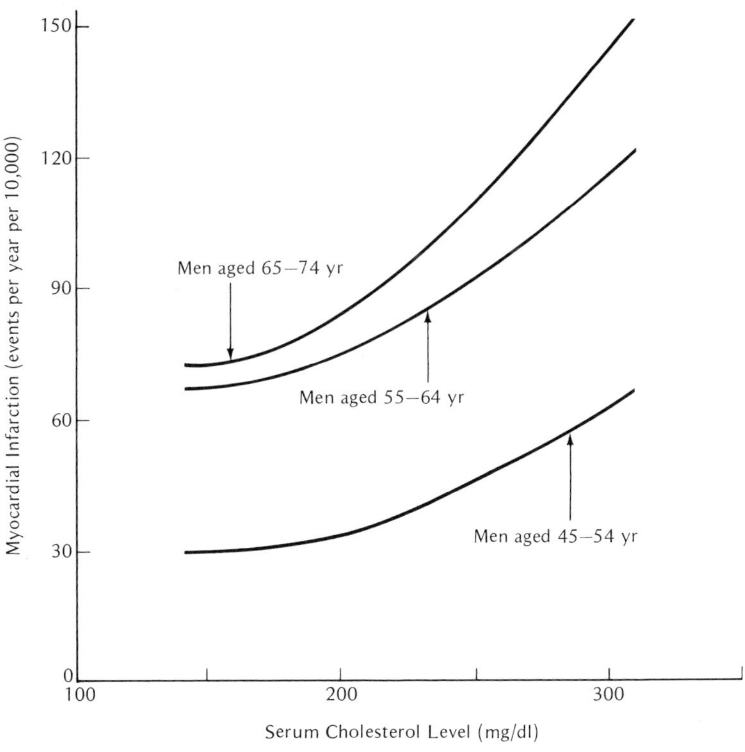

ward. At higher levels of cholesterol, risk changes more with level than it changes at lower levels of cholesterol.

In the past two decades, many other highly creditable population studies have been carried out. Table 2-8 summarizes some findings from 17 of the most significant epidemiologic reports. All but three of these studies strongly confirm the Framingham study's conclusion about the usefulness of cholesterol levels in predicting the incidence of atherosclerotic diseases in individuals. They reinforce the observations that cholesterol has more effect on the risk of myocardial infarction than on other manifestations of atherosclerosis and more effect on people with positive family histories than on those with negative family histories. Some, but not all, of the studies also note the importance of serum triglycerides as a predictor of coronary heart disease.

Three studies are more equivocal, but their inconclusive findings seem more the result of differences in design than of directly contradictory data. In fact, the findings of the "negative" epidemiologic investigations can be reconciled easily with the "positive" other studies.

In the Tecumseh study (Epstein et al., 1965) and in part of the Evans County study (Cassel, 1971a, 1971b; Cassel et al., 1971a, 1971b), the *prevalence* of coronary heart disease was not significantly related to cholesterol levels in all age, sex, and race groups. As the authors note, there are two reasons why prevalence of heart disease is less likely to be associated with high cholesterol than is incidence. First, coronary disease typically has a shorter duration than the follow-up periods of the major epidemiologic studies. Since the prevalence of a disease usually equals its incidence multiplied by its duration, one who records incidence over a long period of time will witness more events than one who records prevalence at a single point in time. Because of the larger number of events recorded, the observer of incidence is more likely than the observer of prevalence to see statistically significant differences as a function of risk factors.

Second, it is possible that cholesterol is particularly associated with those specific forms of heart disease that have short duration. In this case, even if the incidence of heart disease rises with cholesterol level, the prevalence may fall. In the extreme case, suppose that high cholesterol levels rendered any form of acquired heart disease instantly fatal. The prevalence of heart disease among the unlucky people with hypercholesterolemia would be zero, and if we studied prevalence only, we might conclude erroneously that elevations in cholesterol were *protective* against heart disease.

Table 2-8. Epidemiologic studies

Study	*References*	*Subjects at entry*	*Duration of follow-up*	*Positive relationship between cholesterol and CHD*	*Examples of findings*			
I. Studies with positive findings on cholesterol								
Albany	Doyle, 1963	1913 men, 39–55 years	6 years	Yes	Cholesterol	Rate of CHD/1000/yr		
					<200	4		
					200–274	7		
					275	15		
Chicago Peoples Gas Co.	Dyer, 1975	1233 white men 40–59 years	14 years	Yes	Cholesterol	Incidence of CHD/1000		
					<175	43		
					>300	109		
Evans County, Georgia	Cassel 1971a, 1971b; Cassel et al., 1971a; Tyroler et al., 1971	3102 biracial men and women	7 years	Yes, for incidence; no, for prevalence	Cholesterol	Rate/87 mo/1000		
						White male	White female	Black male
					<219	72	21	22
					220–259	109	44	22
					260	95	51	47
					Relative risk highest/lowest	1.3	2.4	2.1
Finland	Pelkonen et al., 1977	1648 men 50–53 years	7 years	Yes	Linear correlation of cholesterol with cardiovascular mortality over all ranges of cholesterol level			

Table 2-8. Epidemiologic studies (continued)

Study	*References*	*Subjects at entry*	*Duration of follow-up*	*Positive relationship between cholesterol and CHD*	*Examples of findings*
Framingham	Kannel et al., 1971a; Kannel & Castelli, 1972; Kannel, 1974	2282 men and 2845 women 30–62 years	14 years	Yes	"The risk posed by every clinical manifestation of coronary heart disease is related to antecedent serum cholesterol values." Relative risks (cholesterol > 265 vs. cholesterol < 220) Age / Men / Women 35–44 / 5.5 / 5.0 45–54 / 2.4 / 1.5 55–64 / 1.7 / 1.3 all / 2.8 / 1.5 Uses "logistic" function to model risk
Israel Ischemic Heart Disease Study	Medalie et al., 1973a, 1973b; Goldbourt et al., 1975	10,000 Israeli men 40 years and up	5 years	Yes	Cholesterol / 5-year incidence of MI/1000 77–189 / 29 190–219 / 39 220–500 / 60 Association was stronger for early MI
Malmö-Kockum Study	Johansson & Persson, 1973	464 men Swedish shipyard employees	17 years	Yes	Cholesterol was associated with higher mortality from any cause

					Group — Mean cholesterol CHD death — 287 Other death — 271 Alive — 252
London Busmen	Morris et al., 1966	700 men	5 years	Yes	Total cholesterol was (with blood pressure) one of the two best predictors of new MI
Los Angeles Heart Study	Chapman et al., 1966, 1971	1503 male civil service employees, median age 47 years	15 years	Yes	Cholesterol level was strongest predictor of MI and sudden death in white subjects. Predictive value was stronger for young men.
Minneapolis-St. Paul	Keys et al., 1971	279 men 47–57 years	23 years	Yes	Risk of "hard" CHD rose by the cube of cholesterol level. Risk of all CHD rose by the square of level. Cholesterol was second to blood pressure as a predictor of risk.
Stockholm Prospective Study	Carlson & Böttiger, 1972; Böttiger & Carlson, 1973	3168 men	9 years	Yes	Ischemic heart disease rates increase linearly with cholesterol level in men under 60 years of age. IHD/1000 = 3.8 + 4.1 (X) in men under 60 years old IHD/1000 = 11.0 + 3.8 (X) in men over 60 years old (where X = cholesterol quintile) Triglycerides were an important independent predictor.
United States Railroad Men	Keys et al., 1972	2404 U.S. railroad men and 8727 European men	5 years	Yes	Uses multiple logistic risk model. (β = .003–.015 for "hard" CHD as a function of cholesterol)

Table 2-8. Epidemiologic studies (continued)

Study	*References*	*Subjects at entry*	*Duration of follow-up*	*Positive relationship between cholesterol and CHD*	*Examples of findings*		
Western Collaborative Group	Rosenman et al., 1967, 1970	3182 men 39–59 years	4½ years	Yes	Cholesterol Level	CHD annual incidence/1000 39–49 yr	50–59 yr
					<220	2.8	9.1
					220–259	6.5	20.5
					>259	13.7	24.6
Western Electric	Paul et al., 1963	1989 white men 40–55 years	4½ years	Yes	Cholesterol level	Relative risk of CHD	
					<200	1.0	
					200–240	2.16	
					250–270	3.46	
					>270	4.26	

II. Studies with negative findings on cholesterol					
San Francisco Longshoremen	Paffenbarger et al., 1977	1665 men 45–74 years had measured cholesterols	12 years for the cholesterol component of the study	No	Blood cholesterol did not distinguish high-risk from low-risk subjects. Physical exercise was the most critical predictive risk factor.
Tecumseh (Michigan)	Epstein et al., 1965	A community of 9500 people, of whom 8641 were examined	Cross-sectional prevalence study	No*	Prevalence of CHD in people with cholesterol > 80th percentile ÷ prevalence in people with cholesterol < 80th percentile Men = 1.5 Women = 1.4
Tromsø Heart Study	Miller et al., 1977	6595 men 20–49 years	2 years (case-control study)	No†	No significant difference in cholesterol levels between cases and matched controls. Cases / Controls Mean cholesterol 248 ± 33 / 229 ± 41 HDL level was a *protective* risk factor.

*Relationship was found in the direction of higher prevalence at higher cholesterol levels but did not reach statistical significance.

†Mean cholesterol was higher in cases than controls, but difference was not statistically significant at the sample size.

The Tromsø heart study of young men, in its first two years, found victims of a coronary event to have cholesterol levels half a standard deviation higher than controls (Miller et al., 1977). This is almost exactly the difference observed in the Framingham study for men of the same age, but because the Tromsø study had only recently begun, there were not enough morbid events to make the difference statistically significant. If the same difference were to persist over the next two years of the study, the four-year results would show those with a coronary event to have significantly higher cholesterol levels than controls. Despite the small numbers of events, high-density lipoproteins were already significantly *lower* for cases than for controls, showing the apparent importance of HDL as a protective risk factor.

In 1961, Paffenbarger et al., (1977) added blood cholesterol measurements to a longitudinal study of fatal heart attacks in San Francisco longshoremen. By that time, the youngest people in their cohort were 45 years old. The observed age-adjusted rate of fatal heart attack was only slightly higher for the high-cholesterol group than for the low-cholesterol group. The authors suggest that this may be due to the age of men studied and the possibility that their physically active lives may offer some protection against the risk of high cholesterol. We calculate that if cholesterol had had the same effect in the longshoremen as in the Framingham subjects, the high-cholesterol group would have had 21 percent more fatal heart attacks than the low-cholesterol group. The difference between this expected ratio and the ratio actually observed is not significant ($p = .15$, one-sided test). In fact, given the Framingham risk estimates, the longshoremen's study had only a 40 percent chance of observing a statistically significant ($p < .05$) difference between the high-cholesterol and low-cholesterol groups.

Despite the difficulty of comparing studies with different designs, the qualitative conclusion from epidemiologic data is remarkably uniform: Knowing an adult's serum cholesterol rank within a population sharing common geography and culture is useful in predicting that adult's risk of subsequent coronary heart disease (especially myocardial infarction and sudden death) as compared with other members of that population. That cholesterol level is a predictive risk factor is no longer subject to doubt.

Cross-cultural studies

Three types of cross-cultural investigation lend support to a hypothesized causal connection between cholesterol levels and coronary heart disease: studies on nonindustrialized cultures, comparisons among industrialized cultures, and observations on migrating ethnic groups.

Nonindustrialized cultures

The incidence and prevalence of cardiovascular disease in primitive and nontechnological societies have repeatedly been found to be significantly lower than that in the developed world. With few exceptions, primitive cultures share low coronary heart disease burdens and low levels of the known risk factors for coronary disease, including hypertension, sedentary life-styles, and elevated serum cholesterol levels (Keys, 1975; Lowenstein, 1964).

Table 2-9 summarizes findings on serum cholesterol levels in different cultures. In general, serum cholesterol levels in infants are similar in all cultures, but the levels in primitive and impoverished people stabilize in childhood, while in Westernized and affluent people, they continue to rise through adult life.

Table 2-9. A sampling of cross-cultural comparisons of cholesterol

Subject group	*Author*	*Example of findings on cholesterol*
South African natives	Bersohn and Wayburne, 1956	Lower levels in native than in European South Africans.
Guatemalan children	Scrimshaw et al., 1957	Lower levels in children in poor families than in wealthy families. Lower levels in rural than in urban poor.
New Guinea natives	Whyte and Yee, 1958	Cholesterol remained at childhood levels in primitive New Guinean natives but rose steadily with age in Australians. Low coronary heart disease in natives.
Polynesians	Hunter, 1962	Lower levels in Westernized Polynesians than in a more primitive group that consumes large amounts of coconut-oil (high in saturated fat)
Pygmies in the Congo	Mann et al., 1962	Very low levels of cholesterol and ischemic heart disease.
St. Kitts islanders	Stuart et al., 1962	Lower levels in islanders, who have vegetarian diets and rigorous life-style. Ischemic heart disease rare.

Table 2-9 Continued

Subject group	*Author*	*Example of findings on cholesterol*
Brazilian Indians	Pazzanese et al., 1964	Very low levels and no detectable ischemic heart disease in very primitive group.
East African children and young adults	Scott et al., 1966	Autopsy study. Less cholesterol deposited in coronary arteries of Ugandan youths compared with age-matched New Yorkers.
South African children	du Plessis, et al., 1967	Cholesterol levels in children of four ethnic groups correlated with coronary death rates characteristic of those groups.
East Africans	Epstein, 1971	Poor have higher cholesterol levels than the wealthy.
Masai men	Mann et al., 1972	Low cholesterol levels in Masai men (despite a diet of milk products and meat).
Mexican schoolchildren	Golubjatnikov et al., 1972	Both cholesterol level and ultimate population risk of coronary disease were lower for Mexican than for Wisconsin schoolchildren.
Rural Jamaican adults	Florey et al., 1973	Lower cholesterol levels for rural Jamaican adults than in populations in developed countries.
Puerto Ricans	Garcia-Palmieri, 1973	Rural men had lower cholesterol levels than urban men (diet, alone, did not account for the difference)
Solomon Islanders (six tribal groups)	Page et al., 1974	Cholesterol levels all low and positively correlated with degree of tribal acculturation to Western life-style.
Nigerian Africans	Taylor et al., 1975	Cholesterol content of cerebral arteries of Nigerian Africans at autopsy much lower than in American Negroes or Caucasians.
Pima Indian children and adolescents	Savage et al., 1976	Cholesterol levels stabilize after childhood at levels much lower than those in Tecumseh, Michigan, which continue to rise with age.

The International Atherosclerosis Project studied over 20,000 autopsies in numerous locations throughout the world, demonstrating wide variations in the prevalence of raised atherosclerotic lesions. Scrimshaw and Guzman (1968) reported on the comparison of atherosclerosis, serum cholesterol, and percentage of dietary calories from saturated fat in 12 of these locations (Table 2-10) and listed striking correlations among these variables, .755, for example, between the atherosclerosis rank order of the autopsy population and the rank order of its serum cholesterol level. The International Atherosclerosis Project concluded, "Severity of atherosclerosis is closely associated with the proportion of total calories derived from fat, and with serum cholesterol concentration."

Masironi (1970) compared diets and atherosclerotic heart disease rates across 37 countries, noting a strong correlation (about .70) between fat consumption and atherosclerotic heart disease death rates.

In some primitive populations, diet alone does not explain low coronary disease incidence or low cholesterol levels. Somali camel herdsmen consume large quantities of camels' milk, which is high in lipids (Shaper and Jones, 1962), and Kenyan tribes who subsist largely on milk, meat, and blood both have low cholesterol levels and are free of coronary disease (Shaper et al., 1963). It is possible that parasitic infections in primitive populations cause malabsorption of fats and thus provide a barrier to the potential hypercholesterolemic effects of high-fat diets. The explanation most frequently proffered, however, is that physical exercise, perhaps by increasing caloric requirements, is protective against hypercholesterolemic effects of a high-lipid or high-saturated-fat diet.

This has been the interpretation of the interesting anomalous case of the Masai tribesmen of East Africa. The Masai have (1) very high cholesterol and animal fat intakes, (2) extensive atherosclerosis, (3) low serum cholesterols, (4) very little pathological evidence of heart disease despite extensive plaques, and (5) coronary arteries of enor-

Table 2-10. Rank order correlations of dietary fat, serum, cholesterol, and atherosclerosis in twelve populations

	Serum cholesterol	*Percentage of calories from fat*
Atherosclerosis index	.755	0.668
Serum cholesterol	—	0.741

Source. N. S. Scrimshaw and M. S. Guzmán, Diet and atherosclerosis. Lab Invest 18: 623–628, 1968.

mous caliber (Mann et al., 1972). Informed observers suggest that the Masai are protected from ischemic heart disease by their extremely vigorous life-styles—that exercise tends to protect against coronary occlusion both by lowering risk factors and by causing the coronary arteries to increase in caliber. This is only speculation, however, and the Masai remain an exception in a field of cross-cultural studies that tend to link Western diet, Western pathology, and Western morbidity in a continuous chain.

Some authors have noted other contributing factors, in addition to physical exercise, that tend to lower cholesterol in primitive groups, such as the predominance of starch in the diets (Groen, 1967) and the deficiency of vitamin C (Bronte-Stewart et al., 1963; Ginter et al., 1970). Furthermore, the low risk of atherosclerosis is attributed not only to low cholesterol but also to low triglycerides (Antonis and Bersohn, 1960), the effects of high dietary fiber content (Burkitt et al., 1974; Trowell, 1972), lower blood pressure (Page et al., 1974), and differences in other risk factors. Neufeld et al., (1973) have studied the variation in coronary artery architecture in childhood as a contributor to the subsequent development of coronary occlusions. Structural changes in the innermost layer of the coronary arteries of children in high-risk Ashkenazy Jewish groups were much more common than aberations in the arteries of children among low-risk Bedouins. Thus, cholesterol is implicated in cross-cultural risk differences, but it is not the only possible culprit.

Western cultures

The large numbers of differences between primitive and Western societies complicate efforts to isolate the effects of cholesterol. Studies among cultures that are more similar to each other can simplify the observations.

Even within the industrialized world, the incidence of coronary heart disease varies widely from society to society. The death rate from coronary heart disease in Japanese men, for example, was noted by Keys in the 1950s to be an order of magnitude lower than the comparable rate in American men.

In the so-called Seven Countries Study, conducted under the leadership of Ancel Keys in the 1950s and 1960s, 11 cohorts of men aged 40 to 59, from seven countries spread throughout the world, were studied prospectively for cardiovascular morbidity and mortality and for the prevalence of risk factors for coronary disease (Keys, 1970; Keys et al., 1966). An enormous quantity of information has been gleaned from these systematic observations, including striking trends relating morbidity, cholesterol levels, and diets. Figure 2-4 illustrates some of the findings. Keys and his colleagues discovered strong correlations between heart disease incidence rates in the populations studied and median serum cholesterol levels, as well as equally strong relationships between disease rates and the percentage of the calories the populations consumed as saturated fatty acids. In the cohorts studied, high saturated fat intake, high serum cholesterol levels, and high coronary morbidity and mortality were closely linked statistically.

Jolliffe and Archer (1959) reported similar conclusions based on a statistical study of coronary disease and environmental factors in 20 nations. Saturated fat intake in the population correlated well (.83) with coronary death rates. Protein intake and ischemic heart disease also correlated with each other (.80).

A study of food consumption patterns in 14 regions of England and Wales reported significant correlation ($r = .60$) between hydrogenated fat consumption and local ischemic heart disease mortality (Thomas, 1975). Similarly, Knox (1977) found positive correlations between ischemic heart disease rates and total animal fats ($r = .69$) and animal protein ($r = .74$) intake in 20 developed nations.

A decrease in coronary heart disease deaths was associated with wartime restrictions on diet, including fats, in Finland (Vartiainen, 1946), Norway (Strøm and Jensen, 1951), the Netherlands (Schornagel, 1953), Greece (Greek Vital Statistics, 1941–1947), and postwar Germany (Jahnke and Breitbach, 1959). Malmros (1950) has shown a strong statistical connection between changes in morbidity and decreases in fat intake.

A careful study of ischemic heart disease and risk factors in 40-year-old men in Edinburgh and Stockholm (Oliver et al., 1975) serves notice again that cholesterol is only one among several probable determinants of risk. Although the risk of coronary heart disease was three times greater in Edinburgh than in Stockholm, the serum cholesterol levels of the two groups were virtually identical. Other factors, including weight, blood pressure, and smoking habits, seemed to play a more important role in risk differences. Similarly, in a comparison of Japanese and American men, Kimura and Keys (1970) found variations in risk factors, including cholesterol, that were insufficient to explain differences in disease rates.

Despite the exceptions, Stamler (1970) finds the cross-national studies highly convincing that "a cause and effect relationship has

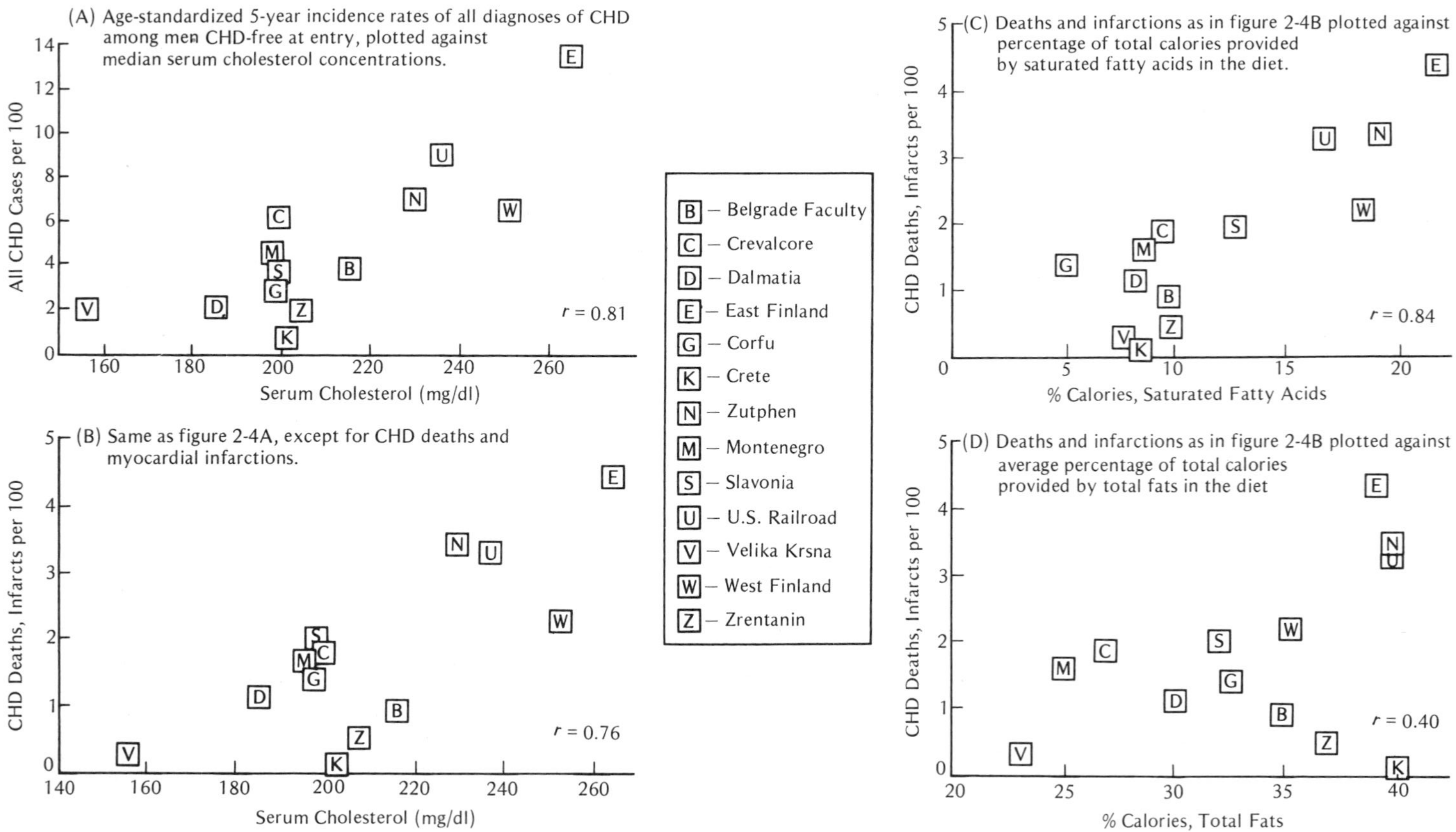

Figure 2-4: Some Results of the "Seven Countries Study." Saturated fat intake, serum cholesterol levels, and death rates from coronary disease were correlated with each other in the "Seven Countries Study." (Reproduced with permission from A. Keys, Coronary heart disease in seven countries. Circulation 41(Suppl 1): 1–211, 1970.)

been demonstrated between dietary lipid (specifically saturated fat and cholesterol) and widespread, premature atherosclerosis, even though substantial direct proof from large-scale long-term mass field trials is still to be obtained."

Migrating populations

The correlation of morbidity indices and serum lipid patterns across cultural groups is tantalizing but does not prove causality. The association of lipid patterns with cardiovascular morbidity may be causal, but both attributes may also reflect characteristics of the populations' gene pools, related to each other by chance or by a third variable instead of by a cause-and-effect connection.

Studies of populations on the move may help us sort out these interpretations. If genetically similar populations come to differ in both lipid patterns and cardiovascular disease incidence when one is transplanted to a new environment, we may be more willing to ascribe the differences to manipulable environmental factors superimposed on genetic endowments. In making our interpretations, we must proceed cautiously. We know that when an individual changes diet, serum cholesterol levels change quickly in response, stabilizing at new levels in a matter of weeks. But atherosclerosis is a process that moves slowly, over years. Bearing this caveat in mind, we may still ask: Do migrating populations share the characteristics of their genetic forebears or of their adoptive environments?

Those who have looked have found the latter. Keys and collaborators (1958) studied Japanese men in Japan, Hawaii, and Los Angeles and found that coronary atherosclerosis, serum cholesterol levels, and percentage of dietary calories from fat varied from one group to the next. Japanese men in Japan were lowest on all three variables, Japanese men in Hawaii next, and Japanese men in Los Angeles highest on all three.

The Ni-Hon-San study (Syme et al., 1975; Nichaman et al., 1975; Robertson et al., 1977) corroborates this result and further notes that second-generation Japanese immigrants in Hawaii have "more Western" levels of cholesterol *and* risk than do first-generation immigrants. In addition, younger Japanese immigrant men have risk levels close to those observed in Western men with similar cholesterol levels, while older Japanese immigrant men have lower risk levels than their Western counterparts with similar cholesterol levels. This lends credence to the speculation that cholesterol level is a good predictor of risk *only* if diet has not changed markedly in the lifetime of the individuals at risk. Elevated risk of coronary heart disease compared with the population of origin has been found as well among Norwegians who migrate to the United States (Epstein, 1971), Italians who migrate to Australia (Epstein, 1971), and Yemenite Jews who have been in Israel for a generation or more (Toor et al., 1960).

Krueger and Moriyama (1967) reviewed census data of foreign-born residents of the United States and compared their mortality from cardiovascular diseases and other causes with death rates in their country of origin and with rates among "native" white Americans. Table 2-11 shows their results for the six countries for which comparison statistics were available (Canada, the United Kingdom, Norway, Sweden, Finland, and Italy). Despite some inconsistencies, the authors concluded cautiously that "there is a substantial amount of support, stronger for males than for females, that death rates for the foreign born from each disease group (cardiovascular-renal and others) tend to become like those of the United States native-born population." Such results must, of course, be interpreted with caution, since emigrants may differ at the outset in important ways from people who remain in their native land.

Special populations

In the field of medicine, one often learns about the ordinary by studying the extraordinary. The unusual subgroups of people most intensively studied for links between cholesterol and cardiovascular disease are victims of myocardial infarction, relatives of these victims, and people with unusually high serum lipid levels. There are two reasons to examine studies in these populations: first, to confirm the findings of large-scale epidemiologic studies and, second, to see whether there are any differences to be observed *within* the population of individuals with high cholesterol levels. The most widespread hypothesis is that while diet, life-style, and genetics all affect cholesterol level, a few individuals may be genetically predisposed to extremely high cholesterol levels. We will return to the question of possible genetic forms of hypercholesterolemia in Chapter 5.

Hyperlipidemia in victims of coronary disease

Survivors of morbid events resulting from atherosclerosis have been studied retrospectively for features that appear to distinguish them from the unaffected population. What do those victims have or lack that makes them different and, by inference, might have contributed to their illnesses?

Table 2-11. Similarity of death rates of foreign-born residents in U.S. to rates of native whites in U.S. and to rates of the country of birth (six countries of origin)*

	Men						Women					
Cause of death	*35–44*	*45–54*	*55–64*	*65–74*	*75–84*	*All*	*35–44*	*45–54*	*55–64*	*65–74*	*75–84*	*All*
Major cardiovascular-renal												
Similar to U.S.	1†	5	4	4	5	19	1	0	3	3	3	10
Indeterminate	2	1	1	0	1	5	5	4	2	2	1	14
Similar to country of birth	3	0	1	2	0	6	0	2	1	1	2	6
All other												
Similar to U.S.	3	4	5	3	3	18	1	2	1	3	5	12
Indeterminate	2	2	0	2	0	6	3	3	3	1	0	10
Similar to country of birth	1	0	1	1	3	6	2	1	2	2	1	8

Source. D. E. Krueger and I.M. Moriyama, Mortality of the foreign born. Am J Public Health 57:496–503, 1967.

*Countries of origin: Canada, United Kingdom, Norway, Sweden, Finland, Italy.

†Table entries are number of nations (out of six studied) whose immigrants in the United States have the indicated patterns of mortality (like the United States, like the country of origin, or indeterminate) for each of six age groups.

Such retrospective studies merit some skepticism. Correlation does not always signify cause and effect, and properties found in common among victims of atherosclerotic disease may be a consequence of the disease or of a treatment for the disease instead of causes of morbidity. Nonetheless, even skeptics can tolerate cautious use of the data, and data abound.

Numerous studies document a higher prevalence of hyperlipidemia among victims of coronary disease than in control groups (Dick and Stone, 1978; Patterson and Slack, 1972; Lewis et al., 1974a, 1974b). For example, in an extensive study of 500 survivors of myocardial infarction under the age of 60, Goldstein and collaborators (1973a) compared lipid levels to those of 950 controls. The results are shown in Table 2-12, which documents the excess prevalence of both hypercholesterolemia and hypertriglyceridemia in the heart attack victim. Table 2-13 summarizes the results of 15 of the most careful retrospective studies of survivors of myocardial infarctions, focusing mainly on younger victims (usually under the age of 50).

These studies usually report the frequency of high cholesterol levels among heart attack victims as compared to the general population. The definition of "abnormal level" is critical in interpreting these studies, and there is wide variation in the choice of cutoff level from one study to another. In some studies, as many as 20 percent of

Table 2-12. Lipid levels in 500 survivors of myocardial infarction

Value (mg/100 ml)	*Percentile** (%)	*Expected*† (%)	*Observed*‡ (%)	*Obs/Exp*
		Cholesterol		
270	88.9	4.3	6.8	1.58
285	93.2	4.4	8.6	1.95
314	97.6	1.6	3.0	1.88
342	99.2	0.8	3.8	4.75
		Triglycerides		
147	88.7	4.1	8.7	2.10
165	92.8	4.2	9.2	2.20
200	97.0	2.0	6.3	3.15
245	99.0	1.0	8.0	8.00

Source. Adapted and revised from J. L. Goldstein et al., Hyperlipidemia in coronary artery disease. J Clin Invest 52:1540, 1973a (Table 4).

*Percentiles are adjusted from the original source assuming log normal distributions of cholesterol and triglycerides.

†Expected = percentage of controls between this value and next higher.

‡Observed = percentage of survivors of myocardial infarction between this value and next higher.

Table 2-13. Lipid levels in survivors of myocardial infarction

Study	*Controls*	*No. of MI survivors Sex:M|F*	*Age range*	*Interval since MI*	*Upper limit of normal cholesterol (mg/dl)*	*Upper limit of normal triglycerides (mg/dl)*	*Percentage with abnormal cholesterol and normal triglycerides*	*Percentage with abnormal cholesterol and abnormal triglycerides*	*Percentage with normal cholesterol and abnormal triglycerides*
Atlas et al., 1975	No	46|4	≤40	2 mo	270	160	22	12	46
Chase et al., 1974	No	58|2	≤55	2–4 yr	age: 20–29 245 age: 40–60 308	age: 20–29 140 age: 30–39 150 age: 40–49 160 age: 50–60 190	12	14	40
Dolder & Oliver, 1975	No	240|0	≤40	6 wk–6 mo	280	200	10	15	20
Engel et al.,* 1974	No	0|17	≤40	Unknown	250	190	76	Unknown	Unknown
Fleischman et al., 1967	No	83|0	30–50	2–2 ½ yr	260	145	24	Unknown	74
Goldstein et al.,† 1973a, 1973b	Yes	401|99	30–89	3 mo	285	165	7.6	7.8	15.6
Gustafson et al., 1972	Yes	229|0	27–55	3 mo	280–300	180	19	10	18
Hatch et al., 1966	Yes	24|0	23–49	6 mo–13 yr	210	150	83	Unknown	40

*5 patients with diabetes mellitus

†44% of patients on diet

Table 2-13. Continued

Study	*Controls*	*No. of MI survivors Sex: M|F*	*Age range*	*Interval since MI*	*Upper limit of normal cholesterol (mg/dl)*	*Upper limit of normal triglycerides (mg/dl)*	*Percentage with abnormal cholesterol and normal triglycerides*	*Percentage with abnormal cholesterol and abnormal triglycerides*	*Percentage with normal cholesterol and abnormal triglycerides*
Leren & Haabrekke, 1971	Yes	318|102	30–64	Variable	275	200	59.0	Unknown	11.7
Mann & Thorogood, 1975	Yes	0|44	25–44	≥6 mo	267	207	29.6	11.4	6.8
Nikkilä & Arö, 1973	Yes	94|7	23–49	6–44 mo	320	210	21.8	9.9	21.8
Oliver, 1974	No	0|32‡	≤45	2–20 yr	270	200	41	33	6
Pagnan et al., 1974	Yes	65|31∮	—	≥3 mo	236	207	27.5	39.9	8.5
Patterson & Slack, 1972	Yes	107|85	—	6–24 mo	325 (men) 311 (women)	212 (men) 130 (women)	9 (control = 3%)	4 (control = 1%)	14 (control = 5%)
Tamir et al., 1972	Yes	64|0	35–41	≥6 mo	250	150	36	17	6

‡48% of a total of 81 women survivors of MI had cholesterol measurements ≥270 mg/dl

∮18 with MI, and 59 with ischemic heart disease.

the controls were defined as abnormal. Despite these methodological problems, it is clear that survivors of early myocardial infarction are at higher risk for hyperlipidemia than are their healthy contemporaries. As seen in Table 2-13, hypercholesterolemia is especially common among *women* who suffer coronary artery disease in early adulthood.

High cholesterol levels do not seem to be particularly characteristic of victims of occlusive peripheral vascular disease but are somewhat associated with cerebrovascular disease. Mathew et al. (1975) found type IV hyperlipidemia in approximately 40 percent of patients with symptomatic large vessel cerebrovascular disease and type II in 9 percent. Serum lipid levels correlate not just with disease incidence but also with severity of disease as determined by coronary angiograms (Berenson et al., 1974; Barboriak et al., 1974; Salel et al., 1977).

Curiously, although early myocardial infarction seems strongly associated with hyperlipidemia, the evidence is mixed on whether lipid levels are good prognostic indicators once coronary disease has appeared. A number of small studies have failed to demonstrate a significant relationship between cholesterol levels and survival subsequent to infarction (Frank, 1968; Little et al., 1965; Shanoff et al., 1970). On the other hand, the Western Collaborative Group Study noted that younger heart attack victims with recurrent infarction more often had elevated cholesterol levels than did victims whose infarction did not recur during the four and one-half year observation period (Rosenman et al., 1970).

Hyperlipidemia in relatives of victims of coronary disease

Victims of coronary heart disease have higher lipid levels than do nonvictims; the same is true of their close relatives. Table 2-14 reviews a number of recent lipid studies of relatives of patients with ischemic heart disease.

In general, children and other first-degree relatives of victims of early coronary artery disease appear to have a risk of hyperlipidemia some three to four times that of the general population and, by inference from epidemiologic studies, at least an incrementally increased risk of developing ischemic heart disease based on their higher lipid levels alone. Our calculations, which are discussed at length in Chapter 5, show that theoretical and empirical results agree: Victims of heart attack under the age of 50 years have mean cholesterol levels about 1 standard deviation above normal, and their first-degree relatives have mean levels about 0.3 standard deviation above normal. Among neonates, cholesterol levels did not differ between children of victims of premature myocardial infarction and a control group, but Kwiterovitch et al. (1973) found elevations of pre-beta lipoprotein to be more common in the infants of parents with the familial form of hypercholesterolemia than in infants of normal parents.

Disease in hyperlipidemic people

Several centers with access to concentrations of people with unusually high lipid levels have followed such people and observed them to be at higher risk for cardiovascular disease than the general population. Such observations are not as reliable as large-scale unselected prospective studies of entire communities, mainly because of the risk of bias toward disease in a group of patients who become known to a medical center, but the papers are widely cited and deserve some cautious examination.

Slack's (1969) study of 78 patients with hyperlipidemia (i.e., cholesterol levels over 325 mg/dl) is the object of much attention. She followed these patients for one to ten years and observed a high risk of ischemic heart disease among men and women with xanthomata. Slack concluded from her data that a type II hyperlipidemic man has a 24 percent chance of suffering from ischemic heart disease by the age of 40, 50 percent by the age of 50, and 85 percent by the age of 60.

Table 2-14. Lipid levels in relatives of victims of myocardial infarction

Author	*Subjects*	*Lipid findings*
Atlas et al., 1975	137 first-degree relatives of hyperlipidemic early MI survivors	45% had type II or IV
Chase et al., 1974	179 children of victims of MI < 50 yr	29% had elevated lipids (15% if proband had normal lipids; 39% if proband was hyperlipidemic)
Deutscher et al., 1966, 1970	89 sons of fathers who died of CHD before age 65	25.8% had ↑ C vs. 21.4% of controls
	74 sons of mothers who died of CHD before age 65	40.5% had ↑ C vs. 17.7% of controls
Førde & Thelle, 1977	846 men aged 20–40 who had one or more first-degree relatives with MI	No significant difference in cholesterol in subjects with positive family history vs. those with negative family history
Glueck et al., 1974	223 children of 70 survivors of MI	31% had ↑ lipids: 15.3% type IIa, 4.5% type IIb, 11.2% type IV

Table 2-14. Continued

Author	Subjects	Lipid findings
Goldstein et al., 1973b	645 adult first-degree relatives of 149 hyperlipidemic survivors of MI	Mean cholesterol 235 mg/dl (±53) compared with 218 mg/dl (±41) in controls
Hennekens et al., 1976	90 children of 39 fathers with premature MI	16.7% had C > 230 mg/dl compared to 4.7% of controls
Nikkilä & Arö, 1973; Arö, 1973	412 first-degree relatives of victims of MI < 50 yr of age	13% had C > 320 mg/dl 6.8% had C > 320 mg/dl and TG > 210 mg/dl 9.5% had TG > 210 mg/dl Controls = 7.3% type IIa 2.7% type IIb 7.3% type IV
Pagnan et al., 1974	339 siblings and children of 77 CHD patients (18 MI and 59 IHD)	36.6% had lipids > 80th percentile 21.1% type IIa 10.2% type IIb 5.4% type IV Controls 27.4% had lipids > 80th percentile 14.7% type IIa 5.1% type IIb 7.6% type IV
Patterson & Slack, 1972	79 first-degree relatives of 23 type II survivors of MI	6 type IIa 4 type IIb 5 type IV
	48 first-degree relatives of 17 type IV survivors of MI	1 type IIa 1 type IIb 1 type III 5 type IV
Tamir et al., 1972	All children of fathers < age 41 who had survived a MI for at least 6 mo	
	47 children of 23 fathers with type IIa	42.6% type IIa
	30 children of 11 fathers with type IIb	30% type IIa
	8 children of 4 fathers with type IV	12.5% type IIa 0% type IV
	55 children of 26 fathers with normal lipoproteins	0% abnormal

Dewailly (1975) conducted a study that followed for ten years a group of 250 patients with type II hyperlipidemia, of whom 50 percent developed either angina pectoris or myocardial infarction. The works of Jensen et al. (1967) and Stone et al. (1974) also showed a greatly increased risk of coronary disease in hypercholesterolemic families with a cumulative incidence of coronary disease in the latter series among type II males of 16 percent by age 40 and 52 percent by age 60. Type II men had a level of risk equivalent to the risk in normal men 20 years older.

Taken together, the retrospective studies of special populations leave little doubt that high lipid levels are significantly more prevalent among victims of ischemic heart disease than among their healthy contemporaries. Prospective epidemiology informs us that the risk of heart disease is relatively high among hyperlipidemics; retrospective study provides the converse observation: Elevated lipid levels are relatively more common among victims of coronary disease and among their close relatives.

MANIPULATION OF CHOLESTEROL LEVELS: CAN THEY BE CONTROLLED?

If cholesterol is to be a lever in primary prevention of cardiovascular disease, it must be susceptible to control. An unchangeable attribute of an individual, such as adult height, may be a superb predictor of some future event and may even be a causative agent, but if we cannot manipulate it, it cannot be our direct tool in prevention or therapy. What we can change, we can use; what we cannot change, we are confined to observe.

The evidence on cholesterol is conclusive on this point: Individual serum cholesterol is not an unalterable personal characteristic but is susceptible to intentional manipulation by changes in diet and behavior. This is the conclusion of dietary experimentation in human infants, children, and adults, which we will review in Chapter 4. For now, let us go on to those studies that used lipid levels as an independent variable, manipulated through diet and drugs, and measured changes in health outcome.

DIETARY INTERVENTION STUDIES

Only experimental studies that test actual lowering of subjects' cholesterol levels by diet can demonstrate finally whether such intervention reduces coronary heart disease. Other studies cannot rule out the possibility that some unknown factor causes both high levels of serum cholesterol and high risk of coronary heart disease, nor can they establish whether the processes by which diet causes clinically manifested atherosclerosis can be reversed or at least slowed in adults. Typically, a cholesterol-lowering diet consists of reducing intake of saturated fats, increasing the ratio of polyunsaturated to saturated fats, and decreasing cholesterol intake in the diet (Bowan et al., 1973; McGandy et al., 1972).

In the last quarter of a century, at least a dozen dietary intervention studies have been reported in medical journals. Numerous reviews of the findings have also been published (Rifkind and Levy, 1974; Blackburn, 1974; Malmros, 1969; Stead, 1969; Committee on Diet and Heart Disease of the National Heart Foundation of Australia, 1974; Stamler, 1971; Stamler and Berkson, 1972; Cornfield and Mitchell, 1969). One excellent review (Cornfield and Mitchell, 1969) provided a helpful summary of the key features of studies as of 1969. Table 2-15 is a modification and extension of their work.

We will divide our discussion into primary (prevention of heart disease in the healthy) and secondary (prevention of recurrence in the sick) interventions. We give primary studies more attention because they relate directly to the programs we will evaluate, programs aimed at the general population. Secondary studies deal with only one particular group, survivors of myocardial infarction, on whom diet may have different effects than in primary prevention—less effect because the interventions are too late, or more effect because the population is at especially high risk.

Primary prevention studies

Three inadequately controlled primary prevention studies found possible beneficial effects of diet. In 1965, Hood et al. reported a retrospective, nonexperimental study of hypercholesterolemics, some with previous disease, most without. In this study, 112 patients had adhered to a strict cholesterol-reducing diet. An equal number of patients who had not strictly dieted were chosen, matched to the dieters by age, sex, blood pressure, degree of vascular symptoms, and initial cholesterol level. Females showed the predicted pattern, with mean serum cholesterol levels in female dieters dropping 20 percent and in controls dropping 6 percent. Male dieters' mean serum cholesterol levels fell 21 percent, but oddly the controls' mean fell 18 percent.

Table 2-15. A summary of findings of dietary intervention studies (drug studies excluded): A review of the design and a sample of the results of 14 prospective trials of dietary therapy to reduce coronary risk

Study site or name	*Major references*	*Number of patients*	*Number of controls*	*Age (years)*	*Sex*	*Clinical setting*
		Primary or mixed primary/secondary prevention				
Copenhagen Geriatric unit	Hansen et al., 1962	133	132	65–90	M	Inpatient
Göteborg, Sweden	†Hood et al., 1965	112	112	20–90	M+F	Outpatient
New York Anti-Coronary Club	*Rinzler et al., 1968	941	457	40–59	M	Outpatient
Los Angeles Veterans Administration	†Dayton et al., 1968	424	422	50–89	M	Institutional
Coronary Prevention Evaluation Programs, Chicago	*Stamler, 1970	519	0	40–59	M	Outpatient
Finnish Mental Hospitals	*Miettinen et al., 1972; Turpeinen, 1978	1273	1022	15–75	M	Institutional
		Secondary prevention				
Seattle, Washington	Nelson, 1956	175	0	Unknown	?	Outpatient
San Jose, California	Lyon et al., 1956	217	0	55	M+F	Outpatient

*Primary prevention only

†Mixed primary and secondary prevention

Average time on diet (months)	Compliance with diet	Mean percent drop in cholesterol		Dropout rate	Sample results on mortality or morbidity
		Patients	*Controls*		
		Primary or mixed primary/secondary prevention			
4.7	Inpatient	13 $N=28$	Unknown	Unknown	Treated: 1.5% (2 of 133) had thrombo-embolism Controls: 11% (14 of 132) had thrombo-embolism
60–204	Dietary recall	16	12	Death only	Treated: 11% dead Controls: 34% dead
120	Adipose tissue analysis	13	0	36%	Treated: 17 new events in 3954 man-years of experience Inactive group: 24 new events in 3207 man-years of experience Controls: 32 new events in 3122 man-years of experience
60–96	49% good	19	7	21%	Treated: 16% had cardiovascular events Controls: 22% had cardiovascular events
60	Records kept	15	—	About 27% per year; cumulative dropout rate of 69% over 7 years	Age-adjusted cumulative coronary heart disease death rate in nondropouts was ¼ as large as in dropouts.
72	Adipose tissue analysis	13	0	12% "turnover" of hospital patients per year	Treated: 1.5% dead from CHD in hospital Controls: 4% dead from CHD in hospital
		Secondary prevention			
50	89% good	15	—	22%	Compliers: 10% (11 of 110) died Noncompliers: 31% (12 of 39) died
48	66% good	Unknown	—	34%	Compliers: 27% (15 of 55) had repeat MI (13 dead) Noncompliers: 41% (51 of 125) had repeat MI (13 dead)

Table 2-15. A summary of findings of dietary intervention studies (drug studies excluded): A review of the design and a sample of the results of 14 prospective trials of dietary therapy to reduce coronary risk (Continued)

Study site or name	*Major references*	*Number of patients*	*Number of controls*	*Age (years)*	*Sex*	*Clinical setting*
		Secondary prevention				
Crenshaw Hospital, Los Angeles	Morrison, 1951, 1960	50	50	32–70	M + F	Outpatient
St. Mary's Hospital, London	Rose et al., 1965	54	52	54	?	Outpatient
Central Middlesex and other hospitals, London	Ball et al., 1965	123	129	65	M	Outpatient
Four district hospitals, London	Morris et al., 1968	199	194	60	M	Outpatient
Oslo, Norway	Leren et al., 1966, 1968	206	206	30–64	M	Outpatient
St. Vincent's Hospital, Montclair, New Jersey	Bierenbaum et al., 1963, 1967, 1973	100	100	30–54	M	Outpatient

Source: Adapted, revised, and updated from J. Cornfield and S. Mitchell, Selected risk factors in coronary disease. Arch Environ Health 19: 382–394, 1969.

The total mortality figures were striking: 9 dieters versus 38 controls, but the result is difficult to interpret because of the anomolous cholesterol changes.

The Anti-Coronary Club Study followed 941 volunteer men aged 40 through 59 at entry (Rinzler, 1968; Christakis et al., 1966) who were placed on a cholesterol-reducing diet, with those overweight also put on weight-reducing diets. Volunteers who kept up the frequent visits for cholesterol determination were deemed active participants. Volun-

Average time on diet (months)	*Compliance with diet*	*Mean percent drop in cholesterol*		*Dropout rate*	*Sample results on mortality or morbidity*
		Patients	*Controls*		
96	—	29	Unknown	Death only	Treated: 44% dead Controls: 76% dead
24	Dietary recall	4	1.2	8%	Treated: 48% dead Controls: 27% dead
36	Records kept	15	10	Death only	Treated: 16% (20 of 123) dead Controls: 19% (24 of 129) dead
24–80	89% good	16 (36 mo)	5	2%	Treated: 31% relapses; 13% dead Controls: 38% relapses; 13% dead
60	84% good	17.6	3.7	2%	Treated: 10% sudden deaths; 17% repeat MI Controls: 8% sudden deaths; 26% repeat MI
120	Dietary recall	9	5	Death only	Treated: 16% had fatal MI Controls: 28% had fatal MI (At 60 mo, 44% of treated patients had experienced a recurrent MI compared with 71% of controls)

teers who lapsed were analyzed separately. A group of cancer clinic volunteers provided the main comparison group.

Active participants' average serum cholesterol level was initially slightly above that of cancer clinic comparisands but fell 13 percent after dieting. After a decade, coronary disease events had occurred at the rate of 430 per 100,000 person-years for active members, 748 for inactive (lapsed) members, and 1025 for comparisands.

The measured demographic and medical differences between the two groups tended to the advantage of the comparisands. Nonetheless, two important problems remain: selection bias and confounding. The active group was constantly losing members, who were relatively obese and young. If these inactive members were disproportionately prone to ischemic heart disease, the shifting composition of the active group created a continuing selection bias compatible with the observed widening gap between heart disease rates. Furthermore, changes in the prevalence of obesity and hypertension confounded the effects of lowered cholesterol.

The Coronary Prevention and Evaluation Project (CPEP) actively sought to make simultaneous changes in diet, exercise, smoking, and hypertensive therapy (Stamler, 1971). The participants were 519 healthy, high-risk men, aged 40 through 59. After five years, the hypercholesterolemics' mean cholesterol levels had fallen 15 percent. Weight loss averaged 7 percent. Fitness and cessation of smoking showed less improvement.

The main reference group was the American Heart Association Pooling Project population, a group with fewer hypercholesterolemics than the CPEP, fewer hypertensives, fewer men with more than two risk factors, the same mean cholesterol levels, lower mean relative weight, but far more smokers. After seven years, one-fourth of the CPEP men had dropped to inactive status. (These inactive men had a higher coronary disease mortality rate and a lower total mortality rate than the Pooling Project men.)

The total mortality among CPEP men, both active and inactive, was 28 percent lower than among comparisands. Among the active men, total mortality was 46 percent lower than among comparisands. Furthermore, coronary heart disease mortality was 75 percent lower and sudden death was 87 percent lower. The CPEP study is particularly confounded by differences in smoking behavior; twice as many comparisands as active men smoked, and smokers had a very high risk of heart disease. If smokers and nonsmokers are considered separately, we find that nonsmokers in the experimental group had a 25 percent reduction and smokers had a 25 percent *increase* in coronary disease relative to comparisands. Although CPEP may have reduced cardiac morbidity, the initial distribution of risk factors obscures any reliable measurement of this reduction.

Semicontrolled trials have also found benefits. Hansen et al. (1962) assigned each ward in a hospital to one of two diets, either a diet using polyunsaturated oils or a control diet. After three months, the dieters' mean serum cholesterol levels had fallen 13 percent. The investigators observed 265 patients for an average of only 4.7 months, noting the occurrence of thrombosis, myocardial infarction, and stroke.

Two dieters and 14 controls had some form of thrombosis. This trial, however, is hardly conclusive, since the assessment of illness was not blind, the assignment of wards was not random, and the patients may have differed in more respects than diet.

Miettinen et al. (1972) (also Turpeinen et al., 1968, and Turpeinen, 1979) studied the entire population of two Finnish psychiatric hospitals. For six years, one hospital served a diet high in polyunsaturated fat while the other hospital served its usual diet. The hospitals then switched diets, and their patients were studied for another six years. During the diet periods, serum cholesterol levels dropped 12 to 18 percent. Overall mortality during the hospital stay was lower for the diet period than for the control period in three of the four hospital-sex groups. The relative risk of coronary death was .47 for male dieters and .66 for female dieters. Unfortunately, both the average observation period per patient and the median age differed between hospitals and between the two stages of the trial. Although mortality rates were calculated to account for the different observation periods and were age adjusted, the differences reduce confidence in the comparability of the control and diet periods.

Hansen and Turpeinen were able to control diet because their subjects were living in institutions. A well-controlled study in the Los Angeles Veterans Administration domiciliary unit shared this advantage. In that study, Dayton et al. (1968, 1969) used random assignment from a single experiment pool and a double-blind protocol (neither subjects nor their doctors knew which regimen they were on). The researchers studied 846 healthy, cooperative men older than 55 for five to eight years, observing deaths and atherosclerotic events, especially sudden death and myocardial infarction. Dieters and controls followed diets containing 40 percent fat: the study diet had mostly polyunsaturated fats, whereas the control diet had mostly saturated fats. Serum cholesterol levels fell 19 percent for dieters and 7 percent for controls.

Total mortality for the two groups was similar. However, 48 dieters and 70 controls died from atherosclerosis—a relative risk for dieters of .68. Furthermore, 66 dieters and 90 controls suffered from a clearly detectable atherosclerotic event, usually heart attack, cerebral infarction, or sudden death—a relative risk for dieters for all events of .37. The relative risk of myocardial infarction alone for dieters was .67.

Apparently, the veterans on the diet who were "saved" from coronary disease died of something else during the study, usually cancer, a finding that sparked an inquiry into possible carcinogenic effects of polyunsaturates. No such effects have been found. The negligible effect on total mortality despite the favorable effect on coronary disease probably resulted from studying a relatively elderly group.

A number of studies exist that attempted prevention through the use of cholesterol-lowering drugs instead of, or in addition to, diet. The most recent of these was a well-controlled six-year experiment on 30,000 men using the drug clofibrate to achieve a 9 percent reduction of cholesterol in the treated group, which experienced 20 percent fewer major ischemic heart disease events than did controls with similar initial lipid levels (Committee of Principal Investigators, 1978). All of the difference in morbidity was attributable to a reduction in nonfatal myocardial infarctions. Although the clofibrate-treated subjects were less likely to die of coronary disease, they were significantly more likely to die of noncardiovascular causes, including malignancy, and the groups therefore did not differ in overall mortality. The possible, but unproven, excess risk of noncardiovascular disease in the pharmacologically treated group increases the attractiveness of dietary therapy as the main component of a cholesterol-lowering effort.

In sum, the studies of primary intervention tend to show evidence that diet can reduce serum cholesterol levels and that chances of nonfatal heart disease or coronary death are probably reduced after adopting a diet that lowers cholesterol. The well-controlled institutional population studies in Los Angeles and in Finland provide the strongest current foundations for believing that a diet that reduces serum cholesterol levels can reduce the incidence of coronary heart disease.

Secondary prevention studies

A large number of secondary prevention studies exist, some of which are included in Table 2-15. Our detailed review of these studies somewhat reconciles their different conclusions. In brief, we note that rates of reinfarction probably fall with dieting, but only when the diet is rather stringent and when the patients are young and have hearts of normal size.

CURRENT PROPOSALS FOR CHOLESTEROL POLICY

The amount of literature on cholesterol and risk testifies to the continuing suspicions that have directed the path of medical research. We find the results convincing enough to worry about the costs of delaying actions, but uncertainties remain. Almost everyone agrees on the value of further study in reducing these uncertainties, but some activists would go further. They argue that the evidence is strong enough and the costs of delay so great that screening and intervention should start now, before all the results are in.

Skeptics point to the relatively small reductions in total mortality that have resulted in the controlled dietary studies. While it is clear that cholesterol and heart disease go hand in hand, it is *not* clear that cholesterol is a lever by which heart disease can be controlled.

Activists look at the same data and conclude that the real problem is in intervening too late—in middle age, when the damage has already been done. From the resulting recommendations—for further study, for intervention, and for screening—come the programs that we will evaluate.

Recommendations for further study

The literature on cholesterol forces any conscientious reader to make discomforting mental notes about important pieces of missing data. Despite disagreement on what to do *now* about cholesterol, consensus is universal on the need for further investigation. Eloquent calls have been issued for large, multifactorial, prospective intervention trials on methods for lowering morbidity and mortality from coronary disease (Blackburn, 1975; Fredrickson, 1968; Wright, 1973). Some of that research has now begun.

In the United States, longitudinal studies of hyperlipoproteinemia in children and in adults are now underway through several Lipid Research Centers and at Specialized Centers of Research in Atherosclerosis. From data to be collected, we will soon learn how well childhood lipid patterns predict adult patterns in individuals. Studies are also in progress to delineate further the modes of inheritance of lipid patterns and to elucidate the genetic defects of hyperlipoproteinemia. At several centers, serial clinical studies of adults on preventive dietary programs will contribute to an understanding of the effect of diet on disease progression.

Community-wide programs to alter life-styles also exist, including the Stanford Heart Study (Farquhar et al., 1975) and the Finnish North Karelia Project (Karvonen, 1974; Puska, 1974; Puska et al., 1978). The programs have yielded estimates of the elasticity of life-styles, including diet, in free-living populations and may ultimately demonstrate the effects of population-wide intervention on patterns of morbidity.

From these efforts will come increased knowledge about how diet, cholesterol, and atherosclerosis interact. Certainty, however, is not to be expected—only new estimates with higher reliability. It is to the rational consumption of these data, both old and new, that our work turns in the subsequent chapters.

Recommendations on screening

Advocates of screening seek to increase the benefits of intervention by first identifying those with the highest risks. The American Medical Association's Council on Foods and Nutrition and the Food and Nutrition Board of the National Academy of Science's National Research Council recommended in 1972 that "measurement of the plasma lipid profile, particularly plasma cholesterol, become a routine part of all health maintenance physical examinations. Such measurements should be made in early adulthood" (Food and Nutrition Board, 1972). Drash and Hengstenberg (1972) have suggested the potential usefulness of screening school-aged children, and Lauer et al. (1975), Hennekens et al. (1976), Kannel and Dawber (1972), Chase et al. (1974), Lloyd et al. (1975), Strong et al. (1975), Lloyd and Wolff (1969), and Fredrickson (1972) have directed attention toward suggestions for screening children who, because of positive family histories for hyperlipidemia or atherosclerosis, may be at especially high risk. Glueck et al. (1971) discuss the possibility of screening cord blood cholesterol or low-density lipoprotein cholesterol levels in such high-risk neonates, and in an editorial, the *British Medical Journal* stated, "Extensive evaluation of cord blood lipoprotein assays is therefore justified for routine screening of babies born to hyperlipidemic parents and to families with a history of early-onset heart disease" (Editorial, 1974). Arguing against *community-wide* childhood screening in recent times are Lloyd (1975), Sackett (1974), North (1975), Schubert (1973), and Motulsky and Boman (1975). Despite misgivings, large-scale childhood cardiovascular risk factor screening programs have been implemented in several settings (Lauer et al., 1975; Kromhout et al., 1977; Williams and Wynder, 1976; Friedman and Goldberg, 1973).

Recommendations on intervention

The high cholesterol levels of affluent societies have caused some scholars to bypass screening and promote population-wide dietary alterations as reasonable and desirable. Keys (1968) noted recommendations from the Medical Boards of Norway, Sweden, and Finland that dietary changes to lower cholesterol should be introduced in the entire population of these nations. Tyroler et al. (1971), reporting on the results of the Evans County, Georgia, study, suggested that " . . . the prevalence of risk factors is so high that interventions should have to include large proportions of the target populations potentially to achieve moderate reduction in incidence [of coronary heart disease]." Several writers suggest population-wide dietary changes in the adult years (Malmros, 1969; McMillan, 1973; Stamler, 1978). Some believe that dietary changes, to be most effective, should begin in childhood (Strong and McGill, 1969).

Dietary intervention in childhood, especially in infancy, seems risky to others, who hold that cholesterol-lowering diets could conceivably do harm to infants (Schubert, 1973). Fomon (1971) writes, "There is little reason to assume that nutritional management appropriate for the adult is desirable for the infant," and Lowe (1972) concurs.

Others have feared the economic dislocation from too rapid a change in the fat composition of the average American diet, with burdensome surpluses of some commodities, such as beef, and inflationary shortages of others (Meyer, 1973).

In 1972, a set of recommendations with an aura of definitiveness emerged from the blue-ribbon Inter-Society Commission for Heart Disease Resources as a report on "Primary Prevention of the Atherosclerotic Diseases." Following an elegant review of the literature, the commission issued strikingly interventionist recommendations:

> (A) That a strategy of primary prevention of premature atherosclerotic diseases be adopted as long-term national policy for the United States . . . (including) . . . changes in diet to prevent or control hyperlipidemia, obesity, hypertension, and diabetes . . . .
>
> (B) That a Special Committee be established at a high level of the Federal Government to develop coordinated plans for large scale, long-term trials to determine the effects of various interventions, particularly diet modification, on the rates of premature atherosclerotic diseases in the United States . . . .
>
> (C) That diets be modified for the general public, and especially those at high risk of CHD to reduce consumption of calories, cholesterol, and saturated fats. [This was to be done through extensive changes in the meat, dairy, and baked good industries achieved by consumer education, research, and labelling reforms.] (Inter-Society Commission for Heart Disease Resources, 1972)

Similar recommendations issued shortly thereafter from the National Heart Foundation of Australia, which encouraged a trend in diet away from high fat and high calories (Committee on Diet and Heart Disease, 1974).

The Inter-Society Commission's recommendations took a long step from the data, and conservative respondents viewed them with alarm. Among these was the American Academy of Pediatrics' Committee on Nutrition, which wrote, "Such dietary intervention [as the Inter-Society Commission proposes] is, at present, experimental and [we] recommend against dietary changes for all children" (American Academy of Pediatrics, 1972). (The committee did endorse treatment for certain hypercholesterolemic children over the age of 1 year.)

Sackett and Holland (1975) believe that such disputes between "evangelists" and "snails" derive more from disagreement on *how to decide* than from differences over particular programs. They argue that the real questions are whether or not we are ready to decide the policy question, and what methods to use for deciding. Debates that leap over these two threshhold issues are doomed to be inconclusive.

Conclusions

The problem of cholesterol policy shares, in our view, major elements with other important social issues, especially other issues in preventive medicine.

First, coronary artery disease is a major killer, a significant enemy, and even small steps toward its solution would have enormous impact—hundreds of thousands of lives are involved. The stakes are high.

Second, information currently available leads reasonable people to tentative conclusions but not to certainty. Today's data lack conclusiveness.

Third, certainty will probably continue to be elusive. Limitations of experimental design in human systems will leave most feasible experiments open to criticism. Furthermore, in childhood intervention to prevent adult disease, even moderately conclusive experiments take decades to bear fruit.

Fourth, both costs and benefits from action are difficult to estimate; they are indistinct, cannot be completely anticipated, and lie in the remote future. The payoffs from preventive efforts are likely to accrue, if at all, not in the next months or years, but decades from now.

Fifth, *not acting* is as much a policy as *acting*. The status quo contains laws, social policies, modes of corporate and personal behavior, and levels of effort that constitute a de facto national policy toward cholesterol, no less than if it were a conscious, centrally coordinated, goal-directed plan. The question is, not whether we should "do anything" about cholesterol levels in Americans, but whether to do anything *different*.

Sixth, interest groups are strong. The food industry, the public health industry, private and semiprivate health organizations, consumer groups, advertising firms—all these and more have significant interest in discussions and initiatives in policy on American diets, and their participation directly moves preventive cardiology into the political arena.

Seventh, the cholesterol problem exists, not in isolation from daily life experiences, but interwoven with the way we live. The issues are at least partially those of life-style and, by inference, of what sort of culture we wish to have.

In the next chapter we will present a method for addressing the question of what our policy on cholesterol should be. We will not sidestep the question of whether more study should precede a decision, although we will cast it in a different light. Our methods will allow us both to examine policy alternatives and to ask the question, "How sensitive is our decision to facts about which we are still uncertain, to unresolved areas that further study may be able to resolve?" Some of the lessons we will learn about cholesterol, we hope, will have meaning by extrapolation to other, similar issues in social health policy.

3. The analytic model

This book presents a method for helping to decide what to do in a matter of health policy when information is imperfect, payoffs are remote, and certainty is elusive. This method, systematic cost-effectiveness analysis, is used to test and critique alternative public policies toward the problem of high cholesterol in the American populace.

The theoretically possible programs to attack cardiovascular disease through altering cholesterol levels range from doing nothing to undertaking a complete restructuring of the life-style of the American citizen. Within these limits, we have selected four plans for further study: (1) doing nothing, (2) screening all children and treating those with high cholesterol levels, (3) screening a limited number of "high-risk" children and treating those with high levels, and (4) attempting to lower lipid levels through population-wide educational interventions without screening. Each of these plans already has advocates in current literature in pediatrics, medicine, and public health. These proposals neither exhaust the choices nor are they strictly mutually exclusive. Our aim is to demonstrate the usefulness of our method by analyzing a few reasonable and representative options.

Public programs can be assessed by many criteria, including four in particular: effectiveness, efficiency, fairness, and feasibility. The latter two criteria, fairness and feasibility, will receive little of our attention hereafter. As long as the selection of beneficiaries is not too limited, we believe that programs to benefit the sick in general are fair.

Feasibility is a more difficult criterion to satisfy, since it depends on details of program design, shifting political climates, and other considerations that lie outside our areas of competence. What we try to provide here is a technical evaluation of the costs and effects of several programs, an evaluation that can be grist for the decisions of those with more political influence and savvy. Our extended discussion will focus on the first two criteria for choice, effectiveness and efficiency.

In the remainder of this chapter, we will describe the general outlines of our analytic approach. In Chapters 4, 5, and 6, we will consider individual program proposals.

THE COST-EFFECTIVENESS METHOD

Our analysis will not provide answers; it will only impose organization on a complex body of information. To use the results of this analysis, a decision maker must know the ground rules under which the analysis was carried out. In this chapter, we will specify the assumptions that underlie our study.

A meaningful comparison of the costs and effects of different programs must set the programs first on common ground. We must specify a single set of measures of cost and effect applicable to all the programs. A traditional cost-effectiveness approach requires a single measure of cost and a single measure of effectiveness, and at times, we will revert to this approach. The problems we are addressing are too complex to be so simply summarized, however, and so we will identify several different types of cost and benefit which we will incorporate into our analysis whenever possible.

We will assess the costs and effects of our proposed programs relative to the status quo. Even though our analysis will encompass four alternatives, we will only need to calculate the *relative* benefits for the three programs that represent changes from existing practices: screening all children, screening children thought to be at high risk, and intervening on everyone without screening. The remaining alternative—doing nothing—provides the base for our calculations, and its relative costs and benefits are therefore set at zero.

The programs we are examining incur costs and harvest benefits over individual lifetimes and, at any one moment, involve people at many different ages. To ensure comparability of the costs and benefits being calculated, we will evaluate all programs over the lifetime of a hypothetical single cohort of children, a method of evaluation that is equivalent to analyzing the annual costs and benefits of a program after it has been allowed to reach "steady state." In fact, instituting any program would involve some "start-up time"—years in which the annual costs and benefits would be quite different from the eventual steady-state conditions. Conversely, when any program ceased operating, benefits would continue to accrue after program costs had ended. The steady-state analysis properly averages these transient effects of starting and stopping programs and gives us the net value of a program over its lifetime.

Measures of benefits

Since the programs we are comparing all claim to reduce cholesterol levels, we might choose changes in cholesterol levels as a direct measure of effectiveness. However, it is not the reduction of serum cholesterol that we, in fact, value. Rather, we are concerned with the health consequences of cholesterol, the most important example of which is increased longevity. This is the primary benefit that we will estimate for each program.

We will measure changes in longevity in terms of average years of life added per person in the cohort—in other words, the change in life expectancy. This measure has become a standard one in evaluating health programs, and it gives a more accurate picture of benefits than the common alternative of "lives saved." Since death cannot be prevented—only postponed—"lives saved" generates an incomplete picture, at best, and is misleading in cases where the same individual's life is allegedly "saved" repeatedly. Choosing added years of life as our primary measure of effectiveness allows us to compare our cholesterol control programs with a broad spectrum of health programs (treating cancer, preventing automobile accidents, and improving ambulance systems, for example), since other authors have evaluated such programs with similar yardsticks.

An important question arises concerning the *quality of life* in the years added by any health program. We would all prefer a program that added active, disability-free years to one that added years of discomfort or restricted activity. In order to account for this preference, some analysts have tried to incorporate a "quality adjustment" into years of life added—to count a year added *after* a stroke as worth half as much as a year added prior to a stroke, for example (Weinstein and Stason, 1976). We have chosen another route: the addition of secondary measures of effectiveness that relate to these quality issues. In particular, we will ask how much cholesterol-lowering programs might postpone the onset of serious illness episodes such as stroke and heart disease. We will calculate "years added *prior* to the onset of heart disease" and "years added *prior* to a first stroke" as collateral benefit measures, qualifiers on our primary measure of effectiveness—changes in life expectancy.

Another benefit attributed to some preventive programs is an ultimate reduction in the cost of medical care. We have not included this as a benefit in our analyses because we are uncertain about the net effect of lowering cholesterol on medical expenses. Lifetime medical costs may decrease or they may increase, depending on which of several competing effects dominates. On one hand, reducing myocardial infarctions and strokes will decrease medical costs in caring for those conditions. Even *postponing* such morbidity represents a cost saving if we have a positive discount rate. (See below for a further discussion of discounting.) On the other hand, if heart disease and stroke are reduced, then other illnesses such as cancer will increase in absolute frequency and may actually be more of a drain on health care resources than the diseases they replace. Furthermore, if people live longer, they will incur routine medical expenses (for colds, arthritis, diabetes, and so on) over a longer period of time, again acting to increase total health care costs. In the long run, preventive measures may increase, not decrease, overall costs to society (Gori and Richter, 1978). Because of the uncertainty involved, and because net changes in medical care costs are likely to be small when compared to program costs, we have chosen not to include medical care costs in our calculations.

A final word about something our analysis will *not* attempt to do: we will not attempt to convert years of life into equivalent dollar values. We feel that such a conversion cannot currently be satisfactory, since the theoretical correct value depends on empirical work that has not yet been done, and the old method of converting years into dollars by using equivalent wages is quite misleading. Moreover, the enterprise of assigning dollar values to life seems, in itself, offensive to some people, and in the current study, we have less emotionally troublesome alternatives.

One promising way to evaluate a lifesaving program in dollar amounts is the so-called willingness-to-pay method. Economic theory states that the value of extra years of life is equal to the amount that the affected people—including the individual whose life is extended, plus family and friends—would be willing to pay for them (Mishan, 1971). Unfortunately, efforts to elicit information on willingness-to-pay through surveys have not been successful. More indirect methods, which attempt to infer this information from observations of government safety programs, market behavior in insurance purchases, or the attitude of people toward risky jobs, have not produced reliable estimates (Acton, 1975). Furthermore, the willingness-to-pay model of the value of life has several corollaries that we find unfortunate and, in some cases, repugnant. For example, the model would have us conclude that a reckless person's life is worth less than that of a cautious person and that a poor person's life is worth less than that of a rich person.

We have also rejected the common tactic of expressing the value of years of life as equivalent wages, because we believe that tactic is misleading on several counts. First, it does not accurately represent the value of life either to the individual or to society as a whole. A person and his or her friends continue to value life even though the person is unemployed, or retired, or employed in some non-wage-earning activity. Second, in theory at least, a person is paid wages by society and receives other governmental benefits in return for what he or she contributes to the society's economy through work and taxes. The economy therefore receives no "net" benefit from a person's continued wage earning and tax payments—what an individual receives balances what that individual produces. According to such a theory, the only losses from premature death that do not balance out in society's ledger are the amounts that a person and his or her family and friends would be willing to pay to prolong that person's life. Since we have no reliable method of discovering this quantity, we are better advised to work directly with years of life instead of attempting a conversion into dollars.

In summary, then, our major measures of benefit will be years of life saved by postponement of fatal events, and secondary estimates will be made as well of years of disease-free life added through the postponement of nonfatal events. Because we do not express all costs and benefits in common units (such as dollars), our product is not, strictly speaking, a cost-*benefit* analysis but rather a cost-*effectiveness* analysis. For the same reason, our work is of less use in deciding whether to implement any program at all than in comparing alternative programs for their *relative* efficiency.

Measures of costs

The principal costs we will consider will be the direct and indirect monetary costs of the programs under evaluation. In screening programs, costs included are those associated with recruiting screenees, performing the test procedure itself, keeping records, and maintaining an administrative structure. The interventions, consisting largely of health education programs, include the direct costs of counseling time, follow-up testing of cholesterol levels, and long-term record keeping.

Indirect costs include the time and inconvenience to the people being examined and treated (and to their parents in the case of children). When adults are required to participate in tests or instruction, time costs may be approximated by applying an average wage rate to the time lost.

Other indirect costs for those treated include the extra expense, if any, of a therapeutic diet, an expense that may be substantial, since such a diet would ideally be maintained throughout much of the person's life. Such expenses may change with altered food-manufacturing technologies, but today, foods to replace those omitted in a cholesterol-lowering diet cost more than the foods replaced.

We do not delude ourselves into believing that the above list of costs and benefits is exhaustive. Many potential costs and benefits that may derive from these programs are intangible, and such costs do not lend themselves easily to the kind of analysis we are performing. In a screening program, these costs may include the pain to the screenee of drawing blood, the psychic pain of being labeled "abnormal," and unwarranted dietary recklessness after being labeled "normal."

Cholesterol-lowering diets generally include reducing the consumption of cream, eggs, and bacon in favor of fish, corn oil, low-fat milk, and oatmeal—a diet that is more palatable to some than to others. Thus, intervention and follow-up programs incur, on the one hand, costs of guilt for failing to stick to the diet and, on the other, costs of dissatisfaction from the sacrifice of desired foods.

These intangibles are most difficult to quantify. One could, in theory, administer questionnaires ("How much would you be willing to pay to be able to eat an egg every day?," etc.) or develop computations based on the responses of consumers to price changes (if egg consumption stays the same despite price increases, then people are perceived to value eggs heavily). However, even if we query individuals about their preferences, we still must find a way to combine *individual* values into a meaningful *societal* index—a virtually impossible task.

If we take the route of economic theory and analyze the effect of price on consumption, we must be prepared to control for concurrent changes in the price and quality of substitute goods. In other words, we must be prepared to analyze the entire food market and industry. And the question would still remain: Have we captured the cost of giving up eggs? If we assign numbers (for the sake of having numbers) to the intangibles and combine these questionable quantities with results that we believe are soundly based, we may contaminate our entire analysis.

We take an admittedly conservative approach, consoling ourselves with two arguments: First, the mere identification of intangible costs is useful. By forcing ourselves to be systematic about listing what we value, we decrease the risk that we may overlook some programmatic effect that, though perhaps unquantifiable, is important. Second, even if we leave certain intangible outcomes of a program unestimated, their identification may help us retain a sense of enlightened humility about the results of our analysis.

We are not ignoring intangibles. Foregone pleasures in forbidden foods may be one of the costliest elements of a cholesterol-lowering program compared with a $5 screening test or a $20 counseling session. We will not quantify these costs, however. Instead, we preface the results of our quantitative analyses with the following statement: This is what we conclude, but remember that we did not assign quantitative values to several of the important intangibles that we identified.

Such a caveat may be unsatisfying to those who would like to view a cost-effectiveness approach to policy questions as an automated "answer machine." We see the role of our analysis as more limited: To organize that which is quantitative into a coherent package, to identify those elements that have not been quantified, and to suggest how the thoughtful policymaker might use our results.

Resource allocation

With measures of cost and benefits in hand, we will address the question of how to distribute a fixed health budget among alternative programs. For programs that do not interact with each other, the greatest effects are achieved by funding projects in order of decreasing cost-effectiveness. However, our programs do affect each other; each reduces the other's expected benefits. For example, if the children at high risk are already on a diet, the value of a media campaign to persuade all children to go on a diet is reduced. Health measures have the greatest effect on the sickly, and as a population becomes healthier, additional programs have less effect. We will discuss further the ways in which the programs we evaluate could interact with each other, but we will not investigate in any detail interactions with other types of preventive medicine programs.

Decisions on the size of the health budget require, in principle, a judgment of whether the least effective funded health program seems more valuable then the least effective alternative program in other sectors of social enterprise, for example, defense, welfare, or education. Such decisions require political judgments about incommensurates and are outside the scope of this book.

Discounting dollars

Pediatric programs designed to prevent adult disease bear a peculiar burden: They expend resources *now* in order to reap benefits *later*. In so doing, they forgo alternative uses of those resources with more proximate payoffs. An evaluation of cholesterol-reducing programs for children must somehow take into account this delay in reaping benefits, and to explain how we do so, we must take a brief detour into the field of economic theory to explore a concept known there as "discounting." Actual calculations using discounting are found in later chapters; in the next few pages, we will examine only the theory.

Delayed gratification earned heaven for ascetics, but today, people seem to prefer consumption now to consumption in the future. By far the most common method for describing this time preference for goods uses a constant *discount rate*. The annual discount rate is the percentage by which a good would have to increase to be worth as much to us in a year as it is worth to us now. If we are indifferent between $1.00 now and $1.07 one year from now, for example, then our discount rate is 7 percent per year.

A benefit postponed is, to economists, a benefit reduced. In deciding between various policies with continuing costs and effects, future benefits and costs must be discounted back to their present value so that goods acquired in different years are commensurate. Thus, a society with a 5 percent discount rate is indifferent between programs that generate $100 of benefits now, $105 next year, $163 ten years from now, or $1167 fifty years from now. The compounding effects of the discount rate make it clear that long-range preventive programs stand or fall with society's valuation of the present compared with the future.

One caution: Discounting is *not* the same as an adjustment for inflation. Clearly, if money is decreasing in purchasing power, a larger nominal amount in the future may, in fact, buy less than a smaller amount now. But even if prices were stable, many rational people would prefer $1.00 now to $1.05 one year from now.

Economists agree that future dollars should be discounted (even after adjustment for inflation), but they stress different reasons for doing so. The major reasons offered are the following:

Productivity of investment. Money can be spent now, or it can be invested to increase productivity, yielding a larger amount later. In choosing between programs that yield benefits at different times, it is not sensible to use a discount rate lower than the return on investments, since earlier benefits can be invested and withdrawn later.

The usual measure of the productivity of capital is the interest rate, the amount the market is willing to pay investors for the use of their money. In a world with friendly banks, perfect information, and no taxes, the discount rate is exactly the rate of interest, since people will invest their money whenever the productive yield of the investment is greater than their wish to consume goods now instead of later.

In the real world, however, the discount rate is *higher* than the inflation-adjusted rate of interest, primarily because of the effects that taxes have on rational investment decisions. When taxes are levied in order to finance public investments (such as a disease-prevention program), less money is available for private investment. Some of that money comes from taxes on individuals who would otherwise have invested it at prevailing interest rates and thereby earned a posttax rate of return somewhat lower than the rate of interest. The rest of the money raised through taxes comes from corporations, and because corporate tax rates are high compared with individual tax rates, corporations invest money only when the pretax rate of return is about double the rate of interest, or more. The rate of return on money raised through taxes, if it had been left in private hands, would have been a weighted average of the rates of return to individuals and to corporations, an average that would have been higher than the inflation-adjusted rate of interest. This higher average is a minimum acceptable figure for a discount rate for public programs, since people in the future can be benefited overall from a tax levy only if the rate of return on public investment financed through taxes is as great as the rate of return on the private investment that the taxes displace.

The proper discount rate for public projects thus depends on productive opportunities and personal desires, which vary over place and time. Recent estimates for the United States have placed this rate at from 7 to 12 percent (Harberger, 1968; Haveman, 1969; Baumol,

1969). Correcting for inflation lowers these estimates to between 5 and 10 percent.

Subjective preference for goods now over goods later. Benefits reaped now can be used in familiar ways or given to familiar people. Future wants are less predictable and less immediate, and so resources to meet those needs are considered less valuable.

In addition, delay means loss of opportunity, for every benefit put off, we forgo the use of current goods. We may be able to buy a better phonograph next year, but by delaying, we lose a year's listening. This argument is particularly apt for such public goods as roads, health, and education, for which present opportunities may be difficult to recapture in the future even if more money is available then.

Finally, many government decisions hinge on how we want to divide resources between ourselves and future generations. Although the next generation will probably be richer than we are, the desire to do something for our progeny is powerful and tends to lower the discount rate. The economists who stress this motive for discounting usually recommend somewhat lower rates than those computed from observed market interest rates (Feldstein, 1964; Marglin, 1963).

Future uncertainty. Unforeseen future events may render a promised payoff less useful than it seems to be now, and we must take account of the possibility of such events in assessing a good's future worth. For example, we may die before we have a chance to receive our withheld good, or a war may occur, or a capricious government may simply withdraw from an agreement with us. In the case of cholesterol screening, future benefits in reduced risk perhaps should be discounted because of the possibility that medical science will discover some simple way to reverse atherosclerotic change or to prevent its complications without altering cholesterol level.

The probability of such dramatic future events is small, but most such developments would tend to reduce the benefits of a preventive program. We have calculated that even with high estimates of probabilities of events affecting a cholesterol screening program, uncertainty increases the annual discount rate by less than half a percent.

Discounting health benefits

The desirability of discounting extends easily to nonfinancial costs and benefits that can simply be converted into monetary terms. However, most of the benefits of health-related programs cannot be stated in dollar amounts. We argue, nevertheless, that health and lifesaving benefits should be discounted just as we discount dollars, and at the same rate. We are *not* thereby suggesting that a child's life is worth less than an adult's life or that we would rather live now than later. Rather, we argue that a year of life should be treated as worth more now than an exactly comparable year of life in the future.

Almost all preventive medical programs incur costs now in order to reap benefits in the future. In a cholesterol-screening program for 10-year-old children, the benefits in reduced cardiovascular disease will not begin to accrue for 30 years or more, when the children we screen reach disease-prone ages. The discounting of future health benefits over such long periods, even at a very low rate, places an enormous burden on such preventive programs. At a discount rate of only 5 percent, for example, a year of life saved loses more than 75 percent of its "value" when delayed for 30 years. In fact, someone with a 5 percent per year discount rate on years of life saved would be indifferent between identically priced programs available for purchase in 1980, one of which would save 100 years of life in 1980, and the other of which would save 432 comparable years of life in the year 2010.

We contend that both years of life and dollars should be subject to the same discount rate. The following example illustrates why.

Suppose we must vote for one of two community lifesaving programs, each of which costs $10,000. Program A uses a mobile resuscitation unit to give prehospital care to victims of myocardial infarction. It will resuscitate 100 forty-year-old male victims of myocardial infarction in the next year, each of whom will live one extra year of normal, healthy life as a result—an addition of 100 man-years to the population, the benefit being realized immediately.

Program B treats 10-year-old boys for a silent disease that kills its victims suddenly at age 40. The treatment at age 10 delays the onset of the fatal episode from age 40 to 41. Program B will add a year of life to 432 boys who would otherwise have died at age 40—an addition of 432 man-years of life to the population, the benefit being realized 30 years from now. Table 3-1 summarizes the hypothetical choice.

Other things being equal, our choice between the programs depends on the discount rate. As the discount rate rises, Program B looks worse and worse, while the value of Program A, whose benefits are more immediate, does not change. If we discount at rates of less than 5 percent, we would prefer Program B; at higher rates, Program A would look more valuable than Program B.

Someone who believes that lives cannot be discounted might argue

Table 3-1. Discounting health benefits: A hypothetical choice*

Program A *Ambulances today*	*Program B* *Heart disease prevention in 10-year-olds*
Cost—$10,000	Cost—$10,000
Benefit—100 man-years (40-year-olds live longer next year)	Benefit—432 man-years (10-year-olds live longer when they reach 40)

*The hypothetical cases include the assumption that the quality of the respective life-years saved is the same for both programs.

that Program B is better, since that program would yield more benefit, regardless of when that benefit accrues.

Such a position, however, leads to a paralytic paradox. If one really does not care when benefit accrues, and always prefers more years of life to earlier payoffs, then one can invest the $10,000 at a real (adjusted for inflation) interest rate of 5 percent. Instead of buying Program B today, he will have $10,500 next year and can purchase 454 years of added life instead of 432. The payoff is delayed by another year, but our imaginary opponent claims that he does not care about delay. Indeed, as long as he can earn real interest on his money, he will delay starting the program because his money, and the payoff, can always grow. Logically, he can never spend any money on a program. Whenever he does, his actions demonstrate a preference for earlier payoffs (that is, a discount rate) at least as large as the real rate of return on productive investment.

In this example, a year of life of a resuscitated 40-year-old is assumed to be as enjoyable as that of the 40-year-old whose life was extended by pediatric intervention. In coronary artery disease, that assumption may not be correct. Still, *other factors* (such as quality of life) *being equal*, there is good reason to discount the value of future years of life gained at the same rate as future monetary costs and benefits.

Empirical work suggests that individuals vary in their valuation of the next few years as compared with years farther in the future. This variation is important for some individual decisions—the choice between surgical and medical therapy for cancer, for example (McNeil et al., 1978). The variation is not so important for our analysis, however, since all the health benefits that accrue to our preventive programs occur several decades after the interventions. Health in "the next few years" is not at issue.

Through the chapters that follow, discounting will recur as the nemesis of pediatric prevention of adult disease, and the policymaker's selection of the discount rate will stand out among the important social policy decisions. Selection of a high rate of discount is not an "antihealth" position but merely indicates that the health budget (of whatever size) should be spent consistently with other societal decisions that balance the present with the future.

Our best guess for the present rate of discount is about 7½ percent, but with deference to those who find any discount rate for health hard to accept, we will use 5 percent as our base case. If our prevention programs seem inefficient with a rate of discount this low, they are surely misguided. For the next few years, we are confident that the appropriate rate of discount to apply will be between 5 and 10 percent.

WHY A FORMAL MODEL?

Formal mathematical models such as we will use are not necessarily the best means to formulate policy. In choosing to use such a model, we have, in fact, rejected several more concrete methods. To explain our choice, we should examine two alternatives to mathematical modeling that deserve particular attention: an experimental approach and decision making via "expert opinion."

An experimental approach to policy formation would involve the implementation of a model program on a small scale, with costs and benefits being measured directly and then extrapolated to operation on a full scale. Such social experiments can be extremely informative, but they tend to be very costly, yield data slowly, and in general allow inferences only about the experimental programs actually observed, not about the dozens of variations that may be under consideration. Indeed, even without alterations in the form of a program, an expansion from an experimental-scale to a full-scale operation may produce distortions and unexpected effects that make extrapolation from the experiment risky.

Another approach resorts to "expert opinions" in the search for reasonable policy. Knowledgeable physicians and scientists can be asked to provide their best estimates of the costs and health benefits associated with screening and intervention programs. If the experts disagree, the Delphi approach or other group feedback techniques can help them to arrive at a consensus. These methods are inexpensive, produce results rapidly compared to experiments, and can be used repeatedly to explore new program options. Unfortunately, techniques for collating expert opinions lack reliability; we have little reason for faith in the answers we get. Those answers are the products of assumptions and reasoning processes that are implicit and, therefore, are not accessible for others to scrutinize. We do not know how opinions would change as different elements of the problem were altered.

We can probably make better use of the expert opinions of others if we break the complex policy problem into less complex parts and then bring the data and the experts to bear on those more manageable pieces. One of the contributions of a formal model is to accomplish just that—to render the unmanageable manageable by dividing a complex whole into simpler subproblems.

In our formal model, we explicitly state hypotheses about how serum cholesterol levels and dietary changes will interact to produce the benefits and costs we care about. For example, how does serum cholesterol level relate to longevity? How does diet affect cholesterol level? How does the childhood cholesterol level relate to the adult level? Our model will spell out the variables and the relationships that we believe to be important. We will use both data and published expert opinions to estimate the qualitative and quantitative forms of these relationships.

Having built the mathematical model, we may then manipulate it more freely than we could experiment with the social process. We will formulate such models for each of the cholesterol-control programs discussed: mass screening, targeted screening, and population-wide intervention. Because we do not have either the computational resources or the data to analyze all possible variables, we will arbitrarily fix some aspects of the programs. We will use the results of our calculations to determine the ideal values for other parameters of the programs, most importantly the cholesterol level above which screened children are selected for intervention. The cholesterol cutoff level for intervention will be chosen so as to allow the hypothetical program to operate as efficiently as possible. Finally, we will deal with our uncertainty about the underlying biological and medical parameters by examining how our estimates of program performance change as these crucial parameters take on different values that reflect the range of our uncertainty, a process known formally as *sensitivity analysis*.

THE VALUE OF SCREENING

Two of the three programs that we will examine involve screening in order to identify a subgroup that would be treated to prevent or delay heart disease. An evaluation of screening implicitly contains two questions, and our model must allow us to address both of them. First, is the proposed *intervention* worthwhile (that is, cost-effective), and if so, is it more valuable to some than to others? Second, is the *screening* worthwhile? Even if the intervention is more valuable to some people than to others, and even if we can identify those people, it still may not be efficient to conduct a screening program.

Our model will allow us to address the first question simply by keeping track of the expected costs and benefits for intervening on different sorts of individuals, men and women, for example, or people at different ages. The desirability of intervention depends ultimately, of course, on deciding whether the benefits are worth the costs, an exercise that we will not carry to completion in this book, since, as noted previously, we will not take the final step of converting all costs and outcomes into a single common unit of measurement.

The second question, about the value of screening, can only be answered if we first clarify several assumptions about the screening programs. We can do this most easily by way of an example.

Why screen?: A hypothetical example

Let us assume for the moment that an intervention is worthwhile on the average; that is, if we apply it to a randomly selected group of individuals, the net benefits are worth the net costs. Suppose, further, that we have been given a fixed budget of $10,000 to deliver this intervention package. Given the costs involved, this $10,000 will allow us to intervene on 1000 individuals. As we are about to begin our intervention program, however, an enthusiast brings a new proposal to our attention, a proposal for a screening program to *precede* intervention.

The new screening proposal is this: Spend part of the $10,000 on widespread administration of an inexpensive screening test. From an individual's results on the test, we can predict the expected benefit he or she will receive from the intervention. Since we will be spending money on screening, it is true that less money will be available for intervention, and therefore a smaller number of people will receive the intervention with screening than without. However, the screening test will allow us to identify a group of individuals who get more than the average benefit from the intervention. Thus the net benefits from spending the $10,000 with a screening program may well be greater than without a screening program.

How should our budget be divided ideally between screening and intervention? If the intervention costs $10 per person and the screening costs $1 per person, our budget would allow hundreds of possible schemes. For some examples, see Table 3-2, Schemes A–E. Or, we might stick with our original plan and not screen at all, as in Scheme F.

In any scheme, the people receiving the intervention should clearly be those who have the largest expected benefits. As may be seen in Table 3-2, the division of funds between screening and intervention is equivalent to selecting a level of expected benefits above which screened individuals will be treated. Which of these options is best will depend on how different the "high-benefit" individuals are from the "low-benefit" individuals identified by the screening test. If screenees in the top 10 percent receive more than twice as many benefits as the average person in the unscreened population, then Scheme B will be better than not screening, even though only half as many individuals get the intervention. If the top 10 percent receive only 1.5 times as many benefits as average, then screening at this level would not be worthwhile, even though screening does identify a group with higher than average benefit.

It is hard to conceive of a realistic situation in which Scheme D or E would be better than no screening, unless the intervention is actually detrimental to a few individuals who are identified through screening. At the other extreme, for a common problem (like high cholesterol), a screening program that is as selective as Scheme A seems unlikely to be wise, since it would treat so few people.

Although we assume in our hypothetical example that the intervention costs remain constant, screening may also be valuable if it identifies individuals for whom intervention costs are especially low, thus increasing the benefits per dollar spent on intervention.

Table 3-2. Some hypothetical budgets for screening and intervention

Shown are a few of the ways in which a fixed budget could be spent on a program including screening and intervention. The optimal allocation depends on properties of the disease and treatment involved.

	Dollars spent for screening	*Number screened*	*Dollars spent for intervention*	*Number who receive intervention*	*Fraction of those screened who receive intervention*
Scheme A	$9,990	9,990	$ 10	1	0.0001
Scheme B	$5,000	5,000	$5,000	500	0.10
Scheme C	$2,000	2,000	$8,000	800	0.40
Scheme D	$1,000	1,000	$9,000	900	0.90
Scheme E	$ 910	910	$9,090	909	0.99
Scheme F	$ 0	0	$10,000	10,000	—

Three elements of our example deserve special emphasis:

1. The intervention budget is fixed and limited.
2. The screening test gives a continuous score that correlates with an individual's expected benefits (instead of identifying a disease state that is simply "present" or "absent").
3. The screening test is used to identify a subgroup of those screened who will receive more benefits per dollar spent on intervention than the average person would in the population as a whole.

These three elements shape our models of the cost-effectiveness of screening for high cholesterol in children. They also influence our decisions about how funds should be divided between screening and intervention.

Criteria for optimal screening programs

How does the model select the screening program with the largest expected benefit for its budget, given all the necessary information about costs and benefits? The problem is one of dividing resources optimally among various subprograms—screening, treatment, and follow-up, for example. A simple economic principle applies to such division—benefits are largest if each subprogram is equally valuable "at the margin". What this means can be seen by example; suppose Scheme B is in operation, and we are given a few additional dollars for the program. We have two different possible ways to use those new dollars. We could use them to screen a few more children and then to intervene on those children whom we find to be in the top 10 percent. Alternatively, we could use the new funds to intervene on a few more of the children already screened; in other words, we could lower the cutoff for treatment. Scheme B is optimal *only* if the additional benefit is the same for those two alternative uses of new dollars: screening more people or treating more people. This is what we mean when we state that "at the margin" the benefits of screening and the benefits of treatment must be equal.

To see why this equality must hold for the optimal program, imagine the contradictory circumstance. Imagine, for example, that our few additional dollars would yield more benefits if a few additional people were *treated* (i.e., if the cutoff level were lowered) than if a few additional people were *screened* (i.e., if the cutoff level remained the same). In that case, even *before* the additional dollars became available, Scheme B could be improved by lowering the cutoff level, that is, by screening somewhat fewer people and treating somewhat more.

The model leads easily to formal expressions of two especially useful ratios:

> The ratio of costs to expected benefits from intervening on children at a given cholesterol level
>
> The ratio of costs to expected benefits from screening a child and intervening *if* his or her cholesterol lies above a given cholesterol level

The model permits determination of both of these ratios at each and every cholesterol level. The most efficient level to use as a cutoff in a screening and intervention program is the level at which the two ratios are equal. That level yields the highest possible expected benefits from the program budget, and the use of that cutoff level for treatment is therefore an optimal strategy under the conditions specified.

At the optimal cutoff level, the proportion of money going to each activity (screening or intervention) is fixed. Thus, with a small budget, many children will not be screened at all. Moreover, since the number of children in the United States available for screening is limited, there is a limit on how much money can be spent on a program. If more money is spent, the children with lower levels of cholesterol can have the intervention, and the cost-effectiveness of the program will fall, although the total benefits will rise.

The cost-effectiveness of the optimal program is useful in comparisons with other health programs. If many other programs obtain higher benefits for the same budget, then cholesterol screening is ill-advised. On the other hand, if cholesterol screening appears much better than many existing programs, we may regard it as a profitable enterprise.

WHAT NEXT?: A PREVIEW OF CHAPTERS 4, 5, and 6

In these first three chapters, we have tried to set the stage for the three chapters now to come. Our conclusions have been general: Preventive medical proposals deserve quantitative analysis, the possible connection of cholesterol to heart disease is a fitting example to explore, and a formal quantitative model is a reasonable tool for that exploration.

Now, we will become more specific. Chapters 4, 5, and 6 will examine three different proposals for attacking heart disease by attacking cholesterol. In each of these chapters, we will follow the same general outline. First, we will describe a representative preventive program, drawing where possible from specific reports in the literature and filling in gaps with reasonable program components. The program discussed in Chapter 4 involves population-wide screening of children for cholesterol levels. In Chapter 5, we will explore the value mainly of targeted screening of high-risk populations of children. In Chapter 6, we will examine the relative merit of omitting screening and engaging instead in population-wide efforts to change diet.

Second, we will use the data now available to make estimates in each chapter of the parameters in the model that affect the efficiency of the program at issue. For example, screening programs assume that cholesterol levels remain relatively constant, at least in rank order, in individuals over time. We will comb the literature to make our best guess at the actual stability of cholesterol rank order, and we will, further, try to specify how confident we are about the accuracy of that guess.

Third, having described a program and estimated the pertinent parameters, we will apply our formal model of cost and benefit, yielding numerical estimates of the health gains to be expected from different levels of functioning of each program. We will include sensitivity analyses to see how dependent our conclusions are on the parameter estimates we use and, by implication, to see what areas of uncertainty in current data are most in need of resolution.

Comparisons among the different programs will be possible at the end, since we will use similar measures of cost and efficacy to evaluate each program separately. This comparative analysis is presented in Chapters 6 and 7.

In the chapters that follow, we have elected to confine the narrative portions to the simplest quantitative discussions. The more complex mathematical underpinnings of our analysis have been relegated to appendices, which are available to the mathematically inclined reader but avoidable by others. No important qualitative conclusion will escape the reader who skips the appendices to Chapters 4, 5, and 6.

4. Universal screening

DESCRIPTION OF A PROGRAM: CHILDHOOD SCREENING

In this chapter, we will perform our first imaginary experiment, constructing, from what we know or suspect, a blueprint for a reasonable program for population-wide childhood cholesterol screening and intervention. We will then build an analytic model to test the costs and benefits of such a program. We make no claim to recommending the best possible program or to being exhaustive in our analysis; we will try to study some reasonable approaches. One ought to leave these pages, and those of the next two chapters, not knowing for certain what program is best but having gained perspectives on what questions to ask. We offer a way of looking at things.

We will refer to the basic program evaluated in this chapter as *Universal Screening*. We choose this name not because *every* child would necessarily be screened—the total number of children who can be screened in a particular program would depend on the budget available—but because, in theory, every child would be a potential candidate for screening. By definition, a Universal Screening program does not preselect children for cholesterol screening based on other risk factors or even on expected cholesterol level. If a budget permitted the screening of, for example, 5000 children, the Universal Screening program would select those children essentially at random, although a real screening program might, for convenience, investigate all the children in a particular school district or geographical area.

In screening children for cholesterol levels, many program parameters come to mind as features subject to choice. We will assign reasonable values to some of those parameters in the attempt to limit the number of unknowns in our optimizing equations later on, and we will leave other parameters open to change as we seek their optimal values.

These are the parameters we will set from the start: age of screening, location of screening, level of enforcement of the program (mandatory versus voluntary), amount of retesting, and the nature and cost of the intervention undertaken with "positive" screenees. Left as an open issue, subject to optimization, is the cutoff cholesterol level above which screenees would be treated and, by inference, the distribution of the program budget between screening and intervention.

Age at screening

If children are being screened, it is probably most efficient to select an age at which several of the following conditions obtain simultaneously. First, we would wish to screen at a time when most children are *accessible* to a public program or to a generally administered private program. Neonatal screening for inherited disease is able to reach a large fraction of all children because it is aimed at an age group that shares a common site of access—the newborn nursery. In contrast, programs which order screening for children who are relatively "invisible" to the public sector or to the health care industry—such as children after the newborn period and before school age—have a difficult time achieving widespread participation. For lipid screening, it seems reasonable to select age groups available for cohort-oriented programs, meaning, for practical purposes, children in newborn nurseries or in school.

Second, since the efficacy of a screening program depends on the expectation of rank order stability—that a person found to have a high level will remain high and that individuals with low levels will remain low—the age at screening should be one at which cholesterol levels are relatively *stable* and reflective of adult rank order. Neonatal cholesterol values may not meet this criterion, and LDL levels, though possibly of higher predictive worth, are expensive to measure with current technologies. As hormonal balances, environmental factors, or both change in puberty, cholesterol levels fluctuate (Starr, 1971, Hennekens et al., 1976), making adolescence a possibly risky time to assess rank orders. If we seek stability of levels, we might do well to measure them at an age of relative developmental tranquility, in the latency-aged child, for example, between 5 and 10 years of age.

Third, dietary intervention beyond early childhood may be most effective at a time when the child's *decisions about food selection* are both consciously made (and so not too young) and still susceptible to adult leadership (and so not too old); when health habits have begun to have meaning, and adolescent rebelliousness has not yet become a modus operandi; and when peer group function can amplify education instead of discrediting it. We should note in passing that the malleability of dietary patterns in childhood is by no means fully known, and further research in this area is badly needed (Leventhal, 1973).

Fourth, if our biological objective is to seek to interrupt the progression of fatty streaks to more advanced plaques, we may wish to intervene prior to the first evidence of that progression, evidence that is frequently present by the end of the second decade of life.

Since we have argued that atherosclerosis may be a process of lifelong evolution, why not begin our screening and intervention as early as possible, with the human infant? After decades of testing the effects of infant diets on infant cholesterol levels, little doubt remains that infant lipid levels could be changed. Cholesterol levels are lower in infants fed evaporated milk with corn oil than in those fed milk without corn oil (Pomeranze et al., 1958), lower in infants on cow's milk than on human breast milk (Pomeranze, 1961; Fomon and Bartels, 1960), and, at 16 weeks of age, lower in infants on prepared formulas with polyunsaturated oils than on either breast or cow's milk (Goalwin and Pomeranze, 1962). Several other studies concur (Woodruff et al., 1964; Lindquist and Malmcrona, 1960; Krasilnikoff and Vesterdahl, 1966). Sweeney et al. (1961) summarized the state of knowledge: "It would be feasible to lower infant cholesterol by diet, if desirable."

But, it may *not* be desirable. Goalwin and Pomeranze (1962) ask the most bothersome question, "Could it be that the higher levels of serum cholesterol found in breast-fed infants and infants fed evaporated milk are more desirable than the lower values which accompany feeding of a corn oil formula?" A troubling issue is raised, the more so since fully 80 percent of infants in the United States are reared from birth on formulas rich in polyunsaturated vegetable oils, and a mere 5 percent are breast-fed beyond the fifth month of life (Fomon, 1975).

Fomon (1971) asks whether a cholesterol dietary "challenge" in early infancy might be necessary to stimulate the development of the metabolic systems responsible for the proper homeostasis, production, and degradation of cholesterol in the body. If so, then the serum cholesterol level of the infant fed vegetable oil is lowered only at the expense of proper cholesterol metabolism in later life. Indeed, in one report, breast-fed children in Paris had marginally lower cholesterol levels as toddlers compared with children who were not breast-fed (Hazemann et al., 1975). In suckling guinea pigs, early weaning from high-cholesterol breast milk to cholesterol-lowering substitute formulas produces mature animals whose cholesterol levels rise far more when challenged with dietary cholesterol as adults than in late-weaned siblings similarly challenged.

The same is seen in suckling swine (Reiser, 1971). Swine fed low-cholesterol diets as sucklings had cholesterol levels 30 to 89 percent higher than those fed high-cholesterol diets when both groups were challenged with dietary cholesterol loads as adult swine. Several studies that have searched for a similar effect by comparing cholesterol levels retrospectively in humans who were breast-fed and formula-fed as infants have so far failed to confirm the findings of these experiments in humans (Friedman and Goldberg, 1975; Hodgson et al., 1976). However, Mann et al. (1972), studying the Masai, who maintain low serum cholesterol levels despite high cholesterol intake (and high atherosclerosis prevalence), make the intriguing observation that the Masai nurse their children on the average until the age of 2 or 3 years and that Masai cholesterol levels *fall* at weaning, declining to adult levels by the age of 4 years.

Schubert (1973) reviews other possible hazards of cholesterol-lowering diets in infancy. In animals, cholesterol is incorporated into the brain very rapidly in the first few days of life, and at least 10 percent of this cholesterol comes from exogenous sources, suggesting an irreducible minimum cholesterol intake necessary in infants for proper brain development. Similar minima appear to exist for some fatty acids, notably the unsaturated fatty acid linoleic acid, whose total absence in human infant diets produces scaliness of skin, growth retardation, hematuria, and susceptibility to infection. Reduction of infantile fat intake in the extreme could produce deficiency of linoleic acid, although no reasonable infant diet reaches this level.

Schubert notes that attempts to lower dietary fat intake below 20 percent of calories (not recommended currently by anyone) would necessitate taking in more calories as protein, presenting high solute loads to immature kidneys, and as sugar, risking diarrhea in the neonate.

Excessive loads of polyunsaturated fatty acids in premature infants increase the requirements for vitamin E through mechanisms not yet well understood. In extreme cases, deficiency of this vitamin would be manifested as edema, irritability, constipation, hemolytic anemia, and a characteristic rash, all reversible upon resupply of the vitamin.

For the present, if there is any area of agreement on dietary prevention of atherosclerosis, it concerns the general use of cholesterol-lowering diets for that purpose in early infancy: The answer is that such diets should *not* be used with infants. Most would agree with Krasilnikoff and Vesterdahl (1966) that the unknowns are too great in infancy and that "for the present, it does not seem justified to start the prevention of atherosclerosis in early infancy." At any rate, we cannot be certain that dietary patterns forced upon infants would survive once individuals reached the ages of conscious choice.

It seems reasonable to select the late latency-aged child as an alternative target for intervention. At the age of 10, children tend to be accessible, being in school; to be in a period of relative hormonal, behavioral, and emotional stability (though we do not yet know how well childhood cholesterol rank order correlates with adult rank order); to be conscious of concepts relating to health and healthful habits; to be agreeably oriented toward adult leadership and reinforcement; and to be free of true atheromatous vascular changes. Compared with infants, their central nervous systems are nearly fully developed and thus less susceptible to the remote effects of dietary manipulation on development.

Location of screening

There is a fundamental decision to make about the "publicness" or "privateness" of a screening program. Should it use the private medical care system, trying to ensure uniform testing through a decentralized delivery system, or should it superimpose a new, publicly run program, bypassing the usual health care system?

The decentralized model, modifying the private system's behavior, has the advantages of preserving inviolate physician-patient relationships and of avoiding new bureaucracies of health care delivery. Unfortunately, it suffers from the deficiencies of any very decentralized system of personal services. For example, the diffusion of policy voluntarily through regular health care delivery channels is often slow, and inequities in the distribution of private health care might exclude from screening those children who lack regular sources of primary medical care.

Indeed, one motivation for selecting the school-aged child as the object of screening is that such children, being in school, are uniformly accessible to a publicly administered health intervention program. Screening in schools can be comprehensive, monitoring of results can be centralized, and quality of care can be standardized. For those who are disturbed by the specter of a "monitored" society, we will discuss the pros and cons further in Chapter 7, but for now, screening in schools seems, at the very least, efficient compared with decentralized screening in the regular health care system.

Level of enforcement

Should a screening program be voluntary or mandatory? The state can lay claim to a special role in protecting the welfare of children, sometimes even in contradiction to parental authority, but is it ultimately desirable to draw blood from a 10-year-old under legislative order against parental wishes or without the consent of the child? There is precedent: Mandatory neonatal screening for phenylketonuria is now the rule in most states, and many school systems both require and dispense immunizations. But how far are we ready to extend such mandates for personal health procedures performed on children in school?

Voluntary screening is arguably more efficient at the onset, since families who do not voluntarily agree to measurement of cholesterol would probably be unlikely to comply with recommendations for dietary change. On the other hand, a mandatory program would be likely to reach and aid some children whose parents, for their own reasons, would otherwise refuse to allow their child to participate, to the child's subsequent detriment.

In the end, the choice between a voluntary and a mandatory program is probably no choice at all but rather the identification of a constraint. We could conceivably mandate screening, and even require dietary advice as a form of health education. But the ultimate behavioral outcomes would remain matters of personal choice, not subject to legal control without unacceptable change in our theories of civil rights and liberties.

We choose a middle ground. Our hypothetical program would offer cholesterol screening to 10-year-old children in public schools, notify parents, and *presume consent* unless parent-initiated opposition is forthcoming. Instead of requiring parental permission, we would thus presume it in the absence of contrary statements. Intervention in hypercholesterolemic children would be voluntary—offered, but not required.

Retesting

When disease is dichotomous, either "present" or "absent," misdiagnosis may be tragic. The phenylketonuric child mistakenly labeled "normal" may be doomed to lifelong retardation; the normal child mislabeled "phenylketonuric" may be needlessly subjected to anxiety and to potentially harmful dietary treatment.

Cholesterol is different. In the borderland on either side of our cutoff value for intervention, a mistake in measurement is less costly than in the case of phenylketonuria. If our ideal cholesterol cutoff value is 220 mg/dl, for example, the child whose real level of 215 is carelessly read as 230 may be "mistakenly" treated but will still reap benefits from the treatment. The reverse error is more costly in morbidity but not in the tragic sense of the missed case of phenylketonuria. What the child suffers by undertreatment is not inevitable tragedy but a slight, though estimable, increment in risk.

To reduce errors in diagnosis, a program could test screenees more than once, but the benefits of such retesting (reducing errors) must be weighed against the added costs. We will later examine more rigorously the effect of retesting on the efficiency of a screening program and on the characteristics of the subpopulation thereby selected for treatment.

We will look at two alternatives in examining our basic screening program: first, a program in which a single measurement of cholesterol is made; and second, a program in which all children are tested twice, basing the determination of who is to be treated on the average of the two tests. When we consider Targeted Screening in Chapter 5, we will examine the possibility of rescreening only those children who are above a certain level on the first test.

The intervention

Screening without treatment and follow-up is mere meddling. Any conscientious screening program must face and resolve the issue of what happens to screenees found "positive." The range of options is broad. At one extreme, "treatment" may consist simply of informing the patient that he or she needs further help or notifying the patient's physician of the test result. At the other extreme are invasive attempts to force the patient into compliance, disregarding rights to privacy and control over one's personal health decisions.

Studies of dietary and drug intervention have tested the efficacy of programs of varying degrees of invasiveness (Gotto et al., 1977; Gross,

1971; Meyer and Henderson, 1974; Rose, 1970; Podell, 1975; Sackett et al., 1975; Sackett and Haynes, 1976; Rosenstock, 1975). The parameters that varied are, among others:

1. Extent of use of the patient's usual source of health care
2. Number and length of physician counseling sessions
3. Number and length of nutritionist counseling sessions
4. Number and frequency of follow-up lipid measurements

We need to know much more about the effects of changes in each of these parameters, but for now, we can choose a reasonable set of options, being prepared to vary them as information becomes available. For a hypothetical intensive program to change the diet of a 10-year-old, we propose the following:

1. The patient's usual source of health care would remain the primary provider for positive screenees, and guidelines would be set for appropriate follow-up by those providers. Where a primary provider is not available, the school health authorities would make arrangements for follow-up.
2. Initial physician counseling sessions would be 30 minutes in length, with subsequent shorter visits at six-month intervals through adolescence, and recommended continuation through adulthood yearly.
3. Nutrition education would be administered through the schools, with general classes for all children and special counseling sessions for hyperlipidemic children and their parents at six-month intervals through the school years.*
4. Lipoprotein typing would be done on all children found to have "positive" cholesterol screens to assist in genetic classification, and serum cholesterol levels would be measured at least once a year in those same children.

Over eight school years following the screening test, hypercholesterolemic children who agree to participate would have the following interventions:

1. Substitution of polyunsaturated oils for saturated fats in the diet
2. Substitution of lean beef, veal, fish, and poultry for fatty red meats
3. Substitution of soy-protein derivatives for bacon, sausage, and other breakfast meats

*The relative usefulness of physician counseling and paramedical counseling is subject to debate. In actual practice, a dietary change program might rely more on nutritionists and less on physicians than we propose.

4. Substitution of skim or low-fat milk for whole milk
5. Reduction of ingested cholesterol by 50 percent, primarily by substituting cholesterol-free products for eggs
6. Reduction or elimination of consumption of commercially processed foods high in saturated fats

This diet parallels several in published reports (Bowen et al., 1973; Conner and Conner, 1972; Ford et al., 1972; Hulley et al., 1977). It aims to achieve a diet with 35 to 40 percent of calories supplied as fat, with a ratio of polyunsaturated to saturated fat of about 1.2, and a daily cholesterol content of under 250 mg/1000 cal.

Since we do not yet know the exact relationship between the intensiveness of an intervention and the resulting change in diet, we will conduct our analysis under varying assumptions about program costs. The intervention just described is the most costly and intensive one we will examine, although truly effective treatment may arguably be even more expensive. Less intensive approaches will be described later in this chapter.

Testing relatives or not

Having identified a hypercholesterolemic child in a screening program, we have thereby opened up a new opportunity for further detection of individuals "at risk"; namely the opportunity to test the child's first-degree relatives. From genetic studies of hypercholesterolemia, we can predict that those relatives will be at greater risk for high lipid levels than is the unselected population (Goldstein et al., 1972). We call this opportunity the "Case-finding" option. Whether or not to use the child as a key to the family is a policy choice about which we will ask more questions in Chapter 5.

THE COST-EFFECTIVENESS MODEL OF SCREENING

Having described the outlines of our program, we are now in a position to build our formal model of the cost-effectiveness of screening. There are three conceptually separate parts to the cost-effectiveness model: (1) a model of the benefits of intervention, (2) a model of the costs, and (3) criteria that allow us to select the optimal cutoff values for screening and intervention programs. The assumptions necessary to the analysis are based as much as possible on the published literature. In parallel appendices, we will explore the details of the studies and of our mathematical approach, but here we will only sketch the rationale behind each assumption, indicating our estimates of relevant parameter values and the confidence that can be placed in the estimate from data currently available.

Model of the benefits of intervention

The model of benefits assumes a causal link between our proposed intervention (screening and changes in diet) and our measures of benefit (years of life added, stroke-free years added, and infarct-free years added). First, we postulate that in the absence of any intervention, the naturally occurring serum cholesterol level influences age-specific mortality and the morbidity of coronary disease and strokes. We then specify the connection between diets that reduce cholesterol levels and reductions in cardiovascular risk, allowing both the diet effect and the risk reduction to depend on the initial cholesterol level. Finally, we examine characteristics of the screening test, that is, how cholesterol is distributed in the population and how this will influence the ideal division of funds between screening and intervention.

Our model of benefits requires that we estimate the values and ranges of uncertainty of six parameters in particular, to which we will now turn our attention. They include (1) the risks attributable to elevated cholesterol levels, (2) the stability of cholesterol levels throughout an individual's life, (3) the impact of a therapeutic diet on cholesterol levels, (4) the amount of compliance to be expected in an intervention program, (5) the "fraction of benefit," relating the risk of an individual with a cholesterol level achieved through therapeutic dieting to the risk of an individual with the naturally occurring same level, and (6) the distribution of cholesterol levels in the population as a whole.

Risks from elevated cholesterol level

Cardiovascular risk and the influence of cholesterol on risk differ greatly between men and women; therefore, our analyses will usually proceed separately for the two sexes.

We assume, supported by the findings of the Framingham study, that the cholesterol level measured at age 30 will be as good a predictor of lifelong cardiovascular morbidity and mortality as any more complicated measure of cholesterol over time (such as an average or a maximum reading) (Kahn and Dawber, 1966). We assume that some causes of death—cancers, accidents, and infections, for example—are unaffected by cholesterol level and that mortality rates from coronary heart disease and stroke increase with increasing levels of serum cholesterol, following the logistic model described in the Framingham study. The logistic model gives us a functional form for the relationship between cholesterol level and risk, which assumes that risk not only increases with cholesterol level but increases exponentially. An example of this relationship was illustrated in Figure 2-3. Thus the *added* risk due to an additional 10 mg/dl of cholesterol will be greater for an individual who starts with a cholesterol of 200 mg/dl than for one who starts at 150 mg/dl.

In the Framingham study's logistic model, the estimated relationship between cholesterol level and risk is summarized for each age-sex group by a single number, "beta." This number, derived from a statistical function that is fitted to the observed results in Framingham, can be interpreted approximately as the change in the natural logarithm of the rate of annual morbid or fatal events for people within the relevant age-sex group whose cholesterol levels differ by 20 percent. The true "beta" for the nation as a whole for any age-sex group may be different from that observed in Framingham for several reasons, including chance variation, systematic differences in morbidity patterns between the Framingham population and the rest of the nation, and deficiencies in the Framingham study's experimental design. A recent comparison of the Framingham "betas" with those of five other large, longitudinal studies shows remarkable agreement (American Heart Association, 1978), so it is unlikely that systematic bias in the Framingham data is a serious problem. In Appendix A, we discuss the impact of chance error in "beta" on our results.

By using the Framingham risk model in conjunction with data from the National Bureau of Vital and Health Statistics, we are able to generate a picture of the lifetime risk of dying at any given age beginning at age 30 for a given cholesterol level. Figure 4-1 shows this relationship for some representative cholesterol levels. An individual with a cholesterol level 3 standard deviations above the mean at age 30 has about a 70 percent chance of being alive at age 60. With an average cholesterol level or a cholesterol level 3 standard deviations below the mean, the corresponding probabilities of survival to age 60 are 78 percent and 81 percent, respectively. Similar graphs can be derived for the lifetime risk of stroke and heart attack. The details of these calculations are presented in Appendix A.

From the survival curves in Figure 4-1, it is a simple matter to relate the remaining life expectancy at age 30 to the cholesterol level at age 30. Remaining life expectancy is found by summing the probabilities

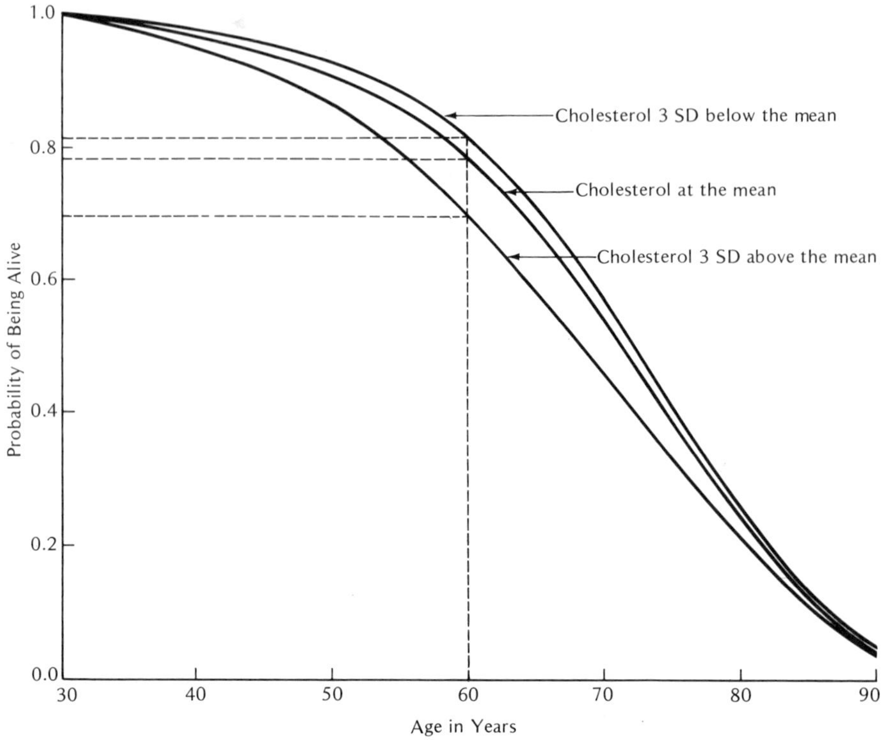

Figure 4-1. The Risk of Cholesterol: Cumulative Survival at Different Levels. Life expectancy decreases more quickly with age for people with high cholesterol levels than for people with low cholesterol levels.

of survival to a given age for every year of age from 30 on. Figure 4-2 shows the remaining life expectancy from age 30 as a function of cholesterol level for males and females.

This view of the added risks associated with elevated cholesterol levels is perhaps the most complex part of our model; yet for all its complexity, it is not complete, for it is based on naturally occurring levels of cholesterol, not artificially lowered levels. We will, nonetheless, accept this risk model as the basis for our calculations.

Figure 4-2 shows that life expectancy not only decreases with higher cholesterol level but actually curves downward, reflecting the exponential form of the risk function. This curvature explains why screening may be desirable. If the benefits were a linear function of cholesterol level, as shown in hypothetical example in Figure 4-3 then diets that lowered all initial levels by the same proportion would give the same benefit to everyone, and there would be no reason to screen.

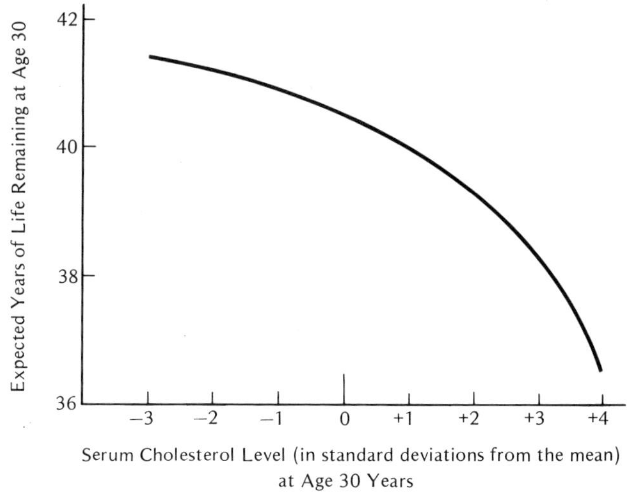

Figure 4-2. Life Expectancy vs. Cholesterol Level (as calculated from Framingham data). For each successive increment in cholesterol level, life expectancy decreases at a faster rate.

Figure 4-3. Life Expectancy vs. Cholesterol Level (from a hypothetical "straight line" risk function). If life expectancy decreased linearly with increasing cholesterol level, then screening to find individuals with especially high levels would not be useful, assuming that the achievable reduction in level did not depend on the starting level.

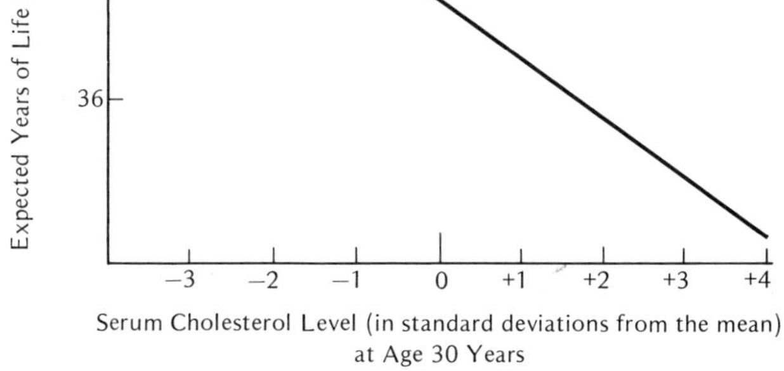

It is the curvature of the benefit function that first suggests the possible usefulness of screening. We will use the curvature in the graph relating life expectancy to cholesterol level as a summary measure of the data in Figure 4-2. Appendix D describes our method for estimating this curvature, which we refer to by the symbol Q, the quadratic component of risk.

Stability of level

Although it is adults with high cholesterol who are at excessive risk for coronary heart disease, we are discussing the screening of children. Such a program assumes that the cholesterol levels of children are closely related to later levels; otherwise, pediatric screening can have little value. In our model, we summarize the long-term stability of cholesterol with a parameter called R.

Figure 4-4 illustrates three possible interpretations of the same hypothetical population trend in the mean cholesterol levels, but with very different stability of level. In Graph A, individuals retain their rank order, and measurements of cholesterol at time I are perfect predictors of rank at time II. In this case, the correlation between measurements is 1.0, a perfect correlation. In Graph B, consistent with the identical trend in the mean, individual levels vary widely with time, and rank order is not preserved. Here, the correlation is zero. In Graph C, an equally valid interpretation of group trends, most individuals vary in rank, but the highest individuals, those who, for example, might be detected in a screening program, retain their rank consistently. If Graph A or C is correct, screening could be valuable, but it would not be valuable if Graph B is correct. In fact, childhood and adult levels do seem to be correlated, but not as perfectly as shown in Graph A. The imperfection in correlation over time results from both short-term and long-term variations in cholesterol levels.

When two samples are taken within a day or two, the correlation is less than perfect because of day-to-day variations in diet, exercise, and hormonal environments. A single measurement of cholesterol has only a correlation of about .8 with an individual's "true" baseline value of cholesterol. In practical terms, this means that very high and very low measurements may contain a large component of noise. A single observed value of X standard deviations above (or below) the mean results in a best estimate of the "true" value of $.8X$ above (or below) the mean. Averaging multiple measurements improves the short-term correlation with the true value; in fact, the "true level" can be *defined* operationally as the average of a very large number of

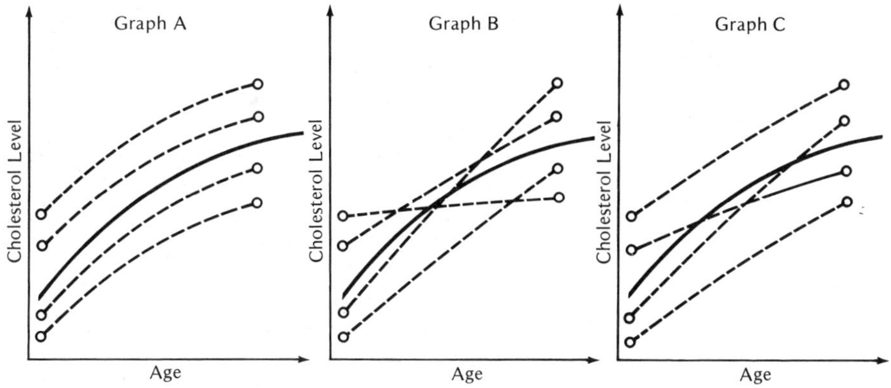

Figure 4-4. Possible Interpretations of a Trend in the Mean. For a screening program to be efficient, rank order must remain somewhat stable from the time of screening to the time for which morbidity is predicted. Reports of the trend in the mean cholesterol level with age are not sufficient to establish the stability of rank order.

measurements in the same individual. Many studies on risk (such as the Framingham study) and on diet are based on single measurements of cholesterol, however, and we will therefore always have to adjust these results so that all of our calculations deal with estimates of true values of cholesterol.

In addition to short-term variation, which we call R_s, the "true" value of cholesterol exhibits some variation from year to year. From the Framingham data, we estimate that the year-to-year correlation in an individual is .98 (see also Lee, 1967, and Jensen and Blankenhorn, 1972). Thus the total correlation between single measurements t years apart (our parameter R) is $(.8)(.98)^t$. We therefore estimate that the correlation between the cholesterol levels we measure in 10-year-old children and their true levels as 30-year-old adults is .54. This estimate is in reasonable accord with recent results from the Muscatine study, which reported a six-year correlation coefficient of .61 for cholesterol levels in children (Clarke et al., 1978). It is this overall long-term correlation coefficient that we refer to as parameter R. We can improve this figure by requiring multiple measurements in the initial screening program. With two measurements in the initial screening, for example, the 20-year correlation rises from .54 to .60. It is also possible that our estimate of year-to-year correlation based on Framingham adults overestimates the real correlation during the hormonally and behaviorally tumultuous years of adolescence. In sensitivity analyses, we will allow this parameter, R, to vary from .33 to .75 (see Appendix B).

The effect of diet on serum cholesterol level

We now turn to the problem of modeling the effects of dietary intervention. What effect does diet have on serum cholesterol level, and how long does it take to achieve that effect? The measured level of cholesterol responds very quickly to diet—in a matter of weeks. The magnitude of the change obviously depends on the kind of dietary changes being prescribed. We assume that *in practice* the recommended dietary changes would include the following: The substitution of polyunsaturated oils for 50 percent of the saturated fats and oils in the average diet; the substitution of veal, fish, poultry, and lean beef for 50 percent of the fatty meats (beef, pork, and lamb); the substitution of skim or low-fat milk for whole milk; and the reduction of ingested cholesterol by 50 percent, mostly through a decrease in egg consumption.

Knowing the current consumption patterns of the American public and the nutritional content of major food products, we can estimate the effect that this diet would have on the average daily consumption of components known to affect serum cholesterol levels, namely polyunsaturated fats, saturated fats, and cholesterol. We can then use an empirical formula developed by Keys et al. (1965a, b, c, d) to estimate the effect on serum cholesterol levels. Keys and associates found that increased ingestion of saturated fats and, to a much lesser extent, of cholesterol increases serum cholesterol levels, while increased polyunsaturates in the diet decrease serum cholesterol levels. The details of these calculations are found in Appendix C. The net result of our dietary recommendations is a projected *average* change in serum cholesterol level of about 22 mg/dl, or a reduction of about 10 percent from the average level in 30-year-olds of 220 mg/dl.

The formula described by Keys gives us a way of estimating the average effect of the recommended diet in a population, but it does not predict the effect a diet would have on a given individual. Since we start with an "average" diet, the formula will underestimate the impact of the diet on an individual whose usual diet is extremely high in saturated fats, while it will overestimate the impact on someone whose usual diet is very low in saturated fats.

The critical question for us is whether the effectiveness of the diet will depend on an individual's initial cholesterol level. On the average, will the intervention produce a larger response in those with high cholesterol levels or in those with low cholesterol levels? Figure 4-5

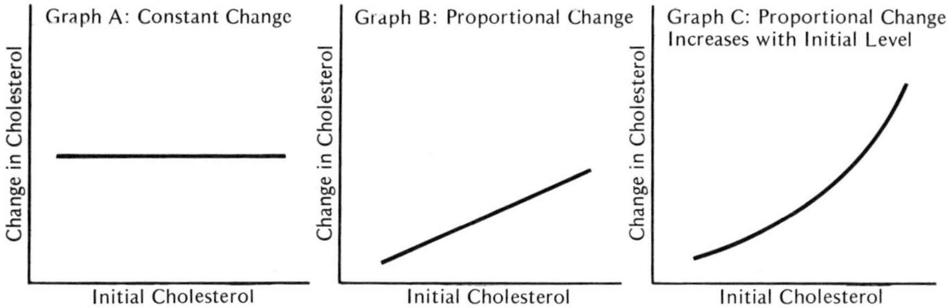

Figure 4-5. How Does Cholesterol Change with Intervention: Three Possibilities. Graph B is the relationship most frequently reported in the literature, although a slight curvature such as in graph C may exist.

illustrates their possible relationships. In Graph A, the therapeutic diet reduces cholesterol by a fixed number of milligrams per deciliter, independent of the initial level. In Graph B, the diet has a constant proportional effect; that is, the serum cholesterol level is always reduced by a fixed percentage of the initial level. In Graph C, the diet has an increasing proportional effect; that is, cholesterol is reduced by a larger percentage of the initial level when the initial level is high.

All other factors being equal, an increasing proportional effect of diet (Graph C) would be most favorable for screening. In this case, the screening program, by identifying those individuals with the highest risk, would also be isolating those with the highest susceptibility to the intervention. A constant dietary effect (Graph A) would be the situation least favorable to screening.

The literature on cholesterol-lowering diets shows, in general, either a constant proportional or increasing proportional effect (Graph B or Graph C). Diet studies usually report change in cholesterol as a constant percentage of initial level, generally between 8 and 15 percent, as in Graph B. Keys et al. (1965a, b, c, d) and McGandy et al. (1972) report results that tend to support the increasing proportionate effect illustrated in Graph C, with reductions of about 8 percent in those with initial levels under 200 and 14 percent in those over 200 (Table 4-1).

In all of these studies reporting the effect of diet, there is a statistical hazard, namely the phenomenon of regression toward the mean. Keys describes the problem in this way:

Caution must be exercised to avoid confusing responsiveness (to the diet) with the operation of the so-called law of regression. Consider a group of men all of whom have the same average serum cholesterol value when their bloods are sampled repeatedly. If a single blood sample is taken from each man, some

Table 4-1. The change in cholesterol with dietary therapy: A summary of 23 experiments

Author	Subjects			Coronary or other disease	Fat
	Number	Sex	Age		
Bierenbaum et al., 1973	100	M	30–50	Post-MI	28%
Brown et al., 1975	17	12M 5F	31–71	Hyperlipidemics	38%
Dalderup et al., 1969	215 (families)			None	42%
Dayton et al., 1968	422	M	54–88	Nursing home	40%
Ederer, 1972	1000	M	—	None	National Diet-Heart Study A, B, and C
Hall et al., 1972	114	M	40–59	"High-risk"	31%
Hatch et al., 1955	10	5M 5F	Mean age 51	Hypertensive	10%
Hodges et al., 1967	6	M	33–46	None	15%
Hood et al., 1965	112	51M 61F	—	Cholesterol over 300	
Leelarthaepin et al., 1974	26	M	Mean age 50	Type II obese	Decrease calories, use margarine
McGandy et al., 1972	63	M	13–18	None	26%
Meyer & Hendersen, 1974	36	—	35–55	"High-risk"	
Morrison, 1960	100	86M 14F	32–70	Coronary heart disease	15%
Nelson, 1956	110	77M 33F	Mean age 56	Coronary disease or stroke	—
Rinzler, 1968	104	M	40–59	"High-risk"	33%
Rose et al., 1965	28	—	Mean age 53	CAD or MI	31%
Sacks et al., 1975	116	73M 43F	16–62	Vegetarians (compared with controls)	
Shorey et al., 1976	55	M	22–30	Over 75th percentile in cholesterol or triglycerides	32%
Sirtori et al., 1977	20	10M 10F	22–68	Type II	
					25–92%

Diet cholesterol	*P/S ratio*	*Initial cholesterol (mg/dl)*	*Changes in cholesterol*			
			Absolute (mg/dl)	*Percentage*		
Limited	0.34	262	−19		−7%	
	2.60	259	−25		−10%	
Limited	1.7	428 (type IIA)	−68		−16%	
		340 (type IIB)	−78		−23%	
(Substitute margarine for butter, only)	1.1	217	−12		−6%	
Limited	—	234	−30		−12.7%	
		242+	—	Diet A	Diet B	Diet C
		210–242	—	−14.9	−15.6	−6.7
		<210	—	−12.4	−12.4	−3.1
				−9.5	−12.2	−0.5
289 mg/day	0.70	277	−34		−12.1%	
30–250	—	217	−26		−12%	
—	1.0	295	−100		−34%	
				Control		Diet
"Strict diet"	—	—	Men	−18%		−12%
			Women	−6%		−20%
	—	307	−71		−23%	
380 mg/day	1.2	200+	—		−15.6%	
		≤199	—		−8.3%	
		overall	—		−9.5%	
Three intervention techniques:	—					
Behavior modification		271	−47		−17%	
Individual counseling		262	−43		−16%	
Physician visits		249	−20		−8%	
50–70 mg/day	—	312	−92		−29%	
—	—	329	−59 ("Lipid responders" only)		−18%	
400 mg/day	1.25	253	−24		−9%	
—	—	263	−20		−8%	
Vegetarian diet		184 (controls)	−58		−32%	
350 mg/day	0.9	242 (type IIA)	−45		−19%	
		263 (type IIB)	−38		−14%	
Soy protein substituted for animal protein		324	−69		−21%	
0	2.7					

Table 4-1. Continued

Author	Subjects Number	Sex	Age	Coronary or other disease	Fat
Tabeqchali et al., 1974	57	—	—	Hyperlipidemics	32%
Turpeinen et al., 1968	234	M	34–64	Mental patients	30–35%
Walker et al., 1960	12	F	17–22	None	36%
Wilson et al., 1971	59	M	Mean age 43	None	40%

men will seem to have relatively high and others low cholesterol values, because single random samples will catch the men at various places in their personal (intra-individual) distributions of cholesterol. If a second sample is then drawn, the inevitable result will be that men who were high in the first sampling will tend to be lower on the repetition; conversely, men low at first will tend to have higher values on the second occasion. . . . To avoid this artifact in, for example, testing the effect of a particular diet or drug, it is necessary to have repeated blood samples in the control condition before concluding what the "treatment" itself actually does. (Keys, 1969)

In fact, although repeated sampling reduces the regression to the mean problem, it does not eliminate it. Adjusting for regression to the mean, we have carefully reviewed several studies that report an increasing proportional effect, such as in Graph C, and we have concluded that if there is such an effect, it must be very small. (That is, if individuals with mean cholesterol levels are lowered by 13 percent, then those at the 95th percentile may be lowered by perhaps 15 percent.)

In our model of dietary effects, we will assume that diet has a constant proportional effect, denoted by the parameter J and qualitatively illustrated in Graph B in Figure 4-5. We are comfortable that this assumption is roughly right, and it has the advantage (over assumptions of increasing proportional effect) of keeping our model simple. Our best guess is that diet lowers cholesterol by 10 percent regardless of initial level; in our sensitivity analysis, we will allow J to vary from 5 to 15 percent.

Table 4-1. Continued

Diet cholesterol	*P/S ratio*	*Initial cholesterol (mg/dl)*	*Changes in cholesterol*	
			Absolute (mg/dl)	*Percentage*
300 mg/day (and drugs if needed)	1.4		51 of 57 achieved cholesterol under 270 mg/dl	
300 mg/day	~1.5	236	−21	−9%
(Substitute vegetable protein for animal protein, holding fat constant)	—	157	−20	−13%
227 mg/day (AHA fat-controlled diet)	1.6	233	−22	−9.6%

Although prospective studies of dietary intervention uniformly show that cholesterol levels can be lowered through diet in individuals, studies of homogeneous free-living populations have generally shown little or no correlation between individual nutrient intakes and observed cholesterol levels in those same populations (Kannel, 1974; Stulb et al., 1965; Nichols et al., 1976a, 1976b; Weidman et al., 1978). Although some writers have taken such evidence to mean that diet and cholesterol level are relatively independent of each other (Mann, 1977), we reach a different conclusion, as do Glueck and Conner (1978) and Jacobs et al. (1979). Our analysis of the results of the Framingham diet-cholesterol study (detailed in Appendix C) shows that the reported results are indeed just as close to the expected effect of diet on cholesterol that is predicted by the Keys' formula as they are to the hypothesis that diet has no effect on cholesterol.

The major reason that the observed effects of diet on cholesterol level are so small in free-living populations is that the variation that is attributable to diet is small when compared with interindividual differences. In effect, the true impact of diet is easily lost in the background "noise." In addition, diet may vary considerably over short periods of time, masking its relationship to observed lipid levels. The negative findings of the Tecumseh study (Nichols et al., 1976a, 1976b), for example, may be due to its use of a rather short time period (24 hours) over which to estimate diet. Several studies (Nichols et al., 1976a, 1976b; and Weidman et al., 1978) further weakened their own ability to detect small effects by using data stratified according to cholesterol levels.

Compliance with treatment

The efficacy of treatment depends not only on the biological potential for lowering cholesterol levels by diet but also on the level of adherence of people to recommended dietary changes. What levels of compliance can be expected?

The most thorough recent review of the literature on compliance with therapeutic regimens is that of Sackett and Haynes (1976). Although the spread of results is wide, most studies of adherence to long-term medications or to dietary regimens (other than cholesterol-lowering diets) showed that between 40 and 70 percent of patients followed the prescribed plan at least moderately well.

A few experiments already in hand give some idea about the levels of compliance with diet in high-risk individuals. The National Diet-Heart Study (1968) of multiple interventions had a dropout rate of 10 percent in its first year. In the Chicago Coronary Prevention Evaluation Program (Stamler, 1971), 63 percent of the 519 men who entered were still participants at the end of seven years. The New York Anti-Coronary Club (Christakis et al., 1966) experienced 36 percent attrition among experimental subjects over a seven-year period, and in Leren's (1966) randomized trial of diets in 206 survivors of myocardial infarction, dieticians who made home visits judged 84 percent to be good or excellent compliers after five years of the study.

Adherence among children, raising different sorts of compliance issues, has been studied by Lloyd (1975), who achieved only a 20 percent response to diet or diet plus drug at the end of two years in a group of hypercholesterolemic children. Glueck et al. (1973b) were somewhat more successful, finding good adherence to diet or diet plus drug in 21 out of 36 type II children aged 7 to 21 years.

The determinants of compliance, thoroughly summarized by Sackett and Haynes (1976), are complex. Foremost among descriptive theories of the behavior of patients is Rosenstock's (1975) Health Belief Model, in which health-related behavior is seen as the product of several psychosocial forces, including health motivation, the perceived susceptibility of illness, the perceived severity of illness, perceptions of the benefits of professional intervention, barriers to taking action, and the patient's level of knowledge of the medical condition and the prescribed treatment. Adherents of this model urge physicians to explain treatments carefully and to be explicit about the properties of the illness and the benefits of treatment. Rose (1970) believes that motivational factors can be expected to be strongest among individuals at the highest risk and that these individuals will be most receptive to advice.

Behaviorists use the language of reward and reinforcement in speculating about effective health interventions. Pomerleau et al. (1975) believe behavior modification to have a central role in preventive medicine, and they cite Meyer and Henderson's (1974) evidence that behavior modification sessions were more effective than physician counseling in changing health habits in a group of high-risk employees.

From a mottled literature, Sackett and Haynes (1976) identify a few factors as "confirmed" in their association with noncompliance with therapeutic regimens. These factors include the complexity, duration, and degree of behavioral change required by a therapy, as well as the patient's inappropriate health beliefs and dissatisfaction with the therapist. Haynes finds that "the majority of studies found no association between patients' knowledge about their disease and compliance" and that "the proportion of patients who fail to comply because they lack knowledge or intelligence is small indeed." For the future, Haynes writes, "Behavioral and combined strategies hold a substantial edge over educational strategies in terms of both increases in compliance and improvements in therapeutic outcomes."

The hypothetical programs whose efficacy we are attempting to evaluate are designed with repetitive "counseling" sessions with both physicians and nutritionists. In this, they parallel intervention studies actually carried out in the past. Just how counseling should occur ideally, and what paradigm of advice or reinforcement should be used, are questions still open to speculation. Our estimate is not of the appropriate intervention strategy but of a reasonable level of expenditure for intervention, no matter what the strategy.

Adherence to diet is a composite estimate of two factors: (1) the compliance; that is, the fraction of people intervened upon who continue with the program (coming in for counseling and annual checkups), and (2) the degree of adherence to diet of those who attempt to comply. The literature on compliance with diet and drug treatment supports the view that dropout rates are somewhere between 20 and 80 percent in conscientious counseling programs and that compliers adhere to diets with good success in the short run and unknown success in the long run. By intervening with children prior to the formation of adult food tastes, we may hope to reset food preferences in stable ways through nutritional counseling and thereby to achieve good long-term compliance.

We expect our screening programs to do better in this regard than mass intervention efforts. It seems likely that screening may *create* compliance, since an individual is more likely to do something about a measured personal risk than about a vaguely perceived population risk.

Our best estimate is that the long-term dropout rate among treated children would be between 75 and 50 percent. In other words, we estimate a compliance fraction, K, of from 25 to 50 percent. We generally assume that noncompliers incur the same intervention costs as compliers, although we also examine the case in which dropouts do not incur these costs.

Compliance is an increasing function of expenditures on intervention. With program costs of $200 to $300 per person intervened upon, we believe that 50 percent long-term compliance is the best that could be expected. Program costs to achieve maximum adherence may be underestimated by a factor of 2, and maximum achievable adherence may be as low as 25 percent or as high as 70 percent. Thus, we will allow K to vary from 25 percent to 70 percent.

The effect of partial adherence to diet by those who do not drop out is more difficult to estimate. To some extent, the shorter term adherence is included in our estimate that diet will reduce level by 10 percent. We do not explicitly include any long-term "slippage" from the diet regimen. This, and other biologic factors that tend to attenuate the actual benefits of screening, can be considered as part of the single parameter, *fraction of benefit*.

Fraction of benefit

In modeling the risks associated with elevated cholesterol levels, we have relied primarily on the Framingham data, which reported risk as a function of naturally occurring levels. The question arises: Does an individual whose cholesterol level is lowered by diet really achieve the risk of someone whose level is naturally at the lower level?

Cholesterol levels respond to diet very quickly (within two to three weeks), while our model of atherosclerosis involves the buildup of deposits over years. If we are considering dietary intervention in adults, then we would be surprised if cardiovascular risk fell as quickly as serum cholesterol levels. In fact, since there is some doubt as to whether an arteriosclerotic plaque is ever reversible, we might think that cardiovascular risk in one whose diet changed late in life may never reach the risk associated with "natural" levels. Depending on when the diet was started and on how much damage had already been done, an adult may be expected to receive some fraction of the benefit (we call this parameter FOB) predicted by our model based on naturally occurring levels. The idea of intervening on children only makes sense if the FOB is higher for them than for adults. Otherwise, we might as well wait until adulthood to screen and intervene.

Data on the reduction of risk by dieting are meager and deal only with diets started on adults. We believe [as does Whyte (1975) in similar calculations] that diets started in childhood may well achieve the full benefit predicted by our model based on natural levels. However, factors other than cumulative damage may act to attenuate benefits—partial compliance with diet, for example. Our best guess at this elusive quantity is that it will be very close to 100 percent in the pediatric programs we are considering. Relevant data on fraction of benefit in adults will be emerging in the next decade from studies now under way.

Distribution of cholesterol levels

The last item we need before we can estimate the benefits of screening is a measure of the expected number of people identified by a screening program with a given cutoff level. If we propose to intervene on all children with cholesterol levels over 300 mg/dl, how many children will that be? In order to be able to answer this question for every possible cutoff level we might choose, we need to know the distribution of cholesterol levels of 10-year-old children. The most careful studies of entire American communities show a log normal distribution of levels. This distribution, an example of which is given in Figure 4-6 from the data of the Tecumseh, Michigan, study, is not symmetric, exhibiting a slight skew to the right. There may be a small second mode at very high levels caused by a rare genetic condition. We will discuss this again in Chapter 5, because it can strongly affect the results of a Case-finding program. For all other programs, this possible second mode will be ignored, because the inclusion of so rare an event as the discovery of a person in this small second population would have little impact on our results. We assume that at every age, cholesterol levels are log normally distributed. For 10-year-olds, the data support a mean level of 165 mg/dl and a standard deviation of ± 30 mg/dl (Table 4–2).

Table 4-2. Twelve major published studies of cholesterol levels*

Author (Study)	No. of S's	Age 1	2	3	4	5–6	7–8	9–10	11–12	13–14	15–16	17–18
						Boys						
Abraham, 1978 (Health & Nutrition Exam Survey)	3192	165	174	170	171	169	174	182	181	171	168	167
Berenson et al., 1978 (Bogalusa Heart Study)	155		158	155	155	158						
Clarke et al., 1970 (Vermont adolescents)	410								169 (±34)	159 (±28)	165 (±38)	169 (±39)
Ellefson et al., 1978 (Rochester, Minn.)	1193					166	170	168	160	158	162	168
Frerichs et al., 1976 (Bogalusa Heart Study)	1142					165 (±30)	161 (±30)	164 (±29)	163 (±26)	154 (±25)		
Friedman & Goldberg, 1973 (Arizona)	1018		151				154			157		
Godfrey et al., 1972 (Australia)	650					160	156	170	163	165	169	177
Hames & Greenberg, 1961 (Evans County)	444					158	167	172	175	184	193	182
Johnson et al., 1965 (Tecumseh, Mich.)	1300					177 (±30)			172 (±28)		166 (±31)	
Kromhout et al., 1977 (Netherlands)	590				166 (±23)	173 (±29)	172 (±27)	186 (±35)	180 (±28)			
Lauer et al., 1975 (Muscatine, Iowa)	2346					175	176	180	185	185	181	175
Milligan et al., 1966 (Utah)	169						181	182	182	174	174	189

								Girls											
Abraham, 1978 (Health & Nutrition Exam Survey)	3159	166	181		178	175		176		181		183		176		171	176		181
Berenson et al., 1978 (Bogalusa Heart Study)	158		162		160	157		155											
Clarke et al., 1970 (Vermont adolescents)	425													165 (±26)		164 (±26)	168 (±27)		178 (±42)
Ellefson et al., 1978 (Rochester, Minn.)	1228							160		164		164		160		155	157		160
Frerichs et al., 1976 (Bogalusa Heart Study)	1030							160 (±28)		165 (±27)		165 (±25)		163 (±27)		161 (±26)			
Friedman & Goldberg, 1973 (Arizona)	1015			153						157						159			
Godfrey et al., 1972 (Australia)	650							163		167		165		169		171	175		186
Hames & Greenberg, 1961 (Evans County)	393							156		166		169		174		185	191		185
Johnson et al., 1965 (Tecumseh, Michigan)	1300							178 (±27)							176 (±31)			173 (±31)	
Kromhout et al., 1977 (Netherlands)	413						175 (±30)		174 (±32)		176 (±27)		187 (±30)		189 (±29)				
Lauer et al., 1975 (Muscatine, Iowa)	2483							175		176		180		185		185	181		175
Milligan et al., 1966 (Utah)	152									195		190		190		178	183		204

*All cholesterol levels expressed as mg/dl (± 1 standard deviation, where available).

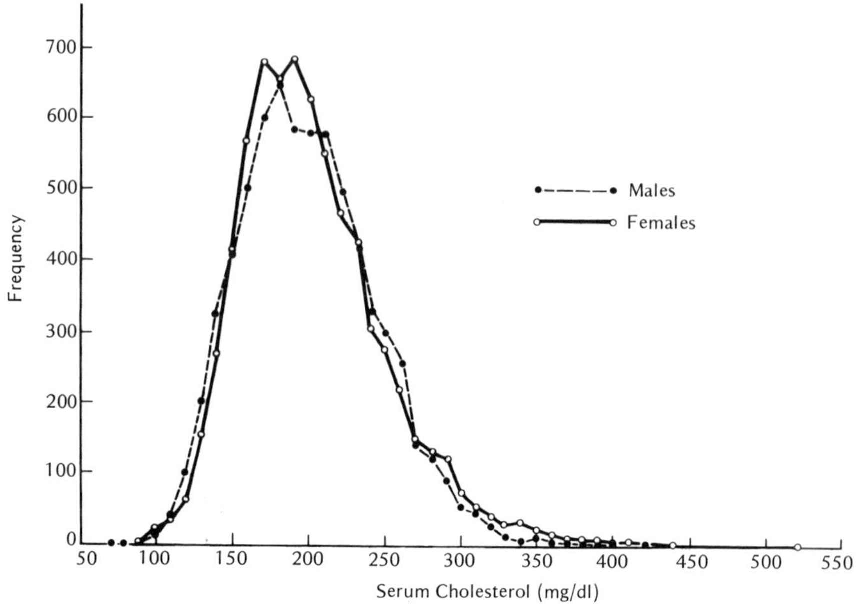

Figure 4-6. Serum Cholesterol Distribution in Tecumseh, Michigan. This graph shows the distribution of serum cholesterol values collected in two rounds of examinations. There were 7076 observations on 4619 males and 7234 observations on 4730 females. People aged four years or less are not included. (Reproduced with permission from C. F. Sing et al., Analysis of genetic and environmental sources of variation in serum cholesterol in Tecumseh, Michigan, Am J Hum Genet 27:333–347, 1975.)

The model of costs

Compared to the model of benefits, the model of costs is a simple one. Estimates of cost components are based on our assumptions about what a "reasonable" program would entail and on some data from similar screening and dietary counseling programs. The rapid inflation of medical costs makes it essential to establish a base year for cost estimates. To facilitate comparison with previous work, we have expressed cost in terms of 1975 dollars.

Cost of screening

Screening costs will depend on the type and organization of the screening program. We have assumed that screening school-aged children would best be done through the public and private school systems. The fixed costs of such a screening program (i.e., the expenses that do not change with the number of screenees) are small compared to the variable costs (i.e., the costs that are incurred each time a new individual is screened). Fixed costs may include rental of facilities and salaries of staff. Variable costs include the costs of supplies used in administering and analyzing each test. We choose to treat all costs as variable costs; thus the total cost of screening is the product of the number of people screened and the cost per screenee. With a single measurement of cholesterol, we estimate the cost per screenee to be about \$1.20, although it may be as little as \$.50 or as much as \$5. Retesting everyone once doubles these costs. Our estimate of screening cost is derived from the experience of large scale programs currently in operation. Efforts such as phenylketonuria and lead screening, for example, incur collection costs of about \$.80 to \$1.00 per sample. We assume that advances will be made in rapid, automated, and inexpensive cholesterol measurements on large numbers of samples, and that \$.20 to \$.50 per sample is a reasonable estimate of achievable costs of such automated chemical analyses.

Costs of intervention

The intervention costs, C_I, will depend on the detail of the intervention, the pattern of compliance, the rate of discount, the age at which intervention begins, and the life expectancy of the individual. We assume that the intervention costs will be based on the following fee schedule in 1975 dollars: initial physician visit, \$15; follow-up physician visit, \$10; nutritionist/counselor visit, \$10; lipoprotein typing, \$20; serum cholesterol measurement, \$1. All deferred costs are discounted at the appropriate rate. If those who fail to comply surface quickly, they will not incur all of these costs. We will look at two bounding conditions: where dropouts incur *no* costs and where they incur full costs. Table 4-3 summarizes the intervention costs for two types of program.

Depending on what kind of food substitutions are used in a cholesterol-lowering diet, the recommended dietary changes may result in increases or decreases in the food costs of those who comply (see Appendix E). Cheaper diets emphasize the use of poultry, fish, beans, and nuts (in addition to lean meat) to replace fatty meats and are up to \$100 per year less expensive than the current "average" American diet. It is likely, however, that noneconomic costs (psychological and cultural factors leading to a preference for beef over beans) would lead most Americans to prefer a more expensive, less healthy diet. More expensive diets (\$15 to \$25 per year more costly than the current "average" diets) replace fatty red meats with costlier cuts of lean red meats and, to some extent, with fish and poultry, without increasing nonmeat protein sources such as legumes. These diets more closely approximate current diets in taste, and thus involve

Table 4-3. Intervention costs*: Two hypothetical programs

Item	*Intensive program*	*Minimal program*
Physician visits—initial	1 @ $15	1 @ $15
Physician visits—follow-up	15 @ $10	2 @ $10
Nutritionist visits	16 @ $10	2 @ $10
Lipoprotein typing	1 @ $25	1 @ $25
Cholesterol tests—follow-up	9 @ $ 1	2 @ $ 1
Added cost of food substitutes	$20/year	$20/year
Total cost excluding food substitutes	$359	$ 82
Total cost including food substitutes	$951	$675
At 5% discount rate		
Total cost excluding food substitutes	$308	$ 80
Total cost including food substitutes	$504	$276

*Costs are expressed in 1975 dollars. Most subsequent analyses are done on the higher figure, the "Intensive Intervention" program.

fewer psychological costs associated with change, but they are more expensive than the diets they replace.

In general, our analysis will exclude food costs, since individuals can choose cholesterol-lowering diets that are no more expensive than current diets. However, we will examine a "worst case" analysis, including an increased food cost of $20 per complier per year. Although it is unlikely that every complier would opt for the most expensive cholesterol-lowering diet, this "worst case" includes some measure of the psychological costs of giving up favorite foods.

The discount rate

The last parameter in our model will be the discount rate, D. Since benefits from the program we are examining are reaped many years after screening and after most intervention costs are incurred, the expected effectiveness of screening will depend crucially on our time preference for money and for life-years saved (see Chapter 3). The discount rate, quantifying this time preference, is thus an especially important variable. We will allow it to take on values from 0 to 12.5 percent.

Summary of the model

Our model of benefits relies heavily on our assumption that the Framingham logistic model accurately describes the risk associated with elevated cholesterol levels. A second fundamental assumption is that the distribution of cholesterol levels in the population is log normal with a mean of 165 mg/dl for 10-year-olds and a standard deviation of 30 mg/dl.

In addition to these two fundamental assumptions, there are several other parameters that we allow to vary during the analysis. These parameters are as follows:

J, the percentage lowering of cholesterol by diet

K, the compliance fraction

R, the long-term stability of cholesterol level

D, the discount rate

C_s, the cost of screening

C_I, the cost of intervention

Table 4-4 shows the range of values tested. We have indicated which single values we believe to be most consistent with data now available.

Our analysis will use these parameter values to prescribe the optimal division of funds between screening and intervention, which is equivalent to saying that we will specify the optimal cutoff level for our screening program, intervening on anyone above that level. Our criterion for selecting this cutoff level, as described in Chapter 3, is that the marginal cost-effectiveness of screening and intervention must be equal. This requires that we select a single measure of effectiveness for choosing the optimal cutoff point. We have chosen "years of life saved" as this primary measure of effectiveness, and other measures of benefit (stroke-free years added and infarction-free years added) will be carried along as secondary measures. The mathematics of our screening model are explored in detail in Appendix F.

We will present our results first for the set of parameter values that represent our best estimates, the so-called base case. We will then allow the parameters to vary in a subsequent sensitivity analysis.

Table 4-4. Parameters, estimated values, and confidence limits

Parameter	*Symbol*	*Range of estimates*	*"Base case" estimate**
Percentage reduction of cholesterol by dietary intervention	J	5–15%	10%
Compliance fraction†	K	0.25–1.00	0.50
Stability of cholesterol rank order over 20 years	R	0.33–0.75	0.54
Short-term stability of cholesterol rank order	R_S	0.40–1.00	0.80
Discount rate	D	0–12.5%	5%
Cost of screening	C_S	\$0.50–\$5.00	\$1.20
Cost of intervention (Table 4-3)	C_I	\$82–\$359	\$82 and \$359
Fraction of benefit	FOB	Unknown	1.00
Curvature of the risk function	Q	(see text, p. 136)	Approximated by Framingham logistic
Linear slope of the risk function	L	(see text, p. 136)	Approximated by Framingham logistic

*"Base case" estimates represent our best guesses about true parameter values. This set of base case assumptions is the one used for most comparisons with other programs in later chapters.

†Our model in general assumes that noncompliers incur the same costs of intervention as do compliers.

RESULTS OF THE MODEL

Cost-effectiveness calculations

For our initial estimation, we choose parameter values that constitute the "base case" figures in Table 4-4. These comprise the best approximations we feel able to make from a review of the relevant literature. To review, these approximations are J = 10 percent, $K = .5$, $R = .54$, D = 5 percent, and C_S = \$1.20. All of the analysis in this section is done for the program labeled "Intensive" in Table 4-3, the more expensive intervention program, but without including the costs of food substitutes in the cholesterol-lowering diet. The intensive program incurs a C_I (intervention cost) of \$359 per person treated (or \$308 when intervention costs are discounted at 5 percent per year).

The first figures present outcomes of the programs as cost per year of life saved, only. More detailed estimates of other health benefits appear later.

Figure 4-7 graphs the cost per year of life saved (YLS) as a function of the cutoff level for treatment in separate programs for men and

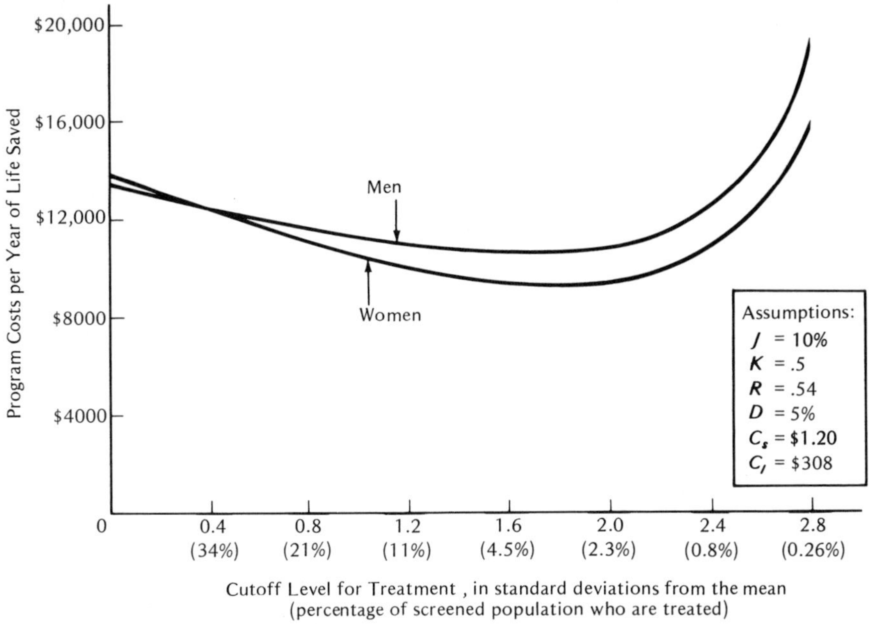

Figure 4-7. Variation of Average Cost per Year of Life Saved with Change in Cutoff Level for Treatment. (Screening of 10-year-old children.) At the lowest points of these cost-effectiveness curves lie the cutoff levels for treatment that result in the most efficient program for each sex. Curves drawn are for the intensive levels of intervention. If the cost of intervention were lower, it would be optimal to treat more people.

women. The most efficient cutoff policy is that at which cost per YLS is the smallest, at the minima of the pictured curves. At higher cutoff levels, so few people are being treated that their gains in life expectancy are exceeded by the extra screening costs. The curves rise steeply in this region (above the optimal cutoff) because high cholesterol levels are so relatively rare. For men at age 40, for example, whose mean level is 220 mg/dl (with a SD of 44 mg/dl), a level 2.8 SD above the mean exceeds that of all but 0.25 percent of people and represents a cutoff value of 375 mg/dl.

At cutoff levels below the optima, although screening costs decrease, benefits decrease more quickly, and so efficiency falls. Note, however, that the slope of the curves at cutoffs below the optima is more gentle than at cutoffs above the optima, reflecting the assumption that most people benefit from treatment no matter what their initial cholesterol level.

We can take note with relief that in the regions of the optima, the curves in Figure 4-7 are quite flat. The optimal cutoff for women, for example, would have us treat about 3 percent of the screenees. If we treat as few as 1 percent or as many as 7 percent, however, the cost-effectiveness of the program remains relatively constant, around $9700 per YLS. The analysis, then, is reassuringly robust. Even if a mistake in our estimates, or a mistake in the operation of the program, results in a large error in estimating the optimal cutoff, we do not lose much in efficiency. The insensitivity of cost-effectiveness to cutoff level in the region between the 99th percentile and the 93rd percentile is largely a result of the continuous nature of the cholesterol-risk relationship. At any level of cholesterol, risk is not very much lower than at the incrementally higher level, and we have adopted this property of continuity in our benefit estimates.

Differences between the curves for the two sexes deserve attention. At most cutoff levels above the population mean, cost-effectiveness for intervention on women is more favorable than for intervention on men, a conclusion contrary to an implicit and pervasive assumption in the literature on preventive cardiology. Even though the overall coronary disease rate for men is higher than for women, it appears from the Framingham data that cholesterol is not as important a relative factor for men as it is for women. Our analysis is for dietary interventions only, and so the contributions of other risk factors are not taken into account here.

The divergence of the cost-effectiveness curves for men and women increases with higher cholesterol levels, reflecting, again, the greater relative role of cholesterol as a predictive factor for women. Only at the lower lipid levels, near the population mean, does intervention on men begin to be more cost-effective than on women.

Because the benefit curve for women is more curved with cholesterol than it is for men, the optimal cutoff level for women is somewhat higher. Under the assumptions listed for Figure 4-7, the optimal cutoff level for treatment of women is 1.89 SD above the mean (treatment of the top 3 percent), whereas for men, the best strategy is a cutoff level of 1.75 SD (treatment of the top 4 percent of men).†

†In the text and figures in this chapter, we have elected to present screening and cutoff levels in standard deviations from the mean, or in percentage of the screened population, rather than in absolute values of cholesterol. We believe that a good estimate of the cholesterol level of 10-year-old American children is 165 mg/dl, with a standard deviation of 30 mg/dl, but there is sufficient variation in mean levels from series to series that the standard scores and percentage treated seem to us less susceptible to misinterpretation.

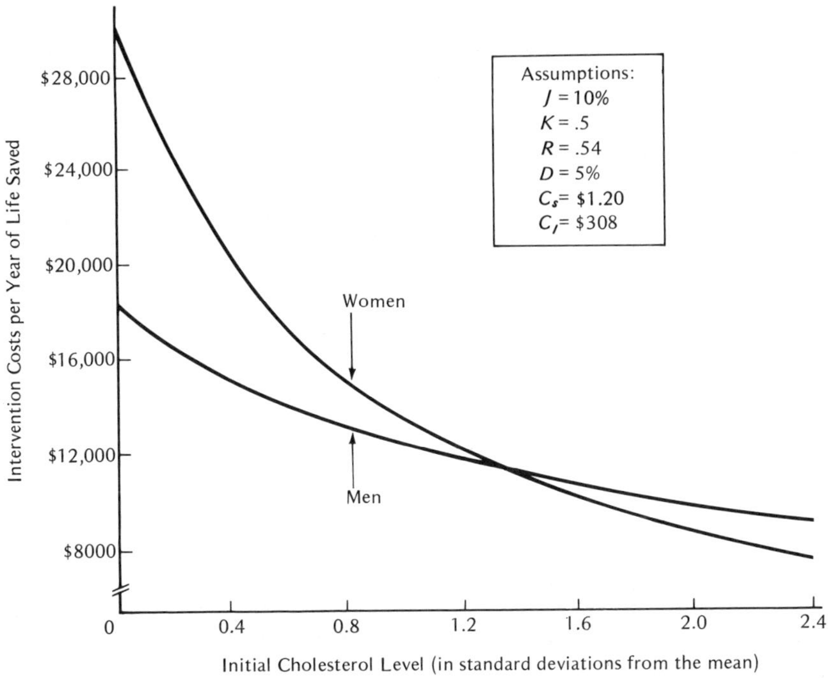

Figure 4-8. Intervention Costs per Year of Life Saved vs. Initial Cholesterol Level. The higher the cholesterol level of a person treated, the lower is the cost per year of life saved.

Figure 4-8 illustrates the cost per YLS for intervention on individuals at different initial levels of cholesterol under the same "base case" assumptions used for Figure 4-7. Note that screening costs play no role in the construction of Figure 4-8.

As expected from the shape of the logistic function, on which our estimates are based, the curves in Figure 4-8 fall continuously with rising cholesterol level. In fact, the equations of the curves are relatively simple, since the benefits of intervention are a linear function of d, the initial level. Each curve is of the form

$$C_I b/(0) + K_o d$$

where b (0) is the benefit of intervening on someone at the population mean (that is, someone with a standard score of zero) and is likewise the benefit of intervening on a random child. K_o is a constant that depends on the assumed parameters.

The steepness of these curves can be judged from the value of d at which $K_o\, d = b$ (0); that is, where the cost per YLS is one-half the cost per YLS at an initial level of 0 SD from the mean. For men, this value is 2.43; for women, it is .82. The cost per YLS falls more quickly for women because benefits to women are more concentrated among high-risk women, the same reason that the program for women is more efficient in Figure 4-7. Without screening, the cost per YLS for women is about $30,000, more than triple the cost achievable with screening. For men without screening, the cost is $17,700 per YLS, about 60 percent higher than the cost with the optimal screening program.

Figure 4-8 seems to raise the plausible idea that we should simply intervene on people with very high cholesterol levels, gaining one YLS for only $7,600, for example, by treating girls with cholesterol levels more than 2.4 SD above the mean. The problem, of course, is that without screening, we cannot know whose level is high. Screening costs are inescapably bound with such intervention decisions, and the actual cost per YLS is $9300, even at the optimal cutoff.

If a budget were fixed, and if screening and intervention costs remained contant over large groups of people, then under the assumptions specified, the greatest number of years of life saved would be achievable by screening only girls and intervening on the top 3 percent of the screenees. If the population of 10-year-old girls were exhausted, and money still remained from the budget, then the next best strategies can be represented by drawing successive horizontal lines across Figure 4-7. At first, such lines intersect only the curve for women, with more and more women being treated at lower cutoff levels and at higher costs. Finally, at a cutoff level of 1.4 SD for women, with 8 percent of women being treated at a cost per YLS of $10,655 for the woman at the borderline, it becomes efficient to screen boys as well. At this level, we would treat boys above 1.75 SD from the mean, or about 4 percent of screened boys, and at an initial cost of $10,655 per YLS, which is the best we can do in a program for males.

The curves in Figure 4-8 cross at $11,900 per YLS, at which level of expenditure we would be treating the same proportion of men and women, about 11 percent of each. Above this expenditure, we would ideally treat more men than women.

The expected benefits of intervention for an average girl (i.e., a girl selected at random) are the same as those for a girl with an average cholesterol level (i.e., a standard score of 0 in our figures). Nevertheless, it is much more efficient to screen the population, even if we were going to treat *everyone* above the average, than not to screen at all. Treating all screenees above the average buys years of life at a cost of $14,000 per YLS (Figure 4-7), whereas treating half the population at random would cost $24,000 per YLS (Figure 4-8). Screening even with such widespread treatment avoids treating those below average, for whom the benefits are smallest.

In making a decision about whether or not to screen a large population, the only critically important information in the above curves are the minima of the curves in Figure 4-7. At these minima lie the points of greatest efficiency for a screening program and, therefore, the cutoff levels at which such a program should operate if it is to exist at all. The average costs elsewhere may be useful in describing the effects of a program but not in deciding how, or if, to run a program in the first place.

At the minima of the curves in Figure 4-7, the *average* cost-effectiveness of intervening on a screenee is exactly equal to the *marginal* cost-effectiveness of intervening on a person whose cholesterol lies just at the cutoff level. Here the marginal efficiency of detecting just one more hypercholesterolemic child through screening is equal to the average efficiency of treating everyone already identified as being above the cutoff level. The optimal cutoff level is thus the point of indifference between finding more and treating more.

Using optima identified in this way, we can calculate the ideal allocation of a budget between screening and intervention costs. Table 4-5 shows the optimal budget, and the effects of a program, applied to children aged 10 years. The assumptions are of the same "base case" estimates as discussed above. (Whereas Table 4-5 excludes the costs of food substitutes, Table 4-6 includes upper bounds on those costs in a similar analysis.)

The cost of screening is the same throughout Tables 4-5 and 4-6, $1.20 per case. The differences in the two tables reflect variations in the cost per intervention and in the proportion of children treated. In all plans, treatment costs are much larger than screening costs, with the fraction

Table 4-5. The optimal allocation of a budget*

Program	*Cost/ screenee*	*Cost/ year of life saved*	*Percentage of screenees treated*	*Percentage of budget for screening*	*Percentage of budget for intervention*
Intensive, men	$13.30	$10,660	4.0%	9%	91%
Intensive, women	$10.10	$ 9,300	2.9%	12%	88%

Assumptions: C_S = $1.20, J = 10%, R = .54, K = .50, and D = 5%.
C_I = $308 for intensive programs.
*Food costs excluded.

Table 4-6. Effect of food costs on total costs*

Program	*Program optimized for . . .*	*Program cost/ screenee*	*Food costs/ screenee*	*Total cost per year of life saved*	*Program cost per year of life saved*	*Food costs (% total)*	*Percentage of screenees treated*
Intensive, men	Program costs only	\$13.30	\$7.80	\$16,930	\$10,660	37%	4.0%
Intensive, women	Program costs only	\$10.10	\$5.90	\$14,740	\$ 9,300	37%	2.9%
Intensive, men	Program *and* food costs	\$ 9.30	\$5.30	\$16,820	\$10,730	36%	2.7%
Intensive, women	Program *and* food costs	\$ 7.10	\$3.90	\$14,620	\$ 9,390	36%	2.0%

Note. Including maximum food costs of \$20 per year for treated individuals raises apparent cost per YLS by about 50% for the intensive programs.
Assumptions: $C_S = \$1.20$, $J = 10\%$, $R = .54$, $K = .50$, and $D = 5\%$.
$C_I = \$308$ for intensive programs.
*Numbers in this table have not been rounded off, as is done elsewhere, so that minor differences may be observed.

of costs going to screening being slightly higher for women than for men.

Table 4-5 can be read as a prescription for a screening program under the assumptions specified. For example, the ideal program for 1000 ten-year-old boys, using the intensive intervention strategy described in Table 4-3, would cost $13,300 or $13.30 per screenee. Of these costs, $1200 should be allocated to screening and $12,100 to intervention. Approximately 4.0 percent of screened boys should be treated, which is equivalent to a cutoff level about 1.75 SD above the mean cholesterol levels. At this level of operation, the program will yield one YLS for each $10,700 spent.

Table 4-6 shows the effect of including the extra costs of more expensive food substitutes in calculating the ideal level of operation for a screening program. These costs represent an upper limit on food costs, since (as shown in Appendix E) cholesterol-lowering diets could also result in decreased food costs under some circumstances. Since the apparent cost of each intervention rises as a result, the ideal number of interventions falls. The effect, analyzed in Table 4-6 only for the intensive program, is not large enough to alter the costs per YLS substantially. (For the minimal program the effect of food costs on cost per YLS would be greater.) Having seen the relatively small effect of the "worst case" food costs, we believe that excluding these costs from further analysis will not distort our conclusions.

As Appendix E explains in detail, the "positive" food costs assumed here represent the costs of substitutes (mainly lean meats for fatty meats) for consumers who adopt a cholesterol-lowering diet but who are unwilling to reduce their intake of meats. For those who are willing to use further substitutions—vegetable protein for meat protein, for example—the cost of a cholesterol-lowering diet may actually be less than the standard American diet. The excess food costs assumed in this chapter thus represent an upper bound on those costs, incurred in an attempt to minimize disruption of dietary patterns.

The health benefits of a program for screening 10-year-old children are summarized in Table 4-7. Since discounting of health benefits is a procedure that has yet to gain widespread acceptance, we have presented these benefits both at their undiscounted levels and at their discounted levels. We believe that the absolute levels are more meaningful for most people but that the discounted levels are more useful for the social planner.

The benefits seem small in most cases. For example, even at a discount rate of zero, prior to screening, a boy may expect, as a result of participation in the program, 5.8 added days of life, 8.4 added days free of nonfatal coronary heart disease, and .5 extra days free of stroke. (The discounted values are .46 days of life, .58 heart-disease-free days, and .04 stroke-free days.) For these benefits, each screenee pays $13.30, of which $1.20 is for screening and $12.10 is for his share of the intervention costs, not including food. If he is "positive" on the screening, and if he complies with treatment, his (undiscounted) gains will be 291 extra days of life, 421 extra heart-disease-free days, and 24 added stroke-free days. (Discounted at 5 percent, his expectations are of 23 life-days, 29 heart-disease-free days, and 2 stroke-free days.)

Benefits for girls are higher than for boys if not discounted. After discounting, however, benefits for girls fall below those of boys. This effect is a consequence of the relatively later onset of cardiovascular disease in females as compared with males, and the consequently greater attenuation by discounting of benefits to females.

Overall, using a discount rate of zero, a boy whose high cholesterol (95th percentile) is detected at age 10 by the postulated screening program, and who is thereby led to adopt a treatment plan, can expect as a result about 10 months of added life and about 14 months extra of life free from the effects of coronary heart disease, as well as 3 weeks free from stroke.

The critical effect of the discount rate is evident in Table 4-7. Benefits are realized, on the average, over 50 years from the time of screening, and the undiscounted benefits per complier are reduced over 15 fold by applying even a moderate discount rate.

Table 4-7. Health benefits from an optimal screening program

	Not discounted (C_I = $359)		*Discounted at 5 percent* (C_I = $308)	
	Boys	*Girls*	*Boys*	*Girls*
Net benefit per screenee				
Added days of life	5.8	7.0	0.46	0.40
Added days free of CHD	8.4	5.5	0.58	0.32
Added days free of stroke	0.5	0.6	0.04	0.04
Net benefit per complier with treatment*	(2.0%)	(1.5%)	(2.0%)	(1.5%)
Added days of life	291	482	23	27
Added days free of CHD	421	380	29	22
Added days free of stroke	24	40	2	3

Assumptions: C_S = $1.20, R = .54, K = .50, J = 10%; noncompliers incur intervention costs.

*Numbers in parentheses are the percentages of screenees who comply with treatment, assuming that 50% of those treated actually comply.

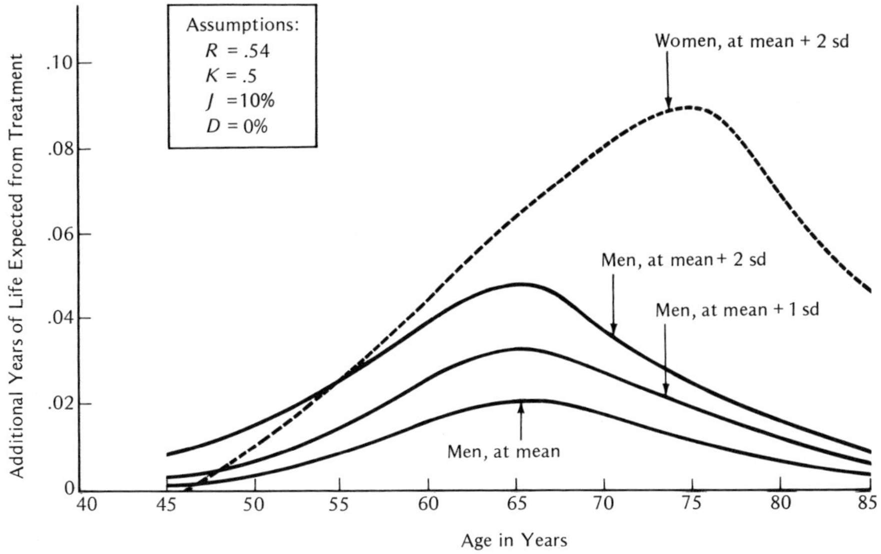

Figure 4-9. Additional Years of Life Expected at each Age from Intervention at Various Cholesterol Levels, Men. The life-years saved for men in a Universal Screening program peak around the age of 65.

The table shows that males acquire more extra days free of coronary disease from the program than do females. This reflects the fact that cholesterol has relatively more effect on fatal than on nonfatal events for females. A program based on preventing nonfatal coronary heart disease rather than on saving years of life would show more favorable results for males than for females even at a 5 percent discount rate. Taking nonfatal disease into account, therefore, we might choose to intervene more on boys than an analysis based on life-years alone would indicate.

The effects of cholesterol-lowering programs on stroke are minimal, reflecting the poor correlation of stroke events with cholesterol level and, in the discounted values, reflecting the relatively later onset of stroke compared with other manifestations of atherosclerosis.

Figures 4-9 and 4-10, for men and women, respectively, show the distribution of undiscounted years of life saved as a function of the age at which those savings accrue. For men, the peak savings accrue to 62- to 67-year-olds, but the benefits are broadly distributed from ages 45 to 80 years. Women, whose coronary disease appears somewhat later, realize their most significant gains after 60 years of age, with peak benefits accruing around age 75. The total undiscounted savings in

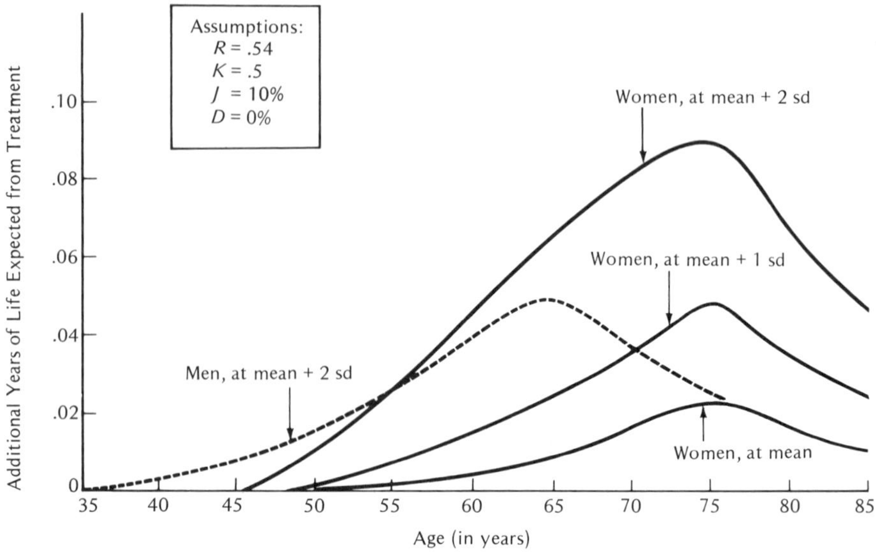

Figure 4-10. Additional Years of Life Expected at Each Age from Intervention at Various Cholesterol Levels, Women. The life-years saved for women come later in life than those for men. This is consistent with the later onset of cardiovascular disease in women.

life-years is represented by the area under each of these curves, the cumulative benefit being, as we already have said, greater for women than for men. At equivalent initial cholesterol levels, life-years accrue *earlier* to men but in *greater amounts* to women. These differences are more exaggerated at high cholesterol levels than at low ones.

Sensitivity analysis

Sensitivity to the estimated risks associated with elevated cholesterol—"beta"

The Framingham study's reports not only provide estimates of the "beta" coefficients relating cholesterol level to heart disease events for each 10-year age-sex group but also give the standard errors of those estimates. Using these standard errors, we may explore the sensitivity of cost per YLS and of optimal cutoff for treatment within specific confidence intervals.

Table 4-8 shows how cutoff level and cost-effectiveness vary within one standard error of our base case estimate of beta. The table entries assume that the error in beta is of the same magnitude and in the same

Table 4-8. Universal screening: Sensitivity to changes in parameters (intensive program, food costs excluded)

		Cost/YLS		*Optimal percentage of initial screenees to be treated*	
Parameter	*Values*	*Men*	*Women*	*Men*	*Women*
Beta	Low	$26,100	$ 18,900	6.2	3.7
	High	$ 6,200	$ 6,400	3.3	2.6
Stability of level	.33	$12,500	$ 12,000	5.3	3.6
(*R*)	.75	$ 9,100	$ 7,500	3.4	2.6
Dietary change in cholesterol	5%	$20,300	$ 17,300	4.2	3.1
(*J*)	15%	$ 7,500	$ 6,700	3.8	2.8
Compliance fraction	.25	$21,400	$ 18,600	4.0	2.9
(*K*)*	1.0	$ 5,350	$ 4,650	4.0	2.9
Cost screening	$0.50	$10,000	$ 8,600	2.0	1.6
(C_S)	$5.00	$12,100	$ 11,000	12.2	8.8
Cost intervention (C_I)	$80	$ 3,100	$ 2,800	11.3	8.2
Discount rate	0	$ 970	$ 620	3.7	2.7
(*D*)	.10	$83,500	$105,000	4.3	3.1
Base Case		$10,700	$ 9,300	4.0	2.9

*Assuming noncompliers incur the full costs of intervention.

direction for all age-sex groups, an unlikely possibility since the estimates of beta for each group are independent.

At high values of "beta," risk is concentrated in people with high cholesterol levels, and this increases the attractiveness of detecting those people and lowering their levels. As a consequence, if beta is high, the cost per YLS is lower (about 50 to 60 percent lower than in the base case) and the cutoff level for treatment is higher, since it is worthwhile to screen more to find especially high-risk individuals. At low values of beta, one standard error below the base case, the cutoff level for treatment is lower, and the cost per YLS is 2 to 2.5 times as high as in the base case. The standard error in the estimated beta for men is larger than for women, and so the "one-standard-error" confidence interval is wider for men.

Sensitivity to the correlation coefficient—R

As expected, the cost-effectiveness of each of the intervention programs improves with increasing stability of cholesterol rank order. The logistic function predicts more benefit from reducing a high initial level than from reducing a lower initial level of cholesterol, and thus any tendency of high screenees to "wander" into lower ranks through random mixing will act to reduce the possible efficiency of targeting intervention efforts at high screenees. In the limiting case of complete mixing (a long-term correlation coefficient of 0), screening would have no advantage (and would cost more) than merely intervening on a random sample of the population. In the range tested (between $R = .33$ and $R = .75$), cost per year of life saved falls by about 25 percent for men and by about 35 percent for women, the steeper slope for women being due mainly to the concentration of risk in high cholesterol women.

As R increases, the optimal cutoff level for intervention rises, and so decreasing percentages of screenees are treated (see Table 4-8). This tendency for cutoff level to rise as R increases is equivalent to a shift of resources from intervention to screening. At high R's, positive screenees are more precise targets, with higher expected benefits, and so it is worth some additional resources to detect them.

Sensitivity to short-term correlation—R_S—and retesting

As we mentioned earlier, it is useful to think of the overall stability of the cholesterol rank order through many years (parameter R) as the product of two kinds of "noise." First, cholesterol rank order may vary over the long run, with a slow wandering of people across percentiles. Second, superimposed on this variation in "cruising altitude," there are more rapid random fluctuations in measured cholesterol levels that result from short-term biologic variation (such as changes in diet, exercise, or health status), diurnal rhythms, and measurement errors. Because of this second type of noise, any single measurement of an individual's cholesterol level at a particular time is only an imperfect estimate of his or her current real "cruising altitude." The correlation of a particular measurement with a person's "true" current cholesterol level we refer to as the *short-term coefficient of correlation,* or parameter R_S. The quantitative relationship of R to R_S is fully discussed in Appendix B. Our best estimate of the long-term component of R, the actual fluctuation in "cruising altitudes," is about .67, based upon the Framingham data. We believe that R_S is about .8, and so we have estimated the resultant R as (R_S) (.67) = .54.

Basic statistical theory predicts that the average of several "noisy" measurements is a better estimate of the true value than is any single measurement. No matter what the value of R_S is, multiple determinations of an individual's cholesterol level provide a better idea of his or her "true" current levels than does a single determination. Specifically, the error of the average of N determinations as an estimate of the true values decreases in proportion to $\sqrt{N}$.

Since we already know that the value of a screening program is enhanced by improving the accuracy of the measurement, would it not be reasonable to use the average of several measurements of a person's cholesterol level, instead of a single measurement, to decide whether or not to institute treatment? Such a "retesting" strategy would give us more confidence that the cholesterol levels we measure do, in fact, reflect the screenees' true levels. The mathematics of retesting strategies are discussed in Appendix G.

Figure 4-11 illustrates the relationship between R_S and program efficiency for two different levels of C_S (\$1.20 and \$0.60), and for "single test" and "retest" (i.e., two test) screening strategies for women. (Results for men are similar.) We note from the figure, as expected, that cost per YLS decreases as R_S increases. This is quite predictable, since random noise must decrease the possible contribution of screening. The usefulness of repeat testing to reduce "noise" depends on the value of R_S. When R_S is low (below about .60), then repeat testing enhances accuracy enough to make the extra testing costs worthwhile in improving efficiency. The effect is not great, however, since so much of the cost of the program lies not in screening but in treatment. If R_S is .40, for example, and C_S is \$1.20, then repeat testing reduces cost per YLS by only 1.5 percent (from \$13,200 to \$13,000).

At slightly higher levels of R_S, retesting actually degrades cost-effectiveness. The crossover points, at which retesting becomes a wasteful strategy, are approximately at $R_S = .55$ when C_S is \$1.20, and at $R_S = .60$ when C_S is \$0.60. Above these values of R_S, the contribution to accuracy made by retesting costs more in added screening expenses than it contributes in extra health benefits. This lack of dependence of cost-effectiveness on test accuracy is largely a consequence of the leveling of the cost-effectiveness curve in Figure 4-8. Around the optimal cutoff levels for treatment, small errors in measurement of true cholesterol are simply not very destructive of efficiency.

Since we believe that R_S in reality is approximately .8, it does not appear that multiple tests hold any advantage over single tests in a Universal Screening program. A more promising variation of the retesting strategy, in which only people with high levels on the first test are tested a second time, will be evaluated in Chapter 5.

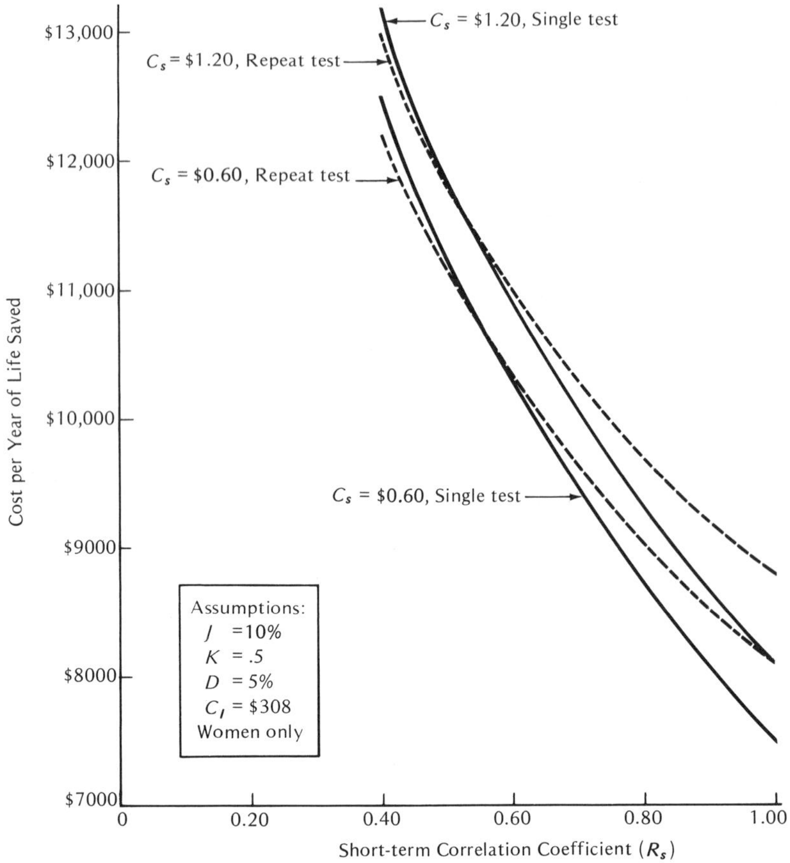

Figure 4-11. Sensitivity of Cost per Year of Life Saved to Short-term Correlation Coefficient (parameter R_s). It is less efficient to use a "noisy" screening test than a highly accurate one, an effect shown here as a rise in cost per year of life saved as the short-term correlation coefficient falls. Repeating the test once, thereby producing a more accurate estimate of true level, increases cost-effectiveness if R_s is less than about 0.55. At higher R_s values, repeating the test wastes resources.

Repeat testing has a profound effect on the cutoff level for treatment. As Figure 4-12 illustrates, a single repeat test nearly doubles the ideal percentage of screenees to treat, no matter what values are assigned to R_S or C_S. The reason for this effect is simple: Retesting doubles the cost of screening. Recall that the optimal cutoff level for treatment is characterized by our indifference between treating another person at that level or screening another person who might have a higher level. Since the curve relating cost per YLS to cutoff level is

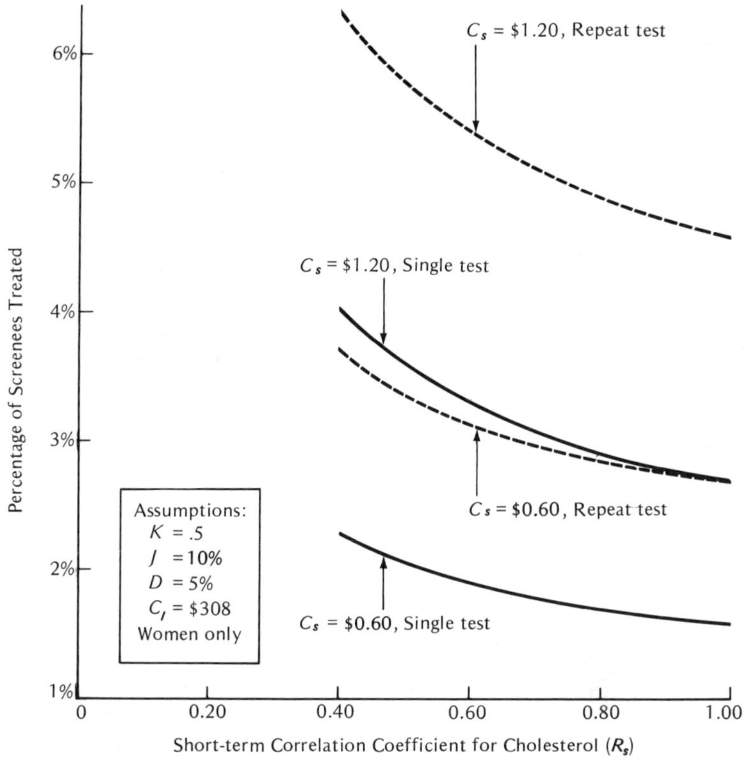

Figure 4-12. Sensitivity of Cutoff Level for Treatment of Short-term Correlation Coefficient (parameter R_s). (Optimal program for 10-year-old children.) Percentage screened depends mainly on the total cost of screening. In addition, the better the test (i.e., the higher R_s), the more of our budget we should be willing to devote to screening.

relatively flat (Figure 4-8), increases in screening costs lead to large increases in the optimal fraction upon which to intervene. The improved precision in identifying high-risk individuals through retesting does act toward decreasing the fraction treated, but only slightly. If R_S is .80, and C_S is $1.20, then we would wish to treat 2.9 percent of screenees using a single test but 4.9 percent of screenees if we test each of them twice.

Sensitivity to dietary change of cholesterol—J

The greater the reduction in cholesterol achieved through a given intervention, the more cost-effective will be the program as a whole. Table 4-8 shows the cost per year of life saved falling (for men) from

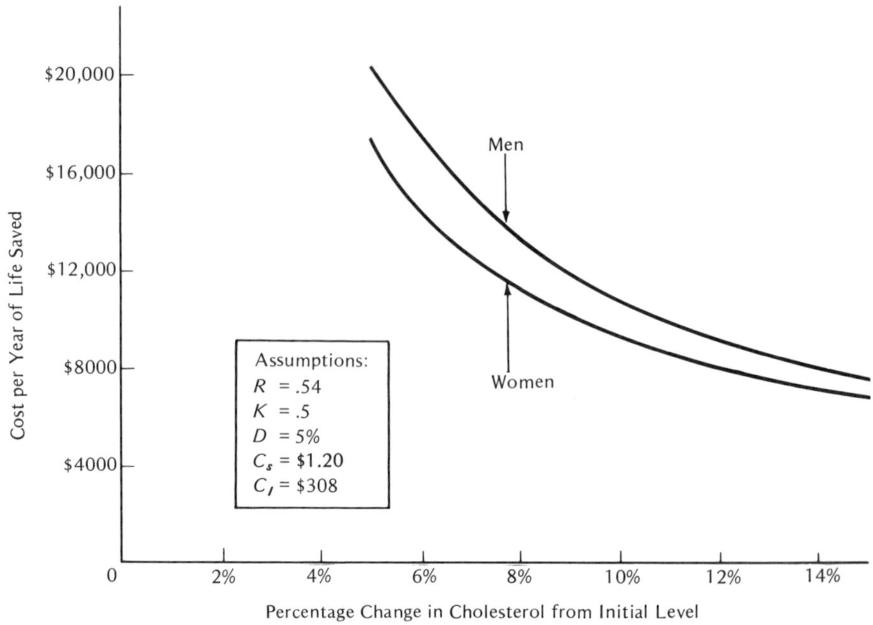

Figure 4-13. Sensitivity of Cost per Year of Life Saved to Percentage Reduction in Cholesterol Level (parameter *J*). (Optimal program for 10-year-old children.)

$20,300 to $7,500 as *J* varies from 5 to 15 percent. The relationship is graphed in Figure 4-13.

Thus, parameter *J* is a powerful determinant of cost-effectiveness, and our current uncertainty about the efficacy of diet permits an error in the estimate of cost per year of life saved as large as 300 percent.

Cutoff levels for treatment, on the other hand, are relatively insensitive to the value of *J* (Figure 4-14). Cutoff levels are more dependent on the way in which cholesterol reduction relates to the initial cholesterol value than on the absolute magnitude of the reduction. If *J* were a fixed absolute number of milligrams per deciliter independent of initial level, we should treat more screenees. On the other hand, if *J* were an increasing percentage of initial level (as some authors believe), we should screen more people and treat a smaller percentage of the screenees than is shown in Table 4-8.

Sensitivity to compliance fraction—K

The exact relationship between cost-effectiveness and compliance depends first on assumptions we make about the behavior of a noncomplier. If a noncomplier is simply a screenee who never partici-

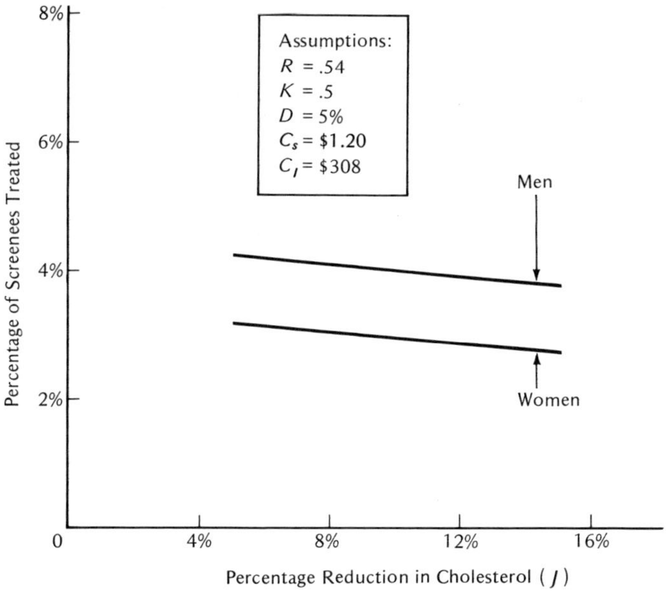

Figure 4-14. Sensitivity of Cutoff Level for Treatment to Percentage Reduction in Cholesterol Level (parameter J). (Optimal program for 10-year-old children.) The more effective treatment is, the more of our budget we would wish to spend on it, and so at higher levels of J, we would treat a higher proportion of screenees.

pates in an intervention program, and who therefore incurs only screening costs and no intervention costs, then the effect of noncompliance is identical to an increase in screening costs. For example, if 50 percent of positive screenees fail to participate in treatment, and thereby fail to incur any intervention costs, then the effect is identical to screening two individuals for every one complier. We may model the effect of this sort of noncompliance by treating C_S as if it were twice as large as the actual amount spent per person screened.

On the other hand, noncompliers might incur all intervention costs (counseling sessions, follow-up cholesterol measurements, etc.) and still fail to adhere to the diet prescribed. (In our model, we need not distinguish between compliance by a portion of the treated population and partial compliance by the entire treated population; the effects on cost and effectiveness are almost exactly the same.) If the latter case holds (i.e., noncompliers do incur intervention costs), then benefits in our model are exactly proportional to K, and as compliance doubles, the cost per year of life saved is cut in half, an effect that is apparent in Table 4-8. Although the cost-effectiveness of treatment changes dra-

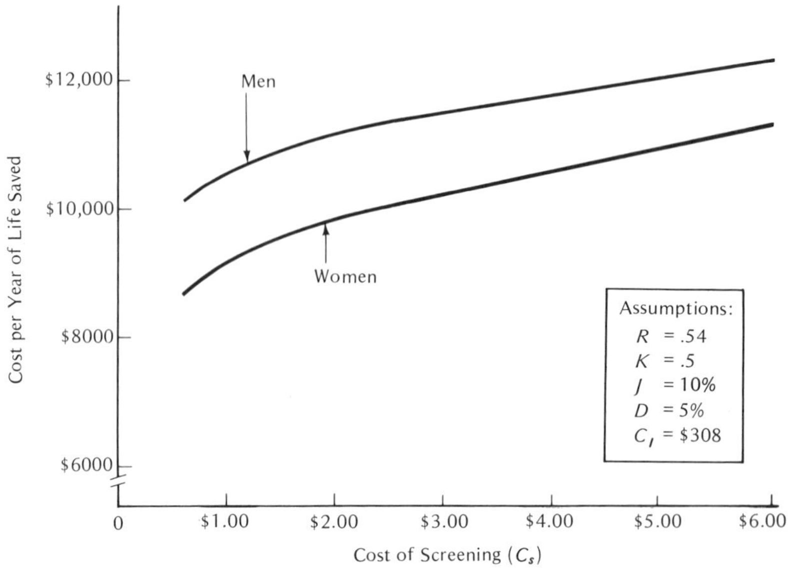

Figure 4-15. Sensitivity of Cost per Year of Life Saved to Cost of Screening (parameter C_S). (Optimal program for 10-year-old children.) Cost-effectiveness is not very sensitive to the cost of the screening test. Most of the program's resources are consumed in treatment, not in screening.

matically with *K*, the optimal cutoff level for treatment does not vary at all. If noncompliers incur all the costs of intervention, our best guess about whom to treat from among the screenees remains unchanged as long as *K* does not depend on the initial cholesterol level.

Sensitivity to cost of screening—C_S

Screening makes a far smaller contribution than intervention to total program costs. As a result, the cost per YLS is relatively insensitive to the cost of screening, C_S. Figure 4-15 shows that even a 1000 percent increase in C_S (from $0.50 to $5.00) results in a change of cost per YLS of only 21 percent for men in the intensive intervention program (from $10,000 to $12,100).

The impact of changes in C_S upon optimal cutoff level for treatment is profound. Figure 4-16 shows that a rise in C_S from $0.50 to $5.00 causes a sixfold increase in the percentage of screenees treated, from 2.0 percent to 12.2 percent for men. The reason for this striking sensitivity lies in the relative gentleness of the slope of the curve relating cost-effectiveness to cutoff level (review Figure 4-8) in the region of the optimal cutoff. At this optimum, we are indifferent between treat-

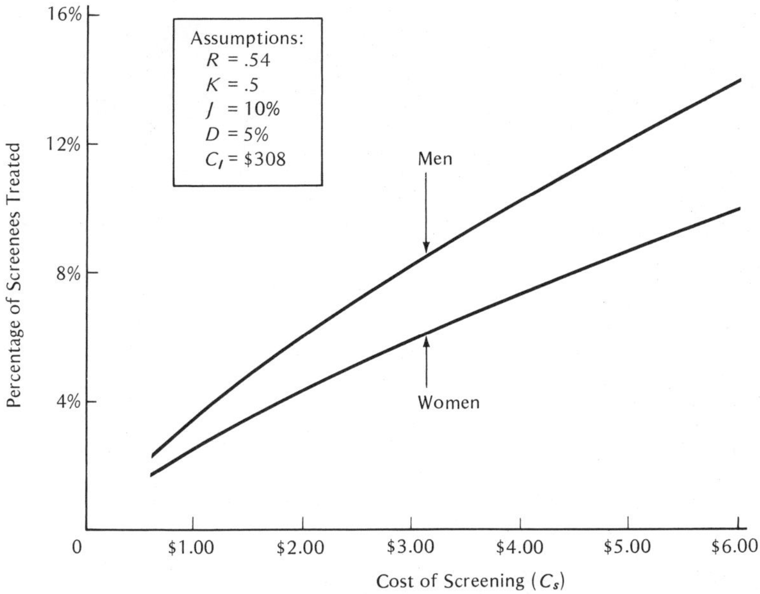

Figure 4-16. Sensitivity of Cutoff Level for Treatment to Cost of Screening (parameter C_S). (Optimal program for 10-year-old children.) The cost of screening dramatically affects the optimal cutoff level for treatment. The more screening costs, the more of our budget should be spent on treatment.

ing an individual with the marginal cholesterol level and screening more people. In the region of the optimal cutoff level, the marginal benefit of treating a person is approximately the same as the marginal benefit of screening another person who might have a higher level. Thus, a small change in screening cost has a large effect on our judgment of whether to screen additional people or to treat additional people; the more expensive screening is, the more money we will reallocate from screening to intervention.

Sensitivity to cost of intervention—C_I

If the costs of intervention are those described under the minimal program in Table 4-3, instead of the intensive intervention we have thus far assumed, then the cost per year of life saved falls dramatically so long as J, K, and other parameters remain the same. With the cost of intervention so low, it becomes worthwhile to treat more than twice as many of the initial screenees, and cutoff levels for treatment accordingly fall dramatically. Table 4-8 shows these effects. Furthermore, with lower program costs, food costs become relatively more important.

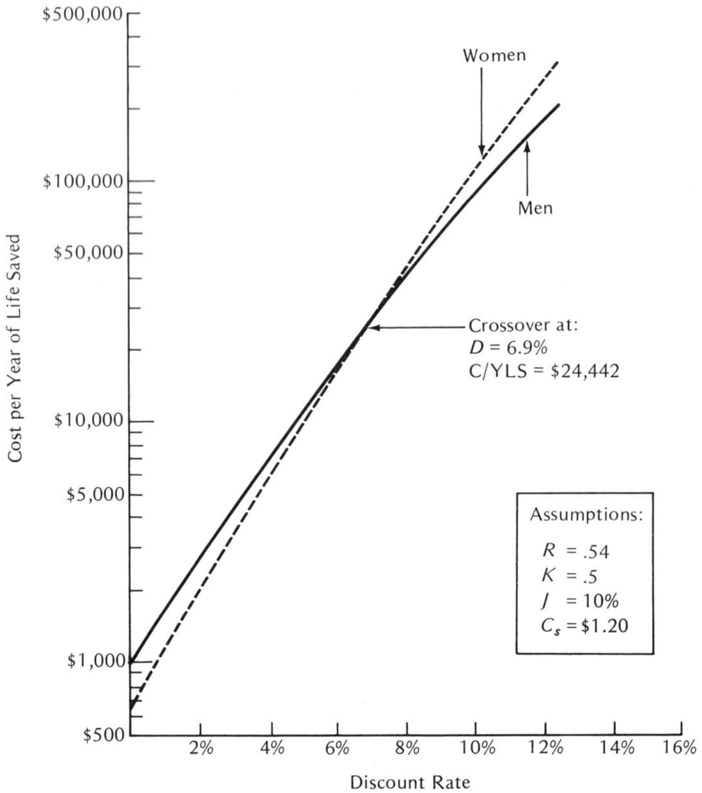

Figure 4-17. Sensitivity of Cost per Year of Life Saved to Discount Rate (parameter D); Intensive program, Food Costs Excluded. (Optimal program for 10-year-old children.) Discounting is the most powerful parameter in determining cost-effectiveness.

Sensitivity to discount rate—D

The rate of discount of dollar costs and health benefits is the parameter to which cost-effectiveness is the most profoundly sensitive in our model.

Figure 4-17 illustrates the dependency of cost per YLS on discount rate. The curves slope sharply upward because a rise in the discount rate results in the decay of apparent health benefits and a consequent increase in cost per YLS.

Since women live longer and incur their cardiovascular diseases later than men, a positive discount rate cuts more deeply into the cost-effectiveness of programs directed at women. Simply put, the discounting process has more time to do its damage on efficiency for women than for men. This increase in attenuation of benefit to women is reflected as a steeper slope of cost as a function of D. The combination of the difference in slope and the lower starting point (higher efficiency at $D = 0$) for women produces a "crossover" discount rate at which the maximum achievable cost-effectiveness for women is the same as for men. This occurs at $D = 6.9$ percent for the intensive intervention program.

By implication, a health planner who believes that the appropriate rate of discounting for health benefits is 5 percent will prefer to administer a program for women, while a planner who makes the same assumptions about the parameter estimates other than D, but uses a discount rate of 8 percent, will consider it more efficient to run a program directed at men. Not only the cutoff level but also the identity of the program's target population is sensitive to the discount rate applied.

The general effect of discounting on cost-effectiveness is enormous, far outweighing the effects of other parameters. Table 4-9 shows the impact of discounting on program options for men and for women under three different assessments of intervention costs: the intensive intervention excluding the extra costs of substitute foods in some cholesterol-lowering diets, the intensive intervention including extra food costs, and the minimal intervention excluding food costs. For men in the intensive program, without food costs included, the cost per year of life saved at a discount rate of 10 percent is 86 times as great as at a discount rate of 0 percent ($83,500 versus $970). For

Table 4-9. Effect of discounting on cost per year of life saved

		Assumed costs of intervention		
Sex	*Discount rate*	*Intensive, food costs excluded**	*Intensive, food costs included*	*Minimal*
Men	0%	$ 970	$ 2,400	$ 250
	5%	$ 10,700	$ 16,800	$ 3,100
	10%	$ 83,500	$114,000	$27,300
Women	0%	$ 620	$ 1,600	$ 165
	5%	$ 9,300	$ 14,600	$ 2,800
	10%	$105,000	$142,000	$35,600
"Crossover" discount rate (where C/YLS for men = C/YLS for women)		6.9%	7.0%	6.4%

*Discounting reduces apparent cost-effectiveness more if excess food costs are excluded from consideration than if they are included.

women, in the intensive program, there is a 170-fold change in the same interval ($105,000 versus $620). Sensitivity is greater for the minimal program and less when food costs are included.

The effect of discounting is greatest for the minimal intervention program, the expenses of which are all incurred within a year of screening and are hence unaffected by discounting. For the intensive intervention (especially when food costs that accrue throughout the patient's life are included), the costs as well as the benefits stretch forward into the future, and so higher rates of discount reduce apparent program costs. Thus, while costs per YLS are higher for the intensive than for the minimal programs (with or without food costs), the cost-effectiveness of the intensive programs are not as responsive to the discount rate. A similar effect is seen when comparing the intensive–no food program to the intensive program with food costs included. For programs with intervention costs extending into the future, the reduction in benefits at higher discount rates is somewhat offset by the reduction in program costs.

The impact of the discount rate on the optimal cutoff level for treatment is far less dramatic than on cost-effectiveness. The results, shown in Table 4-8, reflect two contradictory trends, which tend to cancel each other out. On one hand, discounting reduces apparent intervention costs, even more so when food costs are included than when they are excluded. On the other hand, discounting reduces benefits. The cutoff level in our model is more sensitive to intervention costs than to level of benefits, and so, of the two trends, the former dominates. The net effect is to make intensive intervention look cheaper as the discount rate rises. At higher rates, we therefore would choose to treat a somewhat larger percentage of screenees.

When food costs are excluded, the effect of a rise in discount rate from 0 percent to 10 percent for men in the intensive program is small (3.7 percent treated versus 4.3 percent treated). The addition of food costs magnifies the effect of discounting, with a rise in percentage of men treated from 1.7 percent to 3.3 percent as discount rate goes from 0 percent to 10 percent.

Elasticities—A lens on sensitivity

The foregoing discussion of sensitivities is difficult to digest and use. The reader (and the writer) must perform a perpetual balancing act, remembering what is going up and what is coming down in response to changes in other factors. Not many policymakers will find it simple to recall, for example, that for intensive intervention, as discount rate rises, benefits and screening costs fall, the cost per YLS rises, the cutoff level falls, and the percentage of screenees who are treated rises; or that for minimal intervention, as the discount rate rises the first three effects remain the same and the last two are opposite. A shorthand, or mnemonic, presentation would be helpful, and it exists in the language of economics. Economists generally present results like those above in terms of "elasticities." The elasticity of X with respect to Y is the proportional change in X caused by a small proportional change in Y.‡ With the assumptions in our model, it is a straightforward procedure to compute directly all elasticities graphed in this chapter. (The algebraic formulas are given in Appendix E.)

Table 4-10 shows the results of elasticity calculations for the "base case" parameter estimates. For example, the elasticity of cost per YLS with respect to the cost of screening for men is .09. Thus, a 10 percent increase in the cost of screening results in an increase in the cost per YLS of 0.9 percent§:

$$0.09 \times 10\% = 0.9\%$$

Elasticities offer several advantages for understanding the sensitivity of our results to our assumptions. First, since they compress the information of a graph into one signed number, elasticities can represent sensitivities all on a single page instead of on multiple graphs, making comparisons easier. Thus, if we wish to compare the effects of changes in the cost of intervention with the effects of change in compliance fraction, we note that the former acts to increase cost per YLS (since its sign is positive), whereas increasing compliance reduces the cost per YLS. Moreover, the size of the elasticities shows that changes in the compliance fraction or in the cost of intervention will have large effects on the cost per YLS, whereas changes in the cost of screening will not. To get such information otherwise would require overlaying many different graphs on the same page.

Second, elasticities permit the evaluation of several simultaneous program changes. Suppose we are comparing a current program with a new one that costs 10 percent less for intervention but produces a

‡Technically it is the derivative of $\log X$ with respect to $\log Y$ or $Y\,dx/X\,dy$.

§This is an approximation. Elasticities actually present the change in $\log X$ with respect to a change in $\log Y$, but for small X, $\log X$ is approximately $1 + X$. For larger changes, we must use the log. For example, doubling the cost of screening changes C_S to $2C_S$. Since $\log 2C_S = .69 + \log C_S$, the log (cost/YLS) increases by $.69 \times .09 = .06$, so cost/YLS increases by 6 percent.

Table 4-10. Sensitivity of cutoff and cost per year of life saved to assumptions

Parameter		*Elasticity* of cost YLS with respect to parameter*		*Elasticity of % above cutoff with respect to parameter;*	
		Men†	*Women‡*	*Men†*	*Women‡*
$\frac{1}{1+D} = r$, rate of discount					
Program	Intensive with food	−45	−55	−6	−3.6
	Intensive, no food costs	−46	−56	−2.2	−1.4
	Minimal	−48	−58	.4	.2
C_S	Cost of screening	.09	.12	.8	.8
C_I	Cost of intervention	.91	.88	− .8	− .8
F	Fraction of benefit	− 1	− 1	0	0
K	Compliance: If noncompliers cost C_I	− 1	− 1	0	0
	If noncompliers cost 0	− .09	− .12	− .8	− .8
J	Dietary reduction	− .9	− .9	− .06	− .1
R	20-year correlation	− .5	− .7	− .5	− .4
Q	Curvature of risk	− .4	− .6	− .5	− .4
L	Linear slope of risk	− .6	− .4	.5	.3

*Elasticities provide a summary measure of sensitivity. A negative elasticity indicates that cutoff level or cost per year of life saved *decreases* as the parameter in question increases.

†Assuming for men and women that $F = 1$, $K = .5$, noncompliers pay $C_I = \$308$, $C_S = \$1.20$, $J = 10\%$, $R = .534$, and $D = .05$. In this case, for men $Q = .146$, $L = .218$, the optimal cutoff $d = 1.75$. Then $S = .09$, $b = 2.43$, and $\phi(d)/(1 - \Phi(d)) = 2.15$.

‡The changes for women are $Q = .238$, $L = .151$, $d = 1.89$. Then $S = .12$, $b = .82$ and $\phi(d)/(1 - \Phi(d)) = 2.28$.

compliance rate that is 2 percent lower and a dietary reduction of cholesterol that is 4 percent smaller. We may calculate from data in Table 4-10 that the overall change in cost per YLS (for women) is simply

$$(\eta_{C_I})(\Delta C_I) + (\eta_K)(\Delta K) + (\eta_J)(\Delta J)$$

where η is the symbol for elasticity. Since

$$(0.88)(-0.1) + (-1.0)(-0.02) + (-1.1)(-0.04) = -0.024$$

the new program would decrease cost per YLS by 2.4 percent.

In interpreting the results of sensitivity analysis, we must distinguish between parameters that are outside our control and parameters that we can influence. The former type of parameter, such as the rate of discount (which is set by the economic actions of society) or the curvature of risk as a function of cholesterol (which is a biologic property of the human organism), does affect the value of an intervention program, but its only impact on our actions is to influence our choice of the ideal cutoff level for treatment of screenees. Other variables, such as the cost of screening, the cost of intervention, or the compliance fraction, are, to some degree, controllable, and the way to improve program efficiency is to manipulate these parameters. How to improve these alterable elements of a preventive program is an important subject for health services research. Our sensitivity analysis can help to direct such research toward parameters of especially great importance in determining efficiency.

The data in Table 4-10 allow us to rank variables according to their impact on cost per YLS. The rate of discount is by far the most powerful. Compliance, cost of intervention, dietary reduction in cholesterol, and fraction of benefit all have large effects. The correlation coefficient of cholesterol over time and the curvature of the benefits function are moderately powerful, and the cost of screening and the compliance rate (*if* compliers incur no intervention costs) have very little effect. Increases in the two cost parameters (C_S or C_I) or in the discount rate result in an increase in cost per YLS, but an increase in any other parameter reduces cost per YLS by increasing the benefits. Let us explore the effects of each of these parameters a bit further in terms of elasticity.

Sensitivity to discount rate—D

The elasticity values for the discount rate can be interpreted to reflect the difference in years between payment of the average cost and reaping of the average benefit. Since the average cost is essentially the same for men and women, the higher elasticity for women is a consequence of the lag of about ten years in heart disease mortality for women.

From the computations discussed earlier, we know that programs for men and for women have equal efficiencies at a discount rate of about 6 percent. The higher elasticity for women makes programs for them more attractive at low rates of discount and less attractive at high rates of discount.

Costs

The elasticities for the cost of screening and the cost of intervention are precisely the fractions of program expenditures devoted to screening and to intervention. Since screening costs are only a small part of the overall program costs, changing C_S has little effect on cost per YLS. Even if we use the strategy of repeated testing, thereby doubling the screening costs, the total program expenditures rise only slightly. Nonetheless, the gain in precision that results from repeat testing is not enough to outweigh the added screening expenses, and at the values that we assume for short-term correlation coefficients (R_S), repeated testing even has a slightly negative impact on efficiency.

Compliance, dietary change of cholesterol, and cost of intervention
Compliance (if compliers incur full intervention costs) and dietary reduction of cholesterol are similar in their effects on cost per YLS. The cost of intervention is equally powerful but has effects in the opposite direction. These three variables, K, J, and C_I, constitute the heart of the intervention program, and the major achievable gains in efficiency are found by designing interventions that realize large reductions in cholesterol level with good compliance at low cost. If efficiency is to be held constant, each 1 percent increase in the cost of intervention must be balanced by a 0.9 percent increase in compliance or by a $0.9 \div 0.9 = 1$ percent increase in reduction of cholesterol.

Stability of level, fraction of benefit, curvature of risk, and linear slope of risk
These four parameters, all with moderate effects on cost per YLS, are outside our control, and we can only respond to them by changing the prescribed cutoff level for treatment.

As explained in Appendix F, we have used a quadratic equation to approximate the Framingham logistic risk function. The *average* benefit to individuals from cholesterol reduction is determined in our model by the linear component of this equation, but the differential benefit to individuals depending on their initial cholesterol levels is proportional to the quadratic component (i.e., to the "curvature"). Figure 4-18 shows the discounted added years of life in the base case per complier as a function of the complier's initial cholesterol level. In this figure, the absolute height of the lines (that is, the benefit at the mean cholesterol, zero standard deviation units) is approximately proportional to the linear component of the benefits equation (L). The slope of the lines is proportional to the quadratic component (Q). The relative importance of the quadratic and linear components of benefit can be represented as the ratio of slope to height of the lines in Figure 4-18.

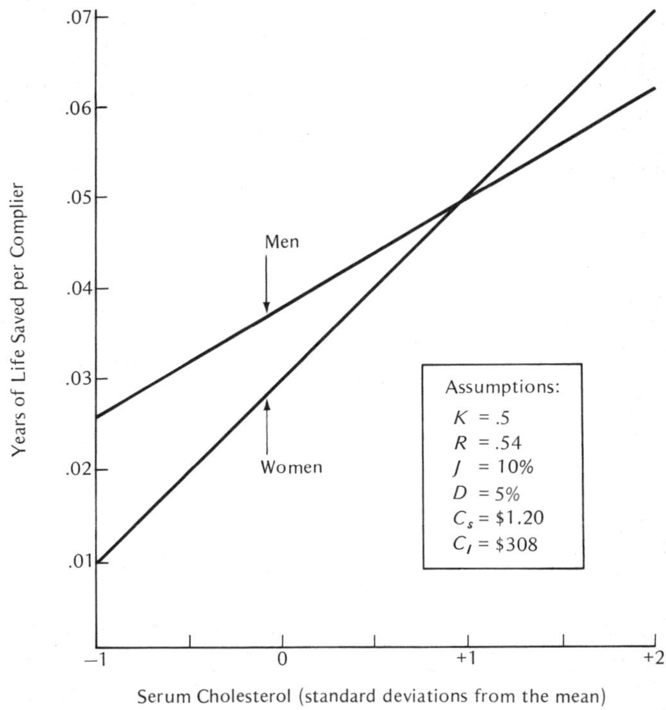

Figure 4-18. Years of Life Saved per Complier vs. Initial Cholesterol Level. A woman with a cholesterol level 2 SD above the mean gains almost 2 1/2 times as much from treatment as a woman whose level is at the mean. A man at the same level gains a little more than 1 1/2 times as much as a man whose level is at the mean.

Because the quadratic component is relatively more important for women than for men—an effect that is seen as a higher ratio of slope to height for women in Figure 4-18—screening is a more efficient procedure for women than for men, and the optimal program for women commits a larger proportion of its total resources to screening than does the optimal program for men. This is equivalent to saying that a smaller proportion of women than men are treated in an optimal program.

Cutoff levels

The choice of how many screenees to treat is the major prescriptive outcome of our formal model. Since most of the budget in a screening and intervention program is used to pay for intervention, the percentage of the population treated has an enormous impact on the overall cost of a program. On the other hand, the efficiency of a program, expressed as cost per YLS, is fairly insensitive to the cutoff level for treatment (see Figure 4-7).

The optimal percentage of screenees to be treated increases when a hypothetical person with average cholesterol level receives a boost in benefits from intervention compared to a person with an unusually high cholesterol level, and also when the costs of intervention fall relative to the costs of screening. All the sensitivity relationships between parameter values and cutoff level for treatment follow from one of these two effects.

The first effect can be thought of as a change in the relative sizes of Q (the quadratic component of risk) and L (the linear component of risk). As Q becomes smaller in relation to L, it becomes less and less worthwhile to search for people with high cholesterol levels, since the benefits they accrue from intervention become less and less distinguishable from the benefits of the same intervention on a person with a lower initial level. The effect would appear in Figure 4-18 as a decrease in the ratio of slope to height of the benefit lines. The value of screening depends directly on the *differential* benefits to people at high and low cholesterol levels.

The second effect, that of the relative cost of screening and intervention, is less complex. As screening becomes more costly, its value compared with intervention must fall, and so we would wish to spend more of our budget on intervention. The discount rate has a much smaller effect on cutoff level than on cost. A change in D from 5 to 4 percent results in a 6 percent decrease in percentage of screenees treated (from 2.7 to 2.54 percent). This decrease is due mainly to the changes in the cost of intervention. The increase in the curvature of benefit, which results from the relatively greater effect of cholesterol on people in their fifties than in later years, has a slight effect on cutoff level in the opposite direction, tending to increase the percentage of people treated as D rises. For the minimal intervention program, treatment costs are all immediate and are therefore not affected by discounting. As a result, the only pertinent effect of a rising discount rate is to increase the curvature of benefits, and so the ideal cutoff point in the minimal program falls as D rises.

Table 4-11 summarizes the effects of the other parameters on cutoff level. An increase in R, by increasing the relative benefits of treating someone with a measured high level, produces a higher cutoff level, with fewer people being treated, and more of a budget spent on screening. An increase in K (if compliers do *not* incur intervention costs) has the same effect as decreasing screening costs.

Table 4-11. Summary of sensitivities

Effect of increases in parameter listed on cost-effectiveness	
Cost-effectiveness increases with rise in:	*Cost-effectiveness decreases with rise in:*
Compliance fraction (*K*) *if* noncompliers incur intervention costs	Discount rate (*D*)
Dietary change in cholesterol level (*J*)	Cost of intervention (C_I)
Curvature of risk (*Q*)	Cost of screening (C_S)
Linear slope of risk (L)	
Correlation coefficient of rank order over 20 years (*R*)	
Compliance fraction (*K*) *if* noncompliers do not incur intervention costs	

Effect of increases in parameter listed on percentage of screenees treated		
Percentage treated increases with rise in:	*Percentage treated remains unchanged with rise in:*	*Percentage treated decreases with rise in:*
Cost of screening (C_S)	Compliance fraction (*K*) *if* noncompliers incur intervention costs	Cost of intervention (C_I)
Linear slope of risk (*L*)		Compliance fraction (*K*) *if* noncompliers do not incur intervention costs
Discount rate (*D*) for intensive programs		Correlation coefficient of rank order over 20 years (*R*)
		Curvature of risk (*Q*)
		Dietary change in cholesterol level (*J*)
		Discount rate (*D*) for minimal programs

Note: Parameters are listed in decreasing order of their impact on cost-effectiveness or cutoff level.

A method for establishing a confidence interval on estimated cost-effectiveness

Although elasticities allow us to explore the sensitivity of our results to simultaneous variation in several parameters, they fall short of providing a clear picture of the range of likely values of true cost-effectiveness. In order to see just how far our base case estimate may be from the true cost-effectiveness of a Universal Screening program, we must combine the results of the sensitivity analysis just presented with some subjective judgments about the confidence intervals we can place around the base case estimates of individual parameters. Our goal is to estimate a subjective standard error around our single "best-guess" point estimate of cost-effectiveness.

If we could safely assume that the errors in each individual parameter were independent of each other, then it would be a simple matter to use the mathematical expressions for elasticities to estimate the variance of the cost-effectiveness. The elasticities are calculated by assuming that the logarithm of the cost per year of life saved may be approximated by a linear combination of changes from the base case for each parameter, as follows:

$$\begin{aligned}\text{Log(cost/YLS)} = C + \eta_1 \log(\Delta \text{ parameter 1}) + \eta_2 \log(\Delta \text{ parameter 2}) \\ + \ldots + \eta_N \log(\Delta \text{ parameter } N)\end{aligned}$$

where η_i is the elasticity associated with parameter i, and C is the logarithm of cost per year of life saved for the base case. When the parameters are independent of each other, the variance of log (C/YLS) is simply the sum of the variances of the individual terms, namely

$$\begin{aligned}&\text{VAR [log(C/YLS)]} = \\ &(\eta_1)^2 \text{VAR [log(parameter 1)]} + (\eta_2)^2 \text{VAR [log(parameter 2)]} \\ &+ \ldots + (\eta_N)^2 \text{VAR [log(parameter N)]}\end{aligned}$$

Unfortunately, the parameters in our model are clearly *not* all independent. While the cost of screening (C_S) and the long-term stability of cholesterol (R) may reasonably be thought of as independent variables, the cost of intervention (C_I) and the effect of the intervention on cholesterol level (J) are almost certainly linked to each other. We have dealt with this problem of independence by partitioning the parameters into five groups. Each *group* is assumed to be independent of every other group, but parameters within a group are not assumed to be independent. The groups are as follows:

1. The cost of screening (C_S)
2. Stability (R)

3. The intervention group, including the cost of intervention (C_I) and the effects of intervention on cholesterol *(J)*
4. The compliance group, including the level of compliance *(K)* and the cost incurred by noncompliers
5. The risk group, including the effects of cholesterol on risk in each sex and age group, summarized in our model by the parameters Q and L.

The first two groups, each containing a single parameter, need no discussion, but the last three groups, involving multiple parameters, must be explained further.

The intervention group includes two parameters (C_I and J), but the first of these, C_I, really represents two sources of uncertainty: the scope of the intervention (the number and kind of visits) and the unit costs of each encounter. The major link between the parameters C_I and J comes, not from the second source (the unit costs), but from the first (the scope of the intervention). Since the scope of the intervention is largely a matter of choice, we will separate the parameters in this group by *defining* the scope of the program to be that described as the "intensive intervention." We will then treat C_I and J as independent parameters, noting that our resulting confidence interval only applies to one specifically defined intervention program.

The parameters in the compliance group may be separated in a similar manner. The costs incurred by noncompliers (full costs, no costs, or some fraction in between) may be viewed as a measure of the vigor with which dropouts are pursued. A vigorous pursuit of dropouts would presumably help to increase the overall level of compliance *(K)*. We will *assume* a program in which dropouts are vigorously pursued and, hence, incur the same intervention costs as compliers. Given this level of effort, we will then estimate the fraction of people who comply. Once again, this will restrict the interpretation of our derived confidence interval to a specific program, but it will allow us to treat the parameter K as independent.

The risk group is more complex than the two groups just considered. Although our model transforms the effects of cholesterol level on life expectancy onto two parameters Q and L, the real source of error lies in our use of the logistic model to link cholesterol level to *annual* risk of heart disease or death and in our use of the Framingham data to estimate the parameters of the logistic model for different age and sex groups. With no attractive alternative to the logistic model, we simply accept it as a reasonable approximation and concentrate on establishing the error in the cost-effectiveness estimate that might result from errors in estimating the logistic parameters. We assume that errors in estimating the parameters for different age and sex groups are independent. We have circumvented the elasticities in this case and have directly evaluated the effect of various combinations of the age-specific logistic parameters on the cost per year of life saved. From this we estimated directly the contribution to the variance of log (C/YLS) which comes from uncertainty in the parameters which make up the risk group.

In estimating the uncertainty in our cost-effectiveness figures, we have assumed several parameters to be fixed. In particular, we have held the discount rate constant at 5 percent, believing that value to be a matter of choice, not chance. In addition, we have omitted food costs and have assumed that the fraction of benefit for complying children is 1.0.

Table 4-12 summarizes the results of these considerations. For each parameter not assumed to be fixed, we have indicated in the table the range that we feel reflects a variation of ±1 standard error. This is equivalent to stating that we believe that the chances are two out of three that the true value of the parameter lies between the indicated limits. We have estimated the contribution of this uncertainty in each parameter to the overall variance of log(cost/YLS). By combining these estimates, we are able to estimate the overall variance of our estimate of cost-effectiveness. For Universal Screening, then, our range estimate for cost-effectiveness, including 1 SD above and below the mean, is $5540 to $20,680 for men and $4930 to $17,670 for women.

SUMMARY OF RESULTS FOR UNIVERSAL SCREENING

For readers who may feel understandably breathless after the gauntlet of numbers they have just run, let us pause to review a few of the more important general results of the analysis of Universal Screening for children.

1. For our base case parameter estimates, including a discount rate of 5 percent, one life-year costs roughly $10,000. We estimate that the odds are two to one that cost-effectiveness lies between $5000 and $20,000 per year of life saved.
2. At discount rates below 6 percent, a screening program for women is somewhat more efficient than a screening program for men; the opposite is true at discount rates above 6 percent.

Table 4-12. Universal screening: Contributions to variance of cost-effectiveness from individual parameters

Parameter	*Best-guess estimate*	*Range of estimate (±1 SD)*	*Contribution to variance of Log(cost/YLS)* *M*	*F*
Cost of screening (C_S)	$ 1.20	$0.70–$ 2.25	.002	.003
Stability of level (R)	.54	.4–.6	.01	.01
Cost per visit	$10.00	$7–$14	.10	.10
Reduction in cholesterol (J)	10%	8–12%	.09	.09
Compliance (assuming noncompliers incur full intervention cost) (K)	.5	.35—.70	.12	.12
Risk (logistic coefficients—beta)				
Men—under age 45	0.63	0.33–0.93		
Men—45 to 54	0.63	0.33–0.93	.12	—
Men—55 to 64	0.48	0.23–0.73		
Women—45 to 54	1.35	0.79–1.91		
Women—55 to 64	1.07	0.70–1.44	—	.09
Women—over 65	0.73	0.37–1.09		
Total variance of log(cost/YLS)			.442	.413
±1 standard deviation of cost/YLS, as percentage of base case estimate			52–194%	53–190%

Note: Dollar values for confidence intervals can be calculated by multiplying the appropriate base case estimate by the stated percentages.

3. If both men and women are to be screened, then for our base case estimates, about 4 percent of men and 3 percent of women should be treated to realize maximum cost-effectiveness. Cost per year of life saved varies by less than 5 percent between the following cutoff points for treatment: 88.5th percentile and 98th percentile for men, 92nd percentile and 99th percentile for women.
4. Since so few screenees are treated, the benefits per screenee in added life and health are small, even at the optimal level of pro-

gram operation. However, screenees who are found to be hypercholesterolemic and who comply with treatment can expect to gain about a year of additional life, a year free from nonfatal manifestations of coronary artery disease, and a month free from stroke. Discounting reduces these benefits by a factor of 10 to 15.

5. Including the current extra costs of substitute foods in cholesterol-lowering diets increases the apparent cost per year of life saved by about 50 percent.
6. Cost-effectiveness is relatively insensitive to the level of compliance (if noncompliers do not incur intervention costs), to the cost of screening, and to the stability of cholesterol rank order. Cost-effectiveness is moderately sensitive to the dietary change in cholesterol level, to compliance (if noncompliers do incur intervention costs), and to the cost of intervention; and it is exquisitely sensitive to the discount rate.

   For an intervention program costing about $350, cost per year of life saved increases by the following factors:

   About 1.2 as C_S goes from $0.50 to $5.00
   About 1.4 as R goes from .75 to .33
   About 1.4 as R_S goes from 1.00 to .60
   About 2.0 as C_I goes from $80 to $300
   About 2.7 as J goes from 15 to 5 percent;
   About 4.0 as K goes from 1.00 to .25 (if noncompliers do incur intervention costs)
   About 86 as D goes from 0 to 10 percent
   (See summary, Table 4-8.)

7. The discount rate is by far the most powerful variable in determining cost-effectiveness. Its influence is greater for women than for men and greater for intervention programs with "one-time" costs than for interventions with ongoing costs.
8. Effort to improve the accuracy of cholesterol measurement through repeat testing reduces cost-effectiveness unless R_S is lower than about .5, and even then the improvement is slight.
9. The optimal percentage of screenees to treat is quite sensitive to costs of screening and intervention, to the decision to retest, and to compliance (if noncompliers do not incur intervention costs). It is moderately sensitive to the correlation coefficient of cholesterol rank order and to beta. It is fairly insensitive to the other parameters in our model.

   Increases in the following parameters result in *more* people being treated at the optimum: cost of screening, and discount rate for programs with ongoing intervention costs. Increases in the following parameters result in *fewer* people being treated at the optimum: cost of intervention, dietary change in cholesterol, compliance fraction if only compliers incur intervention costs, correlation coefficient of rank order, and discount rate for programs with "one-time" intervention costs.

For an intervention program with ongoing costs totaling about $350, the percentage of screenees treated increases by the following factors:

About 6.0 as C_S goes from $0.50 to $5.00
About 1.6 as R goes from .75 to .33
About 1.2 as R_S goes from 1.00 to .60
About 1.1 as J goes from 15 to 5 percent
About 1.7 as K goes from 1.00 to .50 (if noncompliers incur no intervention costs)
About 1.2 as D goes from 0 to 10 percent
(See summary, Table 4-8).

10. The three improvements in program design that can have the largest impact on cost-effectiveness are (a) decreases in intervention costs, (b) increases in compliance (but only if noncompliers incur intervention costs), and (c) improvements in the amount of cholesterol lowering achieved by diet. Reduction in screening costs and improvements in accuracy of cholesterol measurements have little impact on efficiency. Variations in the choice of discount rate overwhelm any such program effects in determining apparent cost-effectiveness.

In view of a body of literature on cardiovascular disease that is strongly biased toward data on men, it may seem particularly surprising that our model suggests that population-wide screening and intervention is somewhat more efficient for women than for men under the base case assumptions. We temper this conclusion with several observations that would make us uncomfortable with focusing intervention on either sex solely.

First, the advantage in efficiency for women depends critically on the accepted rate of discount, with rates over 6 percent favoring men. The selection of a discount rate between 5 and 10 percent is a matter of great uncertainty, and therefore any particular choice is, in large measure, arbitrary.

Second, although intervention in women seems more efficient in life-years saved, men hold a distinct advantage in terms of other, nonfatal outcomes. If we value disease-free years highly, then intervention in men becomes more desirable.

Third, the life-years saved for women occur at older ages than for men. We have eschewed discussion of quality of life gained, but we cannot overlook the possible advantages of gaining life years in the younger decades of life.

Fourth, the effect of concentrating efforts on prevention in women would be, in part, to aggravate an already large sexual differential in life expectancy. We would in effect, be increasing the number of single, elderly women. Instead, the equalization of life expectancy may have some positive social value, arguing in favor of intervention in men.

Fifth, since early cardiovascular death among women is a relatively rare event, extrapolation of predictive curves relating risk to cholesterol levels at young ages in women involves a large amount of uncertainty. In the Framingham study, for example, only six cardiovascular deaths occurred in women under the age of 55, and the resulting estimate of statistical risk must be viewed with special caution. We may wish to avoid formulating a policy aimed solely at preventing disease in women based on such a high level of uncertainty.

With these considerations in mind, we feel confident in proceeding with the assumption that preventive programs compared in this and other chapters ought to include efforts with both men and women.

5. Sequential, targeted, and triggered screening strategies

IMPROVING ON MASS SCREENING: SEQUENTIAL TESTING

The comprehensive screening programs analyzed in Chapter 4 are extremely expensive even under favorable assumptions about the efficacy of treatment. Might it be possible to improve on their performance by making our screening rules more selective and thereby aiming efforts where they may do the most good? We know that the entire population is a mixed bag of people with high and low cholesterol levels, for whom hypothesized benefits will vary greatly with their initial levels because of the shape of the cholesterol risk function. Can we not use some *prior* information about which people would benefit most in order to target expenditures and increase efficiency?

Such targeted programs have occurred to numerous authors (Glueck et al., 1971; Kannel and Dawber, 1972; Chase et al., 1974; Fredrickson, 1972, for example) who have each, at one time or another, commented on the possible attractiveness of selective screening for hyperlipidemia. Aware of the expense and uncertainties of population-wide screening or intervention, these writers have proposed screening adults or children who are known previously to be at high risk—members of families with hyperlipidemia, for example, or with premature atherosclerosis.

Such suggestions for selective screening share in common the use of a *prior* test or criterion, such as a positive family history, before screening of cholesterol levels. They are, therefore, special cases of *sequential* screening strategies, in which the criterion for treatment is positivity on more than one test. They use an initial test like a prospector's pan or a sieve, to wash away less interesting subpopulations, leaving behind a group of special interest for further testing, an enriched subpopulation from which we can expect higher payoffs than if we treated the initial population as homogeneous.

Such a subpopulation may yield higher payoffs for any of three reasons: First, it may include a larger proportion of individuals with higher cholesterol levels than the general population. Second, it may select individuals who will reap higher benefits than the average individual with the same cholesterol level. Third, it may select individuals for whom treatment costs are especially low.

In testing for a dichotomous risk factor, sequential screening can improve efficiency by reducing the proportion of false-positive results, by increasing benefits in the treated population, or by decreasing treatment costs. If the initial test is cheaper than the second screening test, then sequential screening may also improve on test strategy by reducing the number of people who undergo the more expensive test. This is exactly the strategy used in current mass screening programs for neonatal hypothyroidism. Against these gains must be weighed the burdens of an increase in the number of false-negative findings and the added cost of the sequential testing.

For a risk factor that is not dichotomous but rather a continuous variable, like cholesterol, the effects of sequential screening are less discrete then those discussed above. Nonetheless, selective screening might allow identification of a subgroup whose *average* characteristics are especially favorable for subsequent screening or intervention. In the case of cholesterol, a subgroup might have, for example, a higher mean level than the general population, or greater susceptibility to cholesterol-lowering interventions, or more benefit from reduction of cholesterol levels, or more stability of levels over time.

The remainder of this chapter will address three particular strategies for selective screening and, making such assumptions as our consciences will tolerate, will compare their efficiencies with each other and with mass screening as discussed in Chapter 4.

The three strategies are as follows:

1. *Rescreening,* that is, administering a second serum cholesterol test to some part of the original tested population.
2. *Case-finding,* that is, testing siblings of children identified as having high cholesterol levels.
3. *Targeted Screening,* that is, testing children in families that have a history of acquired heart disease at a young age (before age 50, for example).

Rescreening and Case-finding are simple variations in the mass screening programs discussed in Chapter 4. It turns out that results for all of these strategies are quite similar, and we have to report our numerical conclusions to two or three significant figures in order to see differences in performance. Obviously, the uncertainties in the parameters that affect the efficiency of those programs do not permit such a high degree of precision in our results, although we believe that the *direction* and *magnitude* of the *relative* changes we report as we compare programs are reliable. Our analysis is therefore more likely to be of use in deciding which of several alternative programs to implement than in deciding whether to implement any program at all.

THE SIMPLEST STRATEGY: RESCREENING

Limited rescreening

In the programs analyzed in Chapter 4, we have already examined one Sequential Screening strategy: retesting the entire screened population. Testing each child a second time clearly improves the estimate of his or her true cholesterol level. Better estimates improve the focus of the intervention, permit a more accurate prediction of the benefits of the program, and protect against clerical errors and legal liability for errors in screening. As we have seen, however, the cost of the second test outweighs these added benefits under most assumptions. Universal Rescreening does not appear to be a useful strategy.

In retrospect, this result is to be expected. Rescreening everyone *must* be relatively inefficient, since, at the extremes at least, a second test is unlikely to alter the treatment plan. A person whose cholesterol is 3 standard deviations above the mean on an initial screen, for example, is not at all likely to have a screening value that would contraindicate treatment. Nor is a person with an initial cholesterol level of 100 mg/dl likely to be reassigned to a treatment group because of a high second test.

A more efficient strategy might use an initial cholesterol screening value to decide whose cholesterol ought to be remeasured, forgoing a second screen for those whose first levels were very low or extremely high. Such a sequential strategy might be far less costly than the simple and inefficient rule, "screen everyone twice."

In practical terms, however, there is little to gain from omitting a second screen on those whose first levels were very high. First, very few children have such high levels (a consequence of the way cholesterol is distributed in the population), and second, in a real screening program, everyone recommended for treatment is likely to be retested for legal reasons anyway to reduce the number of purely clerical errors that may result in gross misclassification of some individuals. From the point of view of cost-effectiveness, it makes little difference whether we assume that the few children with extremely high levels are rescreened or not. Because it makes our calculations easier, and because it has so little effect on the results, we will assume in the following discussion that *all* children above a certain level on the first test would be retested.

Our results use the "base case" parameter values from Chapter 4, namely, J (the average shift in cholesterol from treatment) = 10 percent, R (the long-term correlation coefficient for cholesterol level) = .54, K (the fraction of positive screenees who comply with treatment) = .50, D (the discount rate for costs and benefits) = 5 percent, C_S (the cost of screening an individual) = \$1.20, and R_S (the short-term correlation coefficient for cholesterol, a measure of "noise") = .8. We first determine the optimal treatment level (based on the average of the two tests) above which all children should be treated. This model is formally presented in Appendix H.

Because the expressions cannot be solved in closed mathematical form, we will test the sensitivity to the two key variables (cost of screening and instability of level) using numerical solutions. We will compare the results of three different rescreening strategies (two of which have already been discussed in Chapter 4), which we will denote by the following labels:

1. *Single Screening*—A program that tests everyone only once; the main type of program examined in Chapter 4.
2. *Universal Rescreening*—A program that tests everyone twice, examined on p. 139.
3. *Sequential Rescreening*—A program that retests a subgroup of the initial screenees.

The three options are shown schematically in Figure 5-1.

Results of the model

Base Case Assumptions

Under the base case assumptions defined in Chapter 4, Sequential Rescreening holds a slight advantage in efficiency over both Single Screening and Universal Rescreening. Table 5-1 shows a comparison of the three programs for women, assuming a discounted intervention cost of \$308 (the "intensive" intervention program). Sequential Re-

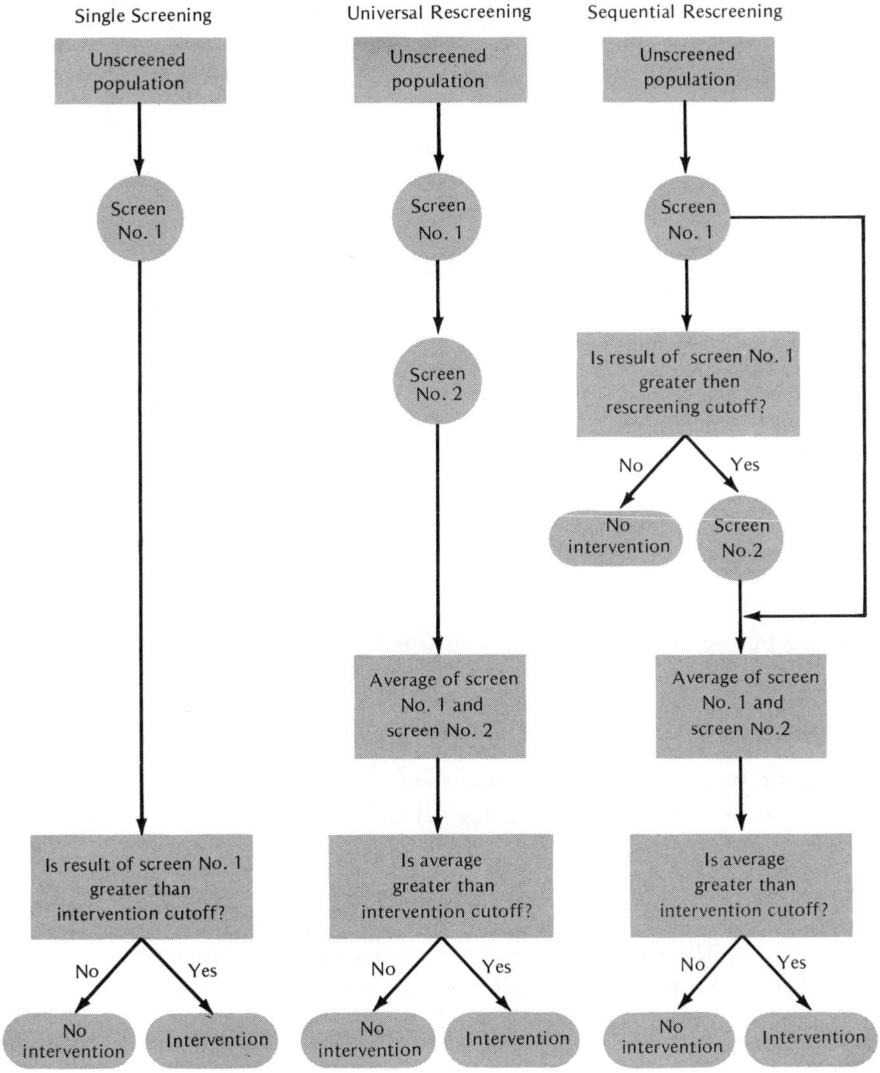

Figure 5-1. Alternative Programs—Single Screening, Universal Rescreening, and Sequential Rescreening. Three variations on a program that screens everyone at least once.

screening lowers the cost per year of added life by about 2 percent as compared with Single Screening.

At its optimum, the Sequential Rescreening strategy would recall about 7 percent of the initial screenees for a second test and, based on the average of the two tests, would refer about 45 percent of these, or 3 percent of the overall population, for treatment. The percentage of the

Table 5–1. A comparison of rescreening strategies

Type of screening program	*Cost/YLS*	*Total percentage treated*	*Final cholesterol cutoff value* (mg/dl)*	*Percentage retested*
Sequential rescreening	\$9120	3.0%	225†	6.7%
Single screening	\$9300	2.9%	230	0%
Universal rescreening	\$9720	4.9%	218†	100%

Note. Sequential Rescreening is about 2% more efficient than Single Screening. Universal Rescreening is about 4.5% less efficient.

Assumptions: C_S = \$1.20, C_I = \$308, D = 5%, J = 10%, K = .5, R = .54, women only.

*Based on 10-year-old mean log cholesterol of 5.1, s.d. of .18 (single measurement).

†Average of both tests.

population treated is slightly higher with Sequential Rescreening than with a single test, indicating a shift of resources from screening to intervention. As we saw in Chapter 4, such a shift toward intervening is to be expected whenever benefits to the treated population improve, and such an improvement is exactly what occurs as a consequence of the better selectivity of the Sequential testing.

In return for the improvement in targeting of interventions, the use of Sequential Rescreening will inevitably omit from treatment a few children whose *average* level on two tests would have been above the cutoff for treatment, but whose level on the *first* test happened by chance to be below the cutoff for retesting. Of course, these children would have been picked up by the Universal Rescreening strategy, but at the price of a decay in overall efficiency. Our analysis shows that only 0.3 percent of all children would be below the cutoff for treatment on the first screen but above the cutoff on the average of two tests. Thus, Sequential Rescreening would detect 90 percent of the children who would, in fact, qualify for treatment if all children were screened twice.

Sequential Rescreening offers less advantage in terms of morbidity than of mortality. Its more accurate determination of cholesterol level adds about 3 percent to the expected discounted gain in days of life per complier (shown in Table 4-7), but it adds only 2 percent for men and 1 percent for women to the expected discounted gain in days free of heart disease. Effects on stroke are so small as to be negligible.

Sensitivity analysis: when is sequential rescreening better than single screening?

Variation with C_S and C_I. Sequential Rescreening improves the focus of treatment at the cost of some additional expenditures on screening.

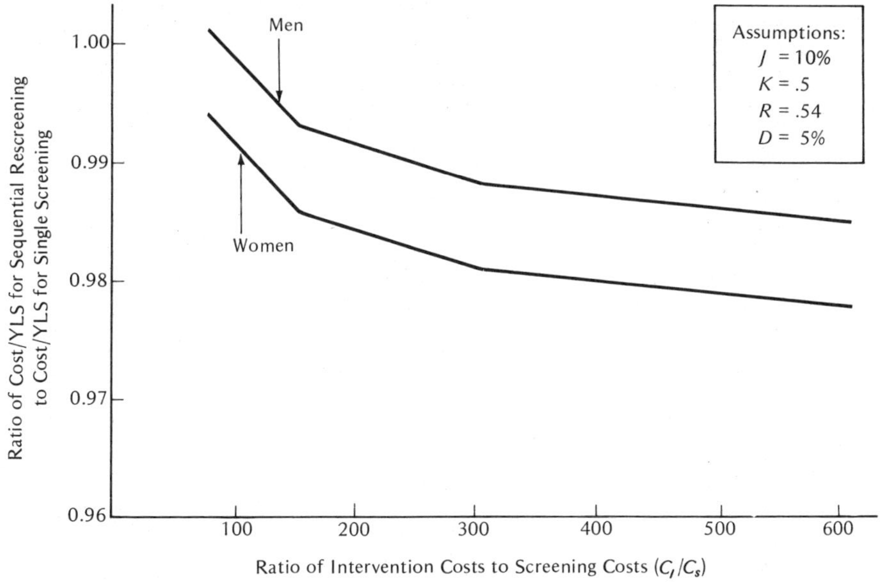

Figure 5-2. Cost-effectiveness of Sequential Rescreening Relative to Single Screening. Rescreening people before treating them (Sequential Rescreening) is more useful at high intervention costs than at low ones. Even at very high interventions costs, however, it improves cost-effectiveness by barely 2 percent over Single Screening.

We will thus not be surprised to discover that its advantage over Single Screening is more apparent when selective intervention is prized (such as when intervention costs are high or when people with high levels receive especially great benefits) or when screening costs are low.

Figure 5-2 confirms our predictions. In this figure, we have graphed the relative efficiency of Sequential Rescreening compared with Single Screening as a function of the *ratio* of treatment costs to screening costs. The pattern is clear and qualitatively as expected. The advantage of Sequential Rescreening grows as the ratio of intervention costs to screening costs increases. Furthermore, the relative advantage of Sequential Rescreening is uniformly greater for women than for men because the increment in risk with cholesterol level is greater for women than for men.

The advantage is small. Even under the assumptions that are most favorable to the Sequential Rescreening strategy ($C_I/C_S = 600$, program for women), it improves the cost per YLS by only about 2 percent. Table 5-2 shows comparative cost-effectiveness in the base case at two levels of intervention costs.

Table 5–2. Relative efficiency (cost/YLS) of sequential rescreening and single screening

Intervention	*Sex*	*Cost/YLS for single screening*	*Cost/YLS for sequential rescreening*	*Change in cost/YLS of sequential rescreening compared with single screening*
Intensive	M	\$10652	\$10527	−1.2%
Intensive	F	\$ 9296	\$ 9119	−1.9%
Minimal	M	\$ 3110	\$ 3115	+0.2%
Minimal	F	\$ 2822	\$ 2804	−0.6%

Assumptions: $J = 10\%$, $R = .54$, $D = 5\%$, $K = .5$, $C_S = \$1.20$.

Using the Sequential Rescreening strategy results in no significant change in the percentage of the population treated. In reality, the programs would not select groups of identical *composition* for treatment, but the *proportion* of screenees treated would be nearly identical.

Variation with R_S. Sequential Rescreening improves our aim by reducing the distortions introduced by short-term fluctuations in cholesterol levels; it makes our estimate of levels less "noisy" by averaging two results. Its relative efficiency thus depends critically on the prevailing "noise" level, which we have denoted in Chapter 4 by the symbol R_S, the short-term correlation coefficient for cholesterol level.

The lower R_S is, the more advantage we can expect from Sequential Rescreening. This is precisely the result illustrated in Figure 5-3, which is constructed for women and for the intensive intervention program.

Sequential Rescreening is nearly 10 percent more efficient than Single Screening at the implausibly low R_S value of .4. At a more realistic level ($R_S = .8$) the difference falls to only 2 percent. Compared with Universal Rescreening, Sequential Rescreening is uniformly about 8 percent better, no matter what the value of R_S.

The effect of changes in short-term correlation upon the percentage of the population treated is shown in Figure 5-4. The differences between the Sequential Rescreening and Single Screening strategies are negligible at all values of R_S. Universal Rescreening, on the other hand, results in the treatment of nearly twice as many people as do the other two strategies, a difference independent of R_S. This added bias toward treatment with Universal Rescreening is a result of the effectively increased cost of screening, which makes treatment seem like a

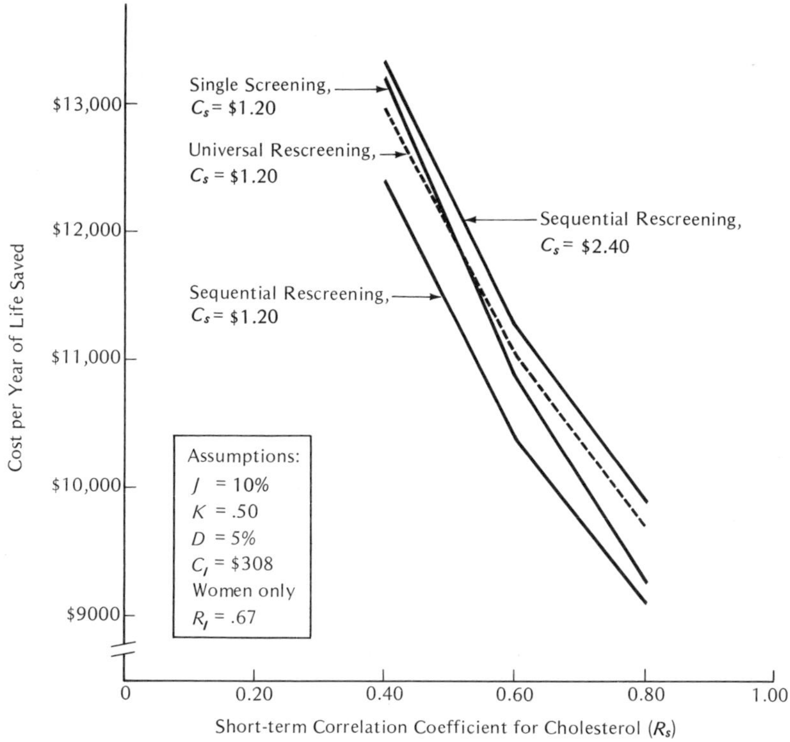

Figure 5-3. Sensitivity of Cost-effectiveness to the Short-term Correlation Coefficient for Cholesterol (R_s) (for various rescreening strategies). The more accurate the screening test is, the more cost-effective is rescreening. In effect, it is better to use a "good" test twice than to use a "bad" test twice.

more attractive bargain. In the limiting case, that is, if screening a person costs just as much as treating him, we should prefer to spend our whole budget on treatment, which would be equivalent to setting the cutoff level for treatment at 0 mg/dl.

When R_S is very low, that is, when the test is a "noisy" one, many more children are selected for rescreening under a Sequential Rescreening strategy. If C_S= $2.40 and R_S = .4, for example, about 18 percent of the original screenees are retested, yielding the 6.4 percent who are finally referred for treatment. Thus, about 30 percent of the rescreened people are treated as compared with 45 percent in the base case example (with C_S = $1.20 and R_S = .8) discussed earlier.

The fixed cost problem. Screening is inexpensive in comparison to intervention partially because of "economies of scale." It can be car-

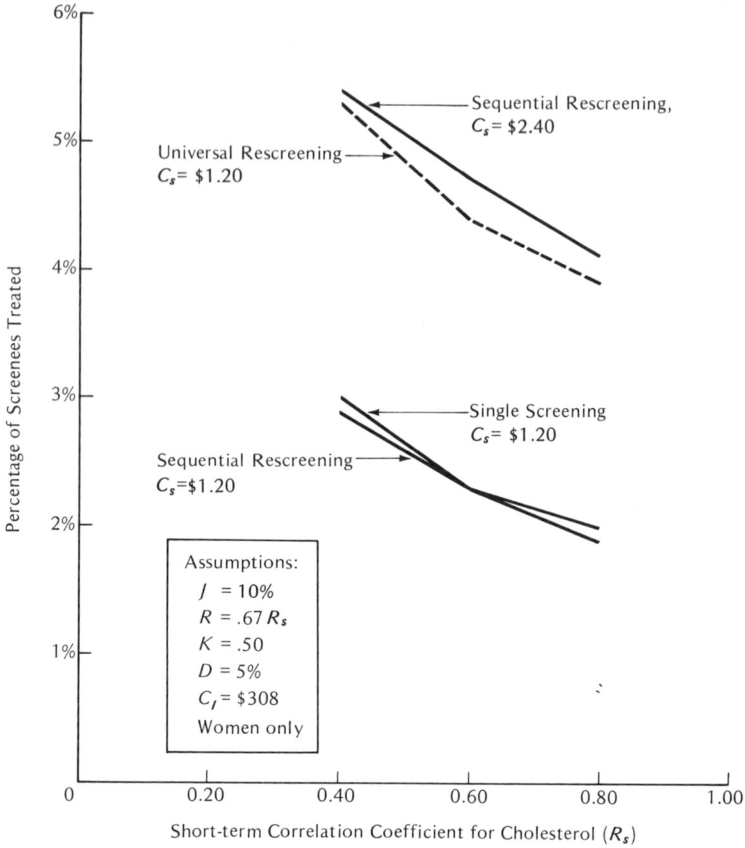

Figure 5-4. Sensitivity of Percentage of Screenees Who Are Treated to the Short-term Correlation Coefficient for Cholesterol (R_s) (for various rescreening strategies). Improving the accuracy of cholesterol measurement by rescreening makes us treat the screenees we already have rather than look for others with higher levels.

ried out in a large scale, on a "production line." Children are already assembled together in school, and a nurse, for example, could presumably work steadily through large numbers of children at a time. The foregoing analysis of Sequential Rescreening has made the tacit assumption that a second test could be done at the same cost per child as the original test. We will pause here a moment and reexamine that assumption with a bit more skepticism.

Suppose that we have determined that 100 children in a school can be screened initially at a cost of $1 per child. Of the $100 thus allotted, however, only a portion represents actual expenditures on *each* child.

The remainder is explained by fixed program costs that may be attributed for accounting purposes to each child but, in fact, would not vary much with the number of children screened. If, for example, it costs $10 for the nurse to get to the school in question and to transport a batch of specimens to the laboratory for analysis, then each of the 100 children screened actually incurs $0.10 in fixed costs and $0.90 in true marginal costs. If that $10 "setup" cost is truly fixed, then the cost of screening one single child would not be $1 but $10.90.

If we ignore fixed costs, the optimal Sequential Rescreening programs retest between 5 and 15 percent of the children, a figure that varies with sex, cost of screening, cost of intervention, and short-term stability of cholesterol level. If we use the figures in the example above, rescreening 10 percent of 100 children would cost $19 in all, or $1.90 per child, instead of the $1 per child we had originally estimated. Fixed costs thus make Sequential Rescreening somewhat more costly and therefore less advantageous. The higher the proportion of costs that are fixed, the worse the conditions are for Sequential Rescreening.

We have calculated the cost per YLS as a function of the proportion of *initial* screening costs that are fixed, and the results are depicted in Figure 5-5. For Single Screening and Universal Rescreening, the cost per YLS does not vary with fixed costs at a particular site (although efficiency *would* improve at large sites compared with small ones). On the other hand, the cost per YLS for the Sequential Rescreening strategy increases steadily with the proportion of costs that are fixed. For the assumptions specified in Figure 5-5, Sequential Rescreening is less efficient than Single Screening when fixed costs exceed 23 percent of the costs of the initial screen. (We assume, of course, that the same fixed costs are unavoidably incurred again at the time of screening.) When fixed costs are less than 23 percent of total initial screening costs, the Sequential strategy is to be preferred.

The percentage of people rescreened rises with fixed costs (Table 5-3), as does the proportion of the group referred ultimately for treatment (Figure 5-6). With high fixed costs, once we have set up to rescreen on a second occasion, we may as well test (and treat) a few more individuals and thereby spread the rescreening costs over more people.

Summary of results of sequential rescreening

Sequential Rescreening, under most assumptions, has distinct advantages over the other two alternatives, but the advantages are small in

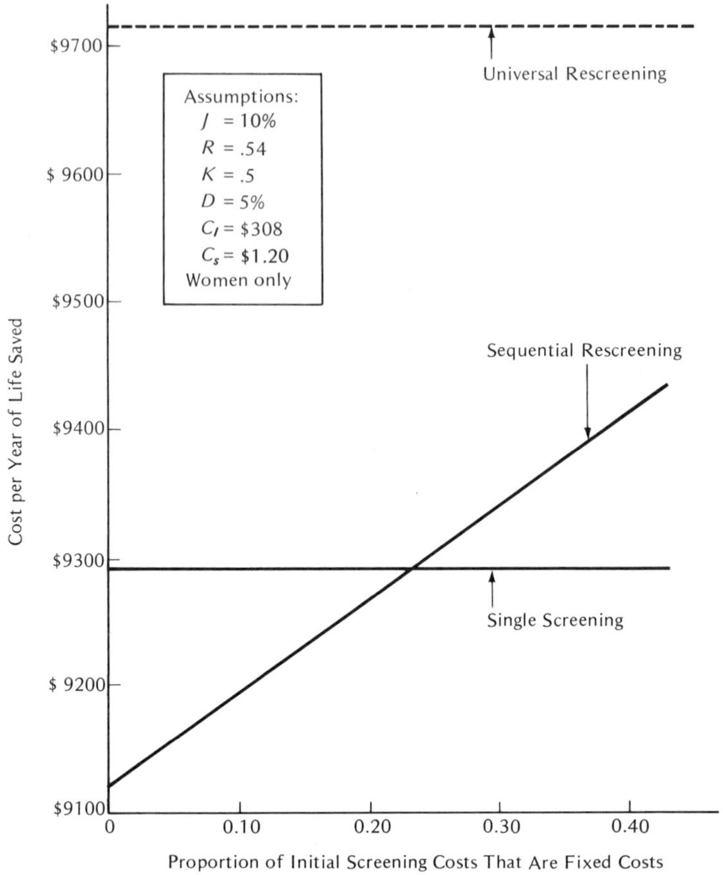

Figure 5-5. Sensitivity of Cost-effectiveness to the Proportion of Initial Screening Costs That Are Fixed Costs (for various rescreening strategies). If fixed costs are high, rescreening a few people is costly and inefficient.

Table 5–3. Percentage of initial population who are rescreened vs. proportion of costs that are fixed

Type of screening program	*Proportion of costs per screenee that are fixed* 0	.1	.2	.3	.4
	Percentage of initial population chosen for rescreening				
Sequential rescreening	6.7%	7.4%	8.1%	8.9%	9.7%
Single screening	0%	0%	0%	0%	0%
Universal rescreening	100%	100%	100%	100%	100%

Assumptions: C_S = \$1.20, J = 10%, K = .5, D = 5%, C_I = \$308, women only.

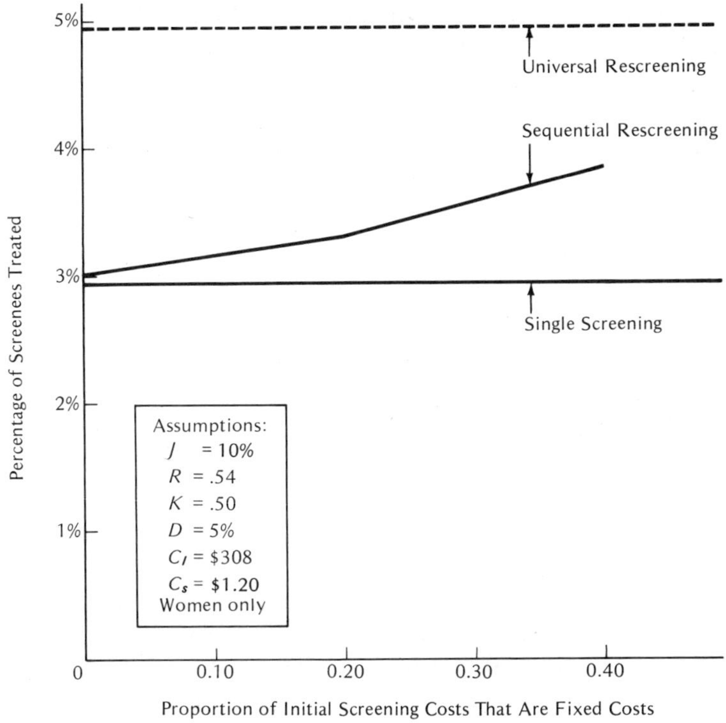

Figure 5-6. Sensitivity of Percentage of Screenees Who Are Treated to the Proportion of Initial Screening Costs That Are Fixed Costs (for various rescreening strategies).

magnitude. Compared with Universal Rescreening, the Sequential strategy avoids wasted expense in rescreening and reaps most of the benefits of a sharpened focus for treatment. Compared with Single Screening, the Sequential method is slightly more efficient unless fixed costs are higher than about 25 percent of the screening costs. As expected, the relative advantages of Sequential Rescreening are accentuated when screening is especially cheap in comparison to intervention and are more noticeable for women than for men. In addition, the advantage is greater in terms of delaying death than in delaying nonfatal morbidity.

OTHER ENRICHMENT STRATEGIES: GENERAL PRINCIPLES

The meaning of "high risk"

Most proposals for selective screening are more complex than the simple test/retest algorithms that we have just evaluated. In general, writers have suggested that cholesterol screening should be limited to (or concentrate on) "high-risk" individuals. We will shortly examine two such strategies, but first we must explore in more depth the meaning of the term "high risk" when applied to cholesterol measurements.

Two meanings are most important. First, "high risk" can refer to those individuals who are *likely to be relatively hypercholesterolemic* (based on information other than their measured cholesterol level), that is, people who are at high risk for elevated cholesterol levels. For example, we have seen in Chapter 2 that the following categories of individuals have higher average cholesterol levels than the general population: victims of early myocardial infarction, close relatives of such victims, and members of families with a known hyperlipidemic member. In fact, as we know from a number of epidemiological studies, the correlation coefficient for cholesterol level among first-degree relatives is positive and statistically significant ($r \cong .3$), and so the simple information that a person has a relative with an elevated cholesterol level tells us that his or her expected cholesterol level is above the population mean.

The second meaning of "high risk" refers not to cholesterol level at all but rather to the *risk of cholesterol-related diseases*. We know from the Framingham data that cardiovascular disease risk is an *accelerating* function of cholesterol level, and the model used in Chapter 4 speculates that the benefits to be achieved from lowering cholesterol levels maintain this curvilinear relation to initial risk. In addition, we know that cholesterol as a risk factor behaves *multiplicatively* with other risk factors. The cigarette smoker or the hypertensive has more to lose from an elevated cholesterol level than does the nonsmoker or the normotensive. If our model holds true, high-risk cigarette smokers or hypertensives also have more to *gain* than their lower risk contemporaries from *lowering* their cholesterol levels, even given the same initial cholesterol level, and even if the "high-risk" individuals continue to smoke and to have high blood pressure. Thus, a sequential screening strategy may be desirable if it focuses efforts on a subpopulation at high risk for heart disease even if that subpopulation is not expected to have unusually high cholesterol levels.

The usefulness of selective screening for those at high risk of having elevated cholesterol levels or for those at high risk of cardiovascular disease depends crucially on the properties of the initial screening test. In most cases, the tests propose to capitalize on the tendency of high cholesterol levels or cardiovascular disease to run in families.

Thus, an initial screening device might be a family history questionnaire, with a positive history of premature atherosclerosis triggering a second screen, namely cholesterol level. Alternatively, a morbid event such as sudden death or myocardial infarction might act as an initial "screening" device, leading to cholesterol measurements among close relatives.

In any case, it becomes critical in predicting the efficiency of sequenced screening to know just how cholesterol and risk are inherited within families, and we will now turn our attention briefly to the understanding of this issue.

The genetics of cholesterol

Correlation coefficients

It has long been known that coronary heart disease runs in families. Early evidence of the link between high cholesterol levels and heart disease came from studies of families with xanthomas and other visible manifestations of severe hypercholesterolemia who were found also to have a greatly increased frequency of early heart attacks.

Family concentrations of elevated cholesterol levels do not prove the existence of a genetic mechanism, since families share culture and environment as well as genes. However, statistical evidence has accumulated that implies a significant genetic influence on cholesterol levels. Correlation coefficients are especially high among monozygotic twins (see Table 5-4).

Correlation coefficients are a statistical measure of how useful one of a pair of numbers is in predicting the other. If the numbers are unrelated, the correlation is 0, and if one number is simply a linear function of the other (i.e., prediction of one from the other is completely accurate), the correlation is 1. Such correlations are quite dependent on the range of environmental variation among and between pairs. Correlations will be larger the more similar the environment shared by members of the same pair and the more diverse the environment between pairs.

The high value for identical twins as opposed to other siblings and the low husband-wife correlation are strong evidence of a genetic influence on cholesterol level. By looking at correlations between people linked in various ways in Tecumseh, Sing and Orr (1978) were able to estimate that about 60 percent of the variance in age- and sex-adjusted cholesterol scores is genetic and another 8 percent comes from environmental effects shared by sibs. Apparently, the shared

Table 5–4. Correlations between cholesterol levels in families

Author	Pair type: Siblings N	Siblings R	Parent-child N	Parent-child R	Spouses N	Spouses R
Brunner, et al., 1971	—	—	90 90	.01[a] .10[b]	90	.06
Garrison, et al., in press	256 283	.269[e] .211[f]	705 707	.202[c] .242[d]	1004	.047
Godfrey, et al., 1972	—	—	942 942	.181[a] .245[b]	—	—
Johnson, et al., 1965	—	—	1194 1175	.255[c] .258[d]	—	—
Martin, et al., 1975						
"S-Leut Group"	12,196	.298	1435 1451	.246[a] .311[b]	298	.085
"L-Leut Group"	11,712	.288	1543 1398	.287[a] .116[b]	315	.023
Schaefer, et al., 1958	123	.370	373 373	.210[a] .365[b]	201	.006
Shear, et al., 1978	720	.28[g]	—	—	—	—
Sing & Orr, 1978	325	.451[j]	210 228	.377[h,j] .459[i,j]	1025	.097[j]

N = Number of pairs
R = Correlation coefficient
[a]Father-child
[b]Mother-child
[c]Father-son
[d]Mother-daughter
[e]Brother-brother
[f]Sister-sister
[g]Whites, only
[h]One offspring compared with midparent cholesterol
[i]Two offspring compared with midparent cholesterol
[j]Same household

environment of parents and children had little effect on level. The other studies are all roughly consistent with these results, and we will use them in our analysis, assuming that the correlation between sibs is .35 and that between other first-degree relatives is .3. Higher and lower values will be tested in sensitivity studies.

Genetic mechanisms

To determine how best to capitalize on the heritability of cholesterol levels in selective screening programs, we might wish to know how many of the relatives of a known hypercholesterolemic can also be expected to have high levels. The answer depends on the genetic mechanism responsible for high cholesterol levels. The two mechanisms most frequently hypothesized are (1) that hypercholesterolemia is a result of a dominant autosomal single gene and (2) that it is a polygenic or quantitative trait (like individual height).

For selective screening based on family correlations, the distinction is extremely important. Let us assume, for example, that a selective screening strategy proposed to focus detection efforts on the first-degree relatives of people already known to have high cholesterol. If the mechanism of inheritance is that of an autosomal dominant gene, then one-half of the first-degree relatives of someone affected by the trait will also be affected. On the other hand, if the condition is polygenic, the proportion of affected relatives will depend upon the cutoff point for definition of the condition and upon the correlation between first-degree relatives. The proportion of affected relatives will be much smaller than 50 percent. For instance, if the correlation is .3 and the top 5 percent of people are called "hypercholesterolemic," then that label will apply to 14 percent of the first-degree relatives of an affected person; if the top 1 percent are called "hypercholesterolemic," then only 5.5 percent of their first-degree relatives will be similarly affected.

There has been a lively debate about the genetic mode of inheritance of severe hypercholesterolemia (HC). Early investigators believed that an autosomal dominant gene was responsible, but their work was marred by ascertainment biases, tautologous classification of hypercholesterolemics, and improper treatment of missing cases. In a survey summarizing and evaluating this work, Jensen and Blankenhorn (1972) proposed instead that a polygenic mode of inheritance fits the data better. Our reanalysis of the 145 survivors of myocardial infarction reported by Goldstein et al. (1973a, 1973b) came to the same conclusion for that group. However, two recent studies have minimized the problems of ascertainment bias by studying large populations of single kindreds and have been able to use more definite classifications and a new statistical method, respectively, to show that a single dominant gene is almost certainly responsible for the observed pedigrees (Schrott et al., 1972; Elston et al., 1975). In addition, as explained in Chapter 2, Goldstein and Brown (1975a, 1975b) have found a biochemical defect that elucidates the specific mechanism of hypercholesterolemia in at least some people who have inherited their condition.

Unfortunately, while such studies prove that monogenic hypercholesterolemia (MHC)* exists, they cannot be used to estimate the proportion of people with MHC in the country as a whole, a proportion that is critical to the analysis of selective screening. The infrequency of MHC, together with the lack of an effective and cheap method of classification, makes the estimation impractically expensive, since the population survey needed would have to be enormous. For example, assuming that the presence of xanthomas is equivalent to MHC, we might use the fact that 6 of the 5127 people screened for the Framingham survey had xanthomas to conclude that 0.12 percent of the population (or about 1 person in 1000) has MHC. However, the standard error of that estimate is 0.05 percent, so that even screening over 5000 people would result in an estimate that is barely significantly different from zero.

In addition, estimation of the prevalence of MHC must confront the several problems mentioned by Jensen and Blankenhorn. First, because of the overlap of cholesterol values between heterozygotes and others, even a statistically determined best possible cutoff using cholesterol levels will give rise to many classification errors.

Second, the use of clinical signs as the diagnostic test may recognize only a subset of people with MHC. For example, although all hypercholesterolemic members of one kindred (Schrott et al., 1972) had arcus cornea by the age of 30 and 80 percent had tendinous xanthomas, only 8 of 40 affected members of the kindred studied by Elston et al. (1975) had arcus cornea, and only 5 had xanthomas.

Third, the use of pedigrees to test whether a given surveyed person with HC is a heterozygote for MHC is made difficult by the fact that some pedigrees of nonheterozygote hypercholesterolemics will look, by chance, as if a single gene is responsible. This problem of false-positive pedigrees is particularly troublesome because even polygenic mechanisms generate positive correlations and because true positives for MHC are so rare. If the true prevalence of MHC were close to the 0.0012 estimated from Framingham, a false-positive pedigree rate of only 1 percent would completely obscure it.

To summarize, MHC exists but is quite rare, and a good determination of its prevalence in the overall population is unlikely to be made.

*To avoid identity with the specific enzyme-defect carriers described by Brown and Goldstein and with the monogenic forms labeled familial hypercholesterolemia by Goldstein et al. (1973b), we have created the designation monogenic hypercholesterolemia to apply to all individuals who are heterozygotes for *any single gene* that causes hypercholesterolemia in the carrier.

For our purpose, we will use three estimates: five per thousand, two per thousand, and zero. The estimate of zero can be justified for most analyses, since, as shown below, people with MHC probably have about the risk of heart disease that their cholesterol levels predict, and we have little information on how they differ from other people with severe hypercholesterolemia in ways that would affect our analysis. In some types of selective screening, however, the actual prevalence of MHC may make a difference. The estimate of 0.002 is derived from three sources: (1) the Framingham value of 0.0012, (2) a value of 0.0014 from the analysis of women in Tecumseh (Sing et al., 1975) (although men there did not appear to have extreme cholesterol scores), and (3) an estimate that the incidence of homozygotes is one in a million, which corresponds to a heterozygote prevalence of 0.002 (Slack, 1979). The estimate of 0.005 is offered as a credible upper limit for the prevalence of MHC.

Because of the classification problems mentioned above, the distribution of cholesterol values in MHC is best ascertained from people we are fairly sure are heterozygous for MHC, namely those from studied large kindreds. In the kindred examined by Schrott et al. (1972), the high cholesterol mode is about at 370 mg/dl, with most age-adjusted values between 320 and 440 mg/dl. This corresponds to a mean log cholesterol about 2.7 SD above normal adult values, with a standard deviation of about 10 percent.

In the report by Elston et al. (1975), the higher group is estimated to have a mean of about 2.3 SD above the usual log cholesterol values. The MHC members in the families studied by Jensen had values about 2.8 SD above normal, but the kindreds were not large, and the 350 mg/dl criterion that they used may have excluded several people with MHC. In our work, we use 2.5 SD as our estimated mean for the heterozygote population, with a standard deviation of 10 percent. This estimate is quite hypothetical, but it would be very difficult to collect the data that would be needed to improve it.

Risk characteristics of severe hypercholesterolemia

It is difficult to separate monogenic from polygenic severe hypercholesterolemia, and most of the studies that give us the data we need to estimate the effectiveness of intervention do not make the distinction. We are therefore forced to limit our inquiry to risk data about severe hypercholesterolemia in general, without regard to the genetics.

For our purposes, the best estimates of risk come from a careful study by Stone et al. (1974) of 239 first-degree hypercholesterolemic relatives of 116 propositi who had xanthomas or affected first-degree relatives. The cumulative incidence of ischemic heart disease was 42 percent at age 50 in men and 25 percent at age 50 in women. By age 60, the cumulative incidence was 65 percent in men and 36 percent in women. These incidence rates correspond in our life-table analysis to cholesterol levels of about 2.6 SD over the mean in men and 2.4 SD over the mean in women. The criteria for selection used by Stone were not based purely on cholesterol levels over 325 mg/dl; the people in their study would have had a mean log cholesterol level of about 2.4 SD over the mean. The agreement between Stone's empirical data and our own more theoretical life-table analysis based on the logistic risk function is not surprising, because even despite the stringent criteria used by Stone, the majority of the relatives studied were probably *not,* in truth, affected by MHC.† Nevertheless, the study suggests that coronary risk in MHC is about what cholesterol levels alone would imply and that a person with MHC is neither more nor less susceptible to disease than another person with an equivalent cholesterol level from a polygenic mechanism. This is the assumption that we make in most of the analysis in this chapter.

The studies by Slack (1969) and by Jensen et al. (1967) give somewhat higher risks for heart disease among heterozygotes than does Stone's study, but they are based on higher cholesterol criteria. The risk of death for MHC family members in Jensen's study is equivalent to a level 3.0 SD above the mean for men and 2.5 SD above the mean for women in our life-table models. Affected men and women in the families reported by Jensen et al. had log cholesterol values averaging about 2.8 SD above normal.

Two strategies that capitalize on the heritability of cholesterol

From the variety of published suggestions for selective cholesterol screening, we have chosen two for more detailed analysis here. The first method we call Case-finding, a strategy that uses the results of an initial cholesterol screening to identify hypercholesterolemics, whose

†We have calculated that, depending on specific assumptions, between 60 and 90 percent of the affected families in Stone's study probably had hypercholesterolemia on the basis of polygenic, not monogenic, determinants, despite their *apparently* positive pedigrees. The relative prevalences of polygenic and monogenic hypercholesterolemia are such that until clear biochemical or clinical markers of the latter are found, even the most careful studies will suffer from the problem of false-positive pedigrees.

relatives are then screened in a second stage. Case-finding capitalizes mainly on the tendency of high cholesterol levels to run in families.

The second strategy to be evaluated here is a form of Triggered Screening, in which a morbid cardiovascular event leads to screening relatives of the victim. This plan attempts to capitalize on the tendency of cardiovascular risk to run in families. Variations on these themes will be mentioned as they arise.

THE CASE-FINDING OPTION

Description of case-finding

Having identified through a Universal Screening program (such as discussed in Chapter 4) an individual with a high cholesterol level, we automatically know about a group of people, the screenee's close relatives, among whom the prevalence of high cholesterol is distinctly greater than in the population at large. An opportunity thus arises. Instead of screening the general population further, why not use what we know to mine richer ore, that is, to screen the members of the family of the identified hypercholesterolemic? Figure 5-7 compares Case-finding diagrammatically with a simple screening program.

Case-finding appears to hold promise for increasing the efficiency of a screening program by focusing screening costs on a particularly high-yield population. Its effectiveness depends on the prevalence and properties of familial hypercholesterolemia in ways that we will discuss shortly. First, however, let us note some general qualitative features of the Case-finding option.

General features of case-finding

Limited lifetime

Case-finding is a Sequential Screening strategy that acts as a supplement to a Universal Screening program. Its potential contribution is limited by its increasing redundancy with the wider screening program. If, for example, we screen 10-year-old children generally and employ Case-finding among the siblings of those found to have high cholesterol, we may expect a reasonably high extra yield, since very few of those siblings would have been detected in the initial screening procedure. As the years go on, however, and more and more people undergo screening at age 10, there would be a decreasing number of undetected hypercholesterolemics among siblings of screenees. Conversely, fewer and fewer hypercholesterolemic 10-year-olds would not have been detected before the age of 10 because

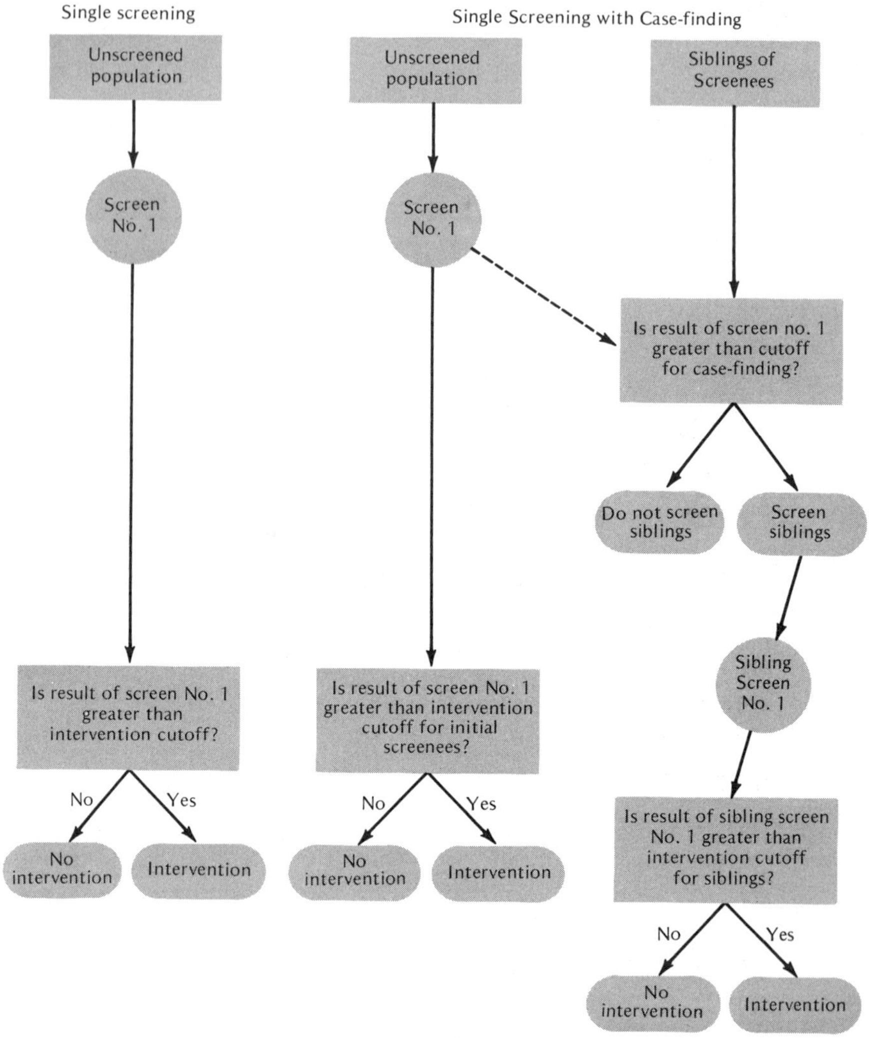

Figure 5-7. Alternative Programs—Single Screening and Single Screening with Case-finding Supplement for Siblings. A schematic diagram of the Case-finding supplement to Universal Screening, in which the siblings of positive screenees are sought. Note separate cutoff levels: one for treating initial screenees, one for Case-finding, and one for treating siblings of initial screenees. At the optimum, these three cutoff levels are *not* necessarily the same.

their hypercholesterolemic older siblings were discovered through Universal Screening.

Thus the productivity of Case-finding would be at a maximum in the first years of operation and would deteriorate to a much lower steady-state level as time passed. It may be best conceived of as an *intermittent* supplement to mass screening—added when productive and withdrawn when its efficiency has decayed so as to make it no longer worthwhile.

Sequential case-finding

In theory, Case-finding need not end with a single iteration. If it is efficient to screen the relatives of a positive screenee, then it may be efficient to screen the relatives of a hypercholesterolemic relative, and so on ad infinitum. The benefit is limited mainly by the administrative difficulty of tracing relatives further and further removed from the propositus.

Such a continuous Case-finding strategy appears clever, but it is probably unrealistic in practice, and we will limit our discussion hereafter to the efficiency of the first iteration, which poses enough administrative obstacles to satisfy even the most aggressive preventive medicine enthusiast.

Effects on the budget

The appending of Case-finding to a Universal Screening program changes the optimal cutoff level for treatment. Specifically, the opportunity to find more high-cholesterol people by screening relatives shifts the preferred cutoff level upward; we choose to treat fewer people and screen more. We forgo treating our bird in the hand to spend money chasing birds in the bush, the latter having predictably more to gain from treatment.

The shift of emphasis from treatment to screening will be reflected in the budget of the program. Of each dollar spent, a larger proportion will go to screening under the Case-finding option than without the option. Later in this section, we will explore just exactly how large the shift in resources should ideally be.

Men and women: When does case-finding make sense?

In our main results in Chapter 4, we estimated that the optimal screening program for women, assuming intervention costs at the "intensive" level, costs about $9300 per year of life saved, whereas the optimal program for men costs $10,660 per YLS. We noted, however, a number of factors that improved the relative attractiveness of programs for men, including our somewhat low estimated discount rate of 5 percent, greater relative effects on nonfatal disease, and larger potential scope of a program for men. For these reasons, instead of restricting our analysis to programs for women, we will examine here the effects of Case-finding on both male and female siblings of the propositus, even though, if improved costs per year of life saved were our only goal, we would screen only females and case-find only their sisters. To make the comparison with the original program (without Case-finding) sharper, we will explore the value of Case-finding when applied to sibs of the same sex as the propositus.

New parameters

In addition to the descriptive parameters estimated in Chapter 4, our model for the evaluation of Case-finding requires that we make reasonable estimates for the following six parameters:

1. The prevalence of monogenic hypercholesterolemia—P_{MHC}

Following the discussion on p. 181, we will use three different estimates of the prevalence of monogenic hypercholesterolemia—0, .002, and .005. We will do sensitivity analysis of the efficiency of Case-finding with respect to this parameter.

2. Distribution of MHC cholesterol values

We assume that the mean log cholesterol among heterozygotes for MHC is 2.5 SD above the population average and that heterozygote levels have a standard deviation one-half as large as that of the normal population. For 40-year-old males, this corresponds to a mean of 354 mg/dl and a standard deviation of 35 mg/dl.

3. The benefit of intervention to a heterozygous hypercholesterolemic—B_{MHC}

Rather than estimate new values of J, R, R_S, K, and risk for the very small percentage of hypercholesterolemics who have the single gene form of the condition, we will make a simplifying estimate of overall relative benefit of treatment to a familial hypercholesterolemic compared with a nonfamilial hypercholesterolemic at the *same cholesterol level.* All the determinants of benefit are thus condensed in a single number, in accord with our ignorance. We let this number vary in sensitivity analysis from a relative benefit of 0.5 to 2.0. The true value is still unknown, and it is even possible that the true heterozygote may benefit *less* from dietary intervention than the nonfamilial hypercholesterolemic at the same cholesterol level. Our "best guess" is that this parameter has a value close to 1.0.

4. General intrafamilial correlation coefficients—R_{SIB} and R_{PAR}

We assume from a relatively consistent literature that observed parent-child correlations are .3 and sib-sib correlation coefficients are .35 for cholesterol level.

5. Siblings per screenee—N_F
Our program will attempt Case-finding only among siblings of the same sex as the positive 10 year-old screenees of the intensive program in Chapter 4. We restrict attention to siblings because of our tentative hypothesis that intervention, if it is to be most effective, should begin in childhood. If the assumption were to be proved wrong, then Case-finding should probably be extended to adult relatives, and indeed, the initial screening, if it is done at all, should be done on adults instead of children to avoid delay in harvesting benefits.

Census data yield a figure of approximately 2.3 siblings per 10-year-old child in the United States. Although this figure may seem high at first glance, it becomes more believable when one remembers that a screening program for children necessarily oversamples larger families and that families with 10-year-olds are nearing the average size of *completed* families, instead of the average size of all families.

6. Cost of case-finding C_F
In addition to the cost of testing siblings, Case-finding incurs an added expense for *locating* and *contacting* these siblings—a cost that may be as low as a single telephone call or postcard or as high as several distant home visits.

That additional cost is unknown, depending on idiosyncrasies of program and subject response that we cannot now predict. For purposes of analysis, we will choose a range of values that we expect contains a realistic figure, letting C_F vary between \$2 and \$40 per relative screened. This range conforms to reported calculations of the cost of retesting positive screenees in a PKU screening program (Bush et al., 1973).

Table 5-5 summarizes the new parameters estimated in analyzing the Case-finding option. "Base case" estimates, our best guesses about the true values, are underlined.

Results of the model

Base case estimates

The heterozygote form of MHC is rare, even when we look within the population of people with high cholesterol levels. We will not be

Table 5–5. New parameters and range of values tested

Parameter	*Symbol*	*Values tested*
Prevalence of monogenic hypercholesterolemia	P_{MHC}	0, .002,* .005
Relative benefit of intervention for a familial hypercholesterolemic compared with a nonfamilial hypercholesterolemic at the same level of cholesterol	B_{MHC}	.5, 1.0,* 2.0
Overall intersib correlation coefficients for cholesterol	R_{SIB}	.25, .35,* .45
Parent-child correlation	R_{PAR}	.3
Same-sex siblings per 10-year-old screenee	N_F	.5, 1.0,* 2.0
Cost of case-finding per relative (includes test costs)	C_F	\$2, \$5,* \$10, \$40

*Underlined values represent our best guess about these parameters and constitute the base case set of assumptions for further calculations.

surprised to find, therefore, that the addition of Case-finding to mass screening will not have a major impact on the overall efficiency of a detection and treatment program. With our expectations thus tempered, let us proceed to see just how much we may gain from the Case-finding supplement. The mathematical derivation of the formal Case-finding model is described in Appendix I.

Our calculations in this section will be mainly for programs directed at women and their female siblings. Improvements in efficiency for men would be slightly smaller. We will use, first, the base case assumptions about the new parameters; namely:

P_{MHC}, the prevalence of heterozygotes for monogenic forms of hypercholesterolemia = .002.

B_{MHC}, the benefits of intervention on a monogenic hypercholesterolemic compared with a polygenic hypercholesterolemic at the same cholesterol level = 1.0.

R_{SIB}, the correlation of cholesterol levels between siblings = .35.

R_{PAR}, the correlation of cholesterol levels between parents and their children = .30.

N_F, the expected number of siblings of a 10-year-old child who are of the same sex as that child = 1.0.

C_F, the cost of locating and measuring the cholesterol level of a single sibling of a 10-year-old screenee = \$5.

The quantitative model for Case-finding must prescribe not only a cutoff level for treatment as in Chapter 4 but also a new cutoff level for Case-finding. The cholesterol level at which we would wish to treat a screenee need not necessarily be the same as the level at which we would find it useful to screen her close relatives. Actual calculations with the base case assumptions show that at the optimum the former cutoff level (for treatment) should be slightly lower than the latter cutoff level (for Case-finding). Specifically, in the base case, we should refer for intervention about 2.7 percent of the 10-year-old girls screened, but only the top 2.1 percent of initial screenees should be used as propositi for Case-finding.

From Case-finding among the top 2.1 percent of screenees, we can expect to detect both heterozygous MHC relatives and non-MHC relatives who happen to have hypercholesterolemia as a result of other causes. Specifically, for every "true" heterozygote found among relatives of a propositus, we will also find about four non-MHC hypercholesterolemics. The comparative yield of "positive" screenees among relatives is strikingly high (about 20 percent) when compared with the yield of the initial screening program (2.7 percent), but the *absolute* yield is quite small, equivalent to only 0.41 percent of the initially screened population.

We might conceive of the yield of the Case-finding program as nonetheless an excellent bargain. Instead of identifying 2.7 percent of screenees at a cost of \$1.20 per screenee (a screening cost of \$44 per positive), Case-finding gives us a 20 percent yield at a cost of \$5 per screenee (a screening cost of \$25 per positive). With such a bargain available, why would we not wish to case-find among a larger proportion of our initial screenees?

The answer is that the productivity of Case-finding decays very quickly with decreasing cholesterol level. As the cholesterol level of the propositus—that is, the cutoff level for Case-finding—falls, the probability also falls that Case-finding will uncover a sibling who will benefit more than a person already screened whose cholesterol level is just below the cutoff for treatment. Below the 98th percentile, almost no relatives with the heterozygous form of hypercholesterolemia remain to be discovered. (In our model, the theoretical limit on the percentage of MHC in the unscreened population of relatives is 0.1 percent, since half of people with MHC will have 10-year-old sibs *without* hypercholesterolemia and hence would never be sought after.) This decay in prevalence of MHC among relatives is to be expected, since the probability that any given propositus from the initial screen has MHC falls steeply with the cutoff level. With our base case assumptions, a person at the 99.9th percentile has about an 11 percent chance of being a heterozygote for MHC, whereas a person at the 97.7th percentile has only a 1 percent chance of being a heterozygote. Figure 5-8 shows the proportion of people at each cholesterol level between +2.0 and +3.5 SD above the mean who would, in fact, have the monogenic form of hypercholesterolemia, assuming that the overall prevalence of heterozygotes is .002.

If we assume, as we do here for the moment, that the benefits from treating a person with MHC are the same as the benefits from treating a nonheterozygote at the same cholesterol level (i.e., that $B_{\mathrm{MHC}} = 1.0$), then any improvement in cost-effectiveness that may result from Case-finding will be attributable solely to the increased yield of treatable cases per screening dollar, not to a change in benefits. As expected, the increment in efficiency is very small, the cost per YLS for women falls about 0.6 percent. The additional cost of Case-finding is $5 × 2.1 percent, or 10 percent of screening costs, which is about 1 percent of the overall program budget. When we discuss Case-finding, therefore, we are in fact considering only a very modest change in the cost, effectiveness, and scope of a mass screening program.

Besides a cutoff for treatment and a cutoff for Case-finding in the initial population screened, a model for Case-finding should generate a third prescription that need not coincide with either of the other two; namely at what level of cholesterol should hypercholesterolemic relatives of propositi be treated? The added information that the secondarily detected relative has a sibling (the propositus) with a high level should make us more confident that the relative's *true* cholesterol level is high. The effect of this added piece of information is similar to a reduction in R_S—the measured level has, in effect, less "noise" in it. Since we are more confident of the accuracy of our measurement, we have higher expectations about the benefits to be expected from treating the detected relative, and therefore, we should be more willing to commit resources to treatment. This logic leads to a reduction in the optimal cutoff level for treatment of case-found relatives compared with the cutoff level for treating initial screenees. For 10-year-old girls for instance, making the usual base case assumptions, our model would prescribe the following cutoff levels: 232 mg/dl for treatment of initial screenees; 237 mg/dl for initiating Case-finding among same-sex siblings; and 224 mg/dl for treating siblings detected through Case-finding.

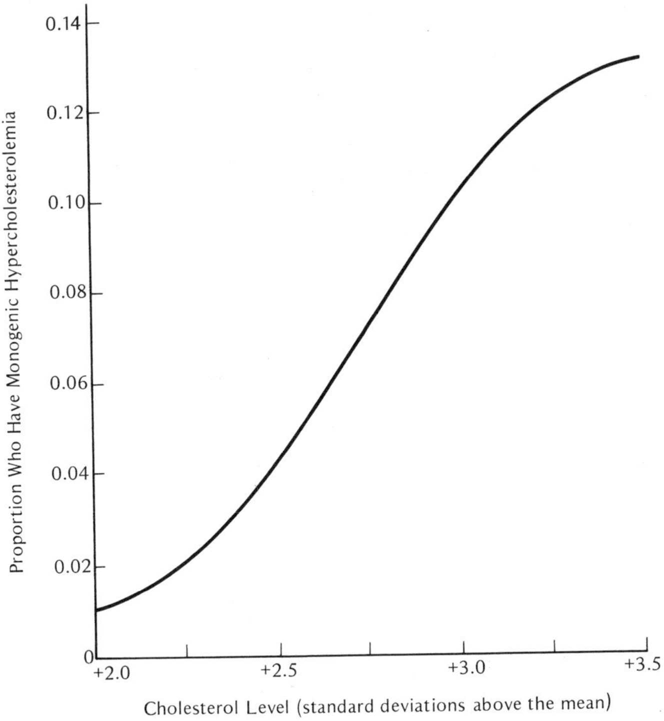

Figure 5-8. Proportion of People at Each Cholesterol Level Who Have Monogenic Hypercholesterolemia. Most people with hypercholesterolemia do not have the single-gene form of the condition. This graph is drawn assuming $P_{MHC} = 0.002$, that is, that the frequency of the gene is about one in 1000.

It may be enlightening to take a brief look at Case-finding as if it were a totally separate and distinct screening program in which the "screening" costs are the Case-finding costs. As we saw above, these costs are about 40 percent lower than the initial screening costs ($25 instead of $44 per positive screenee). Because the screened population is relatively rich in people with MHC, the benefits to be expected by each screenee in the Case-finding program are about 1 percent higher than the benefits per screenee in the programs examined in Chapter 4. Using the figure 0.12 as the elasticity of cost per YLS with respect to the cost of screening (see Table 4-9), we can calculate the change in cost per YLS for the Case-finding program compared with mass screening. Specifically

$$\begin{aligned} \Delta \text{ Cost/YLS} &= \Delta \text{ benefits} + (\Delta\, C_S)\ (\text{elasticity } C_S) \\ &= -1\% + (-40\%)\ (0.12) \end{aligned}$$

$$= -1\% + (-5\%)$$
$$= -6\%$$

Thus the program of screening and intervention among relatives is about 6 percent less costly per YLS than the initial screening program.

Unfortunately for our program's efficiency, the above calculation assumes an unlimited (or very large) supply of relatives of propositi. In fact, since the potential scope of Case-finding (given our assumptions) is limited to one sibling per propositus, its impact on cost per YLS is much smaller. The reduction in cost per YLS is proportional to the percentage of all treated people who come from the Case-finding part of the program. As we saw above, about 2.7 percent of initial screenees would be treated, whereas the people who reach treatment through Case-finding would amount to only 0.41 percent of the initially screened population. The improvement in cost per YLS is thus only

$$6\% \times \frac{0.41}{2.7 + 0.41} \cong 0.8\%$$

If there were two siblings per propositus on the average ($N_F = 2.0$), then cost per YLS would fall 1.6 percent as a result of Case-finding. If $N_F = 0.5$, then cost per YLS would fall only 0.4 percent.

The above figures have referred in general to programs for women. Similar analyses for men, for whom targeting of treatment is less critical, show that Case-finding could reduce cost per YLS by 0.3 percent (half the improvement for women). At optimal levels of operation, about 1.7 percent of initially screened men would be used as propositi for Case-finding efforts.

Case-finding has a smaller effect on morbidity than on mortality. The discounted gain in days of life per complier (as in Table 4-7) is increased 0.6 percent for men and 0.9 percent for women by Case-finding, and the discounted gain in disease-free days is increased only 0.3 percent for men and 0.4 percent for women. Both Case-finding and Sequential Screening identify a population of people with a somewhat higher expected cholesterol level than the general population, and cholesterol as a risk factor has a greater impact on death than on non-fatal disease.

Among the base case assumptions made above is the selection of a high C_I, ($C_I = \$308$); that is, we have done our calculations for the "intensive" intervention program only. For the less expensive "minimal" intervention program, Case-finding offers no advantage, since that program, at its optimum, treats about 10 percent of initial

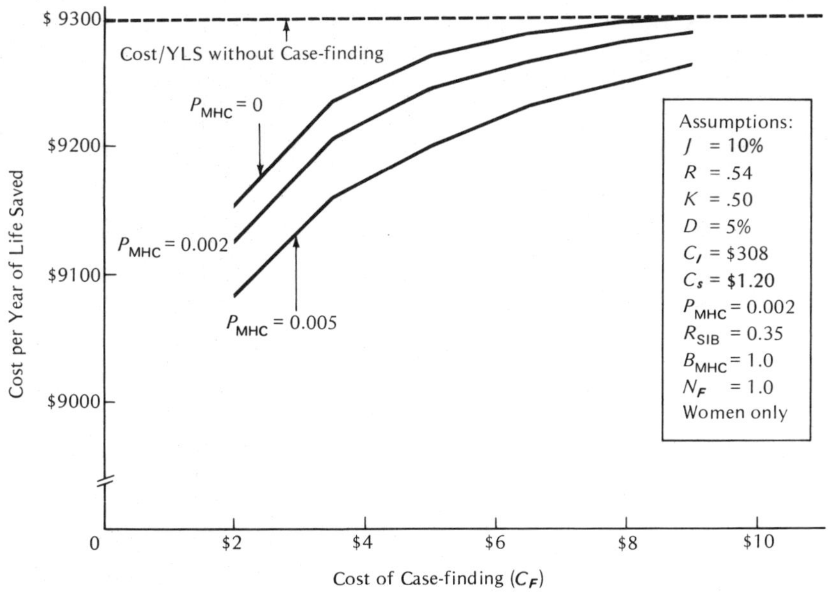

Figure 5-9. Sensitivity of Cost-effectiveness of Screening with Case-finding to the Cost of Case-finding (C_F) at Various Prevalence Levels for MHC. Case-finding works better if the heterozygotes are more prevalent. If the cost of finding siblings is over $12, however, it offers no improvement over Universal Screening *without* Case-finding.

screenees, thereby demonstrating little interest in highly focused targeting of intervention efforts.

Sensitivity analysis

Sensitivity to cost of case-finding, C_F. As we have seen the improvement in efficiency from Case-finding is most clearly related to the impact of the strategy on the screening cost per positive screenee, which accounts for about three-fourths of the reduction in cost per YLS. As the cost of Case-finding, C_F, rises, this advantage is quickly lost, and the benefit of the strategy decays rapidly. As Figure 5-9 shows, Case-finding offers little advantage when C_F approaches a value of $12 (or ten times the cost of initial screening in the base case). In programmatic terms, we would be well advised, therefore, to limit the complexity of Case-finding procedures, attempting to hold down C_F by restricting our search to relatives who, for example, are enrolled in the same school as a propositus or who can be reached with little additional expenditure of time or money.

As C_F rises and as the efficiency of Case-finding falls, the optimal cutoff cholesterol level for Case-finding changes as well. In particular, as Case-finding becomes more expensive, we would wish to use it on fewer and fewer of the initial screenees. As Table 5-6 shows, if C_F doubles from $5 to $10 for example, the ideal percentage of initial screenees to refer for Case-finding falls by a factor of 5, from 2.1 percent to 0.4 percent of the initial population. The proportion of relatives who are chosen for treatment, incidentally, rises, from about 20 percent of relatives (0.41/2.10) to 25 percent (0.10/0.40), since we would now lean more toward treatment than toward additional (and expensive) screening.

Sensitivity to relative benefit, B_{MHC}. In the base case, we assumed that a heterozygote for MHC who has a cholesterol of 300 mg/dl, for example, has neither more nor less to gain from treatment than a person who has a cholesterol level of 300 mg/dl but is *not* a heterozygote. We have virtually no data on the validity of this assumption, and there are acceptable arguments for believing that B_{MHC} is in fact greater than 1.0 and less than 1.0.

Sensitivity analysis (see Table 5-7) shows that higher estimates of B_{MHC} do improve the expected efficiency of Case-finding. Case-finding, when added to a mass of screening program for women, reduces cost per YLS by 0.6 percent (from $9296 to $9244) if $B_{MHC} = 1.0$,

Table 5–6. Sensitivity of cost per YLS and cutoff to the cost of case-finding (C_F)

C_F	*Cost/YLS*	*Percentage of screenees referred for case-finding*	*Yield of case-finding**
$2.00	$9127	10.7%	1.08%
$3.50	$9205	4.3%	0.65%
$5.00	$9244	2.1%	0.41%
$6.50	$9266	1.3%	0.30%
$8.00	$9279	0.7%	0.19%
$10.00	$9290	0.4%	0.10%
$20.00	(less efficient than no Case-finding)	<0.001%	~0%

Note. The cost of Case-finding must be relatively low if the Case-finding supplement is to be worthwhile.

Assumptions: J = 10%, R = .54, K = .5, D = 5%, C_I = $308, P_{MHC} = 0.002, C_S = $1.20, R_{SIB} = .35, B_{MHC} = 1.0, N_F = 1.0, women only.

*Yield expressed as equivalent percentage of initially screened population.

Table 5–7. Sensitivity of cost per YLS and cutoff to the relative benefits to the heterozygote (B_{MHC})

B_{MHC}	*Cost/YLS*	*Percentage of screenees referred for case-finding*	*Yield of case-finding**
B_{MHC}			
(If P_{MHC} = 0.002…)			
1.0	$9244	2.1%	0.41%
2.0	$8963	3.0%	0.46%
(If P_{MHC} = 0.005…)			
1.0	$9203	2.5%	0.54%
2.0	$8461	3.9%	0.59%

Note. We believe it to be unlikely that the value of B_{MHC} is very far from 1.0.
Assumptions: $J = 10\%, R = .54, K = .5, D = 5\%, C_I = \$308, C_S = \$1.20, C_F = \$5, R_{SIB} = .35, N_F = 1.0$, women only.
*Yield expressed as *equivalent* percentage of population initially screened.

but the same program reduces cost per YLS by 3.6 percent (from $9296 to $8963) if $B_{MHC} = 2.0$. The improvement is more striking at higher prevalence estimates for MHC.

Despite the sensitivity of efficiency to B_{MHC}, the Case-finding program remains, even under the most favorable assumptions, one of limited scope, accounting for only about 20 percent of the treated group and only 1 to 2 percent of overall program costs.

Sensitivity to prevalence of MHC (P_{MHC}) and to intersibling correlation coefficient (R_{SIB}). Increasing either the prevalence of MHC or the degree of correlation of cholesterol levels among family members has the same effect on the desirability of the Case-finding strategy. Both tend to increase the titer of hypercholesterolemic people among the relatives of positive screenees, and both therefore increase the attractiveness of using propositi to detect affected relatives. We would, under these circumstances, desire to make Case-finding a larger part of our overall program and would thus reduce our cutoff threshold for Case-finding. Figures 5-10, 5-11, and 5-12 show that the expected impact on cost per YLS, although in the expected direction, turns out to be rather small within the range of uncertainty in P_{MHC} and R_{SIB}. Indeed, from the set of assumptions least favorable to Case-finding ($P_{MHC} = 0$, $R_{SIB} = .25$) to the set most favorable to Case-finding ($P_{MHC} = .005$, $R_{SIB} = .45$), cost per YLS changes by only 1.5 percent (from $9296 to $9153) in the optimal programs.

On the other hand, the parameters in question profoundly influence our cutoff level for initiating Case-finding. Between the same two sets

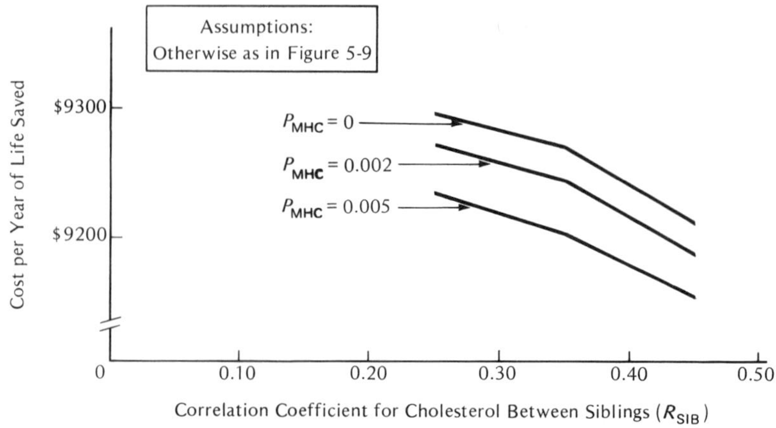

Figure 5-10. Sensitivity of Cost-effectiveness to Intersibling Correlation Coefficient (R_{SIB}) (for various MHC prevalences). Case-finding performs more efficiently if the intersibling cholesterol correlation coefficient is high.

Figure 5-11. Percentage of Initial Screenees Referred for Case-finding vs. Intersibling Correlation Coefficient (for various MHC prevalences). The higher the intersibling correlation of cholesterol, the more siblings we would wish to screen.

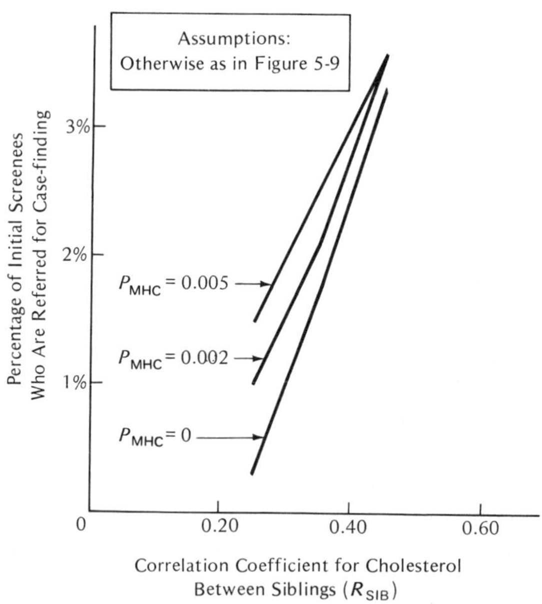

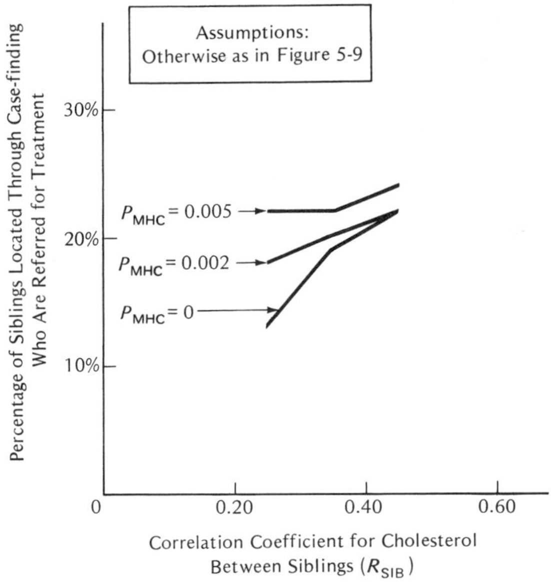

Figure 5-12. Percentage of Siblings Located Through Case-finding Who Are Referred for Treatment vs. Intersibling Correlation Coefficient (for various MHC prevalences). A larger proportion of siblings are treated than of initial screenees at the optima. If P_{MHC} is 0.002, and R_{SIB} is 0.35, then we would wish to treat nearly one sibling in five of those we screen.

of assumptions ($P_{MHC} = 0$, $R_{SIB} = .25$, and $P_{MHC} = .005$, $R_{SIB} = .45$), the percentage of the population referred for Case-finding increases 12 fold (from 0.3 to 3.6 percent). Thus increases in P_{MHC} and R_{SIB} would have relatively little impact on the efficiency of a screening program but relatively great impact on the administrative form of the ideal program (at least when C_F is low, i.e., below about $10).

Final comments on case-finding

Although we have restricted our view to programs for women, we believe, as argued in Chapter 4, that Case-finding for men may offer advantages of a similar (small) magnitude. The expected yield of any program for men, with or without Case-finding, is linked strongly both to the discount rate and to the relative weight we attach to postponement of *morbidity* (which is great for men) compared with postponement of *mortality* (which our model predicts is greater for women).

The rationale for Case-finding (and screening) to be "coeducational" is further strengthened by the reasonable assumption that compliance with diet may increase as more members of a family are advised to use the same diet.

Our analysis of Case-finding seems to lead to two major conclusions. First, as a supplemental strategy, Case-finding is of very limited potential value and scope under most reasonable estimates of the critical parameters. It is useful, but only marginally so. Second, what little usefulness Case-finding has depends crucially on the cost of the supplementary screening, C_F. An administrator who hoped to improve a mass screening program through the addition of a Case-finding strategy would be well advised to use all means at hand to reduce C_F, or alternatively, to forget the whole idea.

SCREENING BY FAMILY HISTORY

Types of selectivity

Case-finding uses an initial test, screening cholesterol in 10-year-olds, as a filtering device to select from among siblings of 10-year-old children those who ought to have their cholesterol levels measured. Case-finding can be viewed as a selective screening strategy that "asks" all children, "Do you have a 10-year-old sibling whose cholesterol level was found to be over x mg/dl?," where x is the cutoff level for Case-finding. Those who answer "yes" to this first test are then screened; those who answer "no" (either because they have no 10-year-old sibling or because their sibling's level was below x) do not undergo the second test.

This is therefore a rather peculiar example of one type of selective screening strategy, which we call Targeted Screening. A more commonly proposed form of Targeted Screening would use a family history questionnaire as an initial screening device, trying to locate children whose families have members with a history of early atherosclerosis or a high risk of coronary heart disease. Children who have a positive family history would undergo the second test, serum cholesterol measurement.

Our focus on preventive intervention in 10-year-old children impairs the efficiency of such a preliminary screening algorithm, since even high-risk parents of 10-year-old children are usually too young to have experienced coronary morbidity. Grandparents are more likely to have had their ischemic heart disease diagnosed, but the usefulness of Targeted Screening, which depends on heritability of risk through *two* generations (grandparent to child), is thereby diluted. In addition, although several risk factors besides cholesterol run in families, intervention on those other factors ought probably to be directed at adults, not children. Nevertheless, family history is so important a prognostic factor that such screening might still be worthwhile in comparison to alternative programs.

A second form of selective screening is called Triggered Screening. This device involves a program of ongoing surveillance for events that should initiate screening among a group of people who are identified by the event. For example, the occurrence of a myocardial infarction in a man under 55 years of age could trigger cholesterol screening of his children and/or grandchildren. The accuracy of ascertainment would presumably be higher than that derived from a family history questionnaire, and feasible administrative mechanisms for surveillance, through hospital intensive care units, for example, are not difficult to formulate.

A family history questionnaire program: Targeted screening

In our hypothetical Targeted Screening program, all 10-year-olds would be given a questionnaire to take home asking about the family history of heart disease. In particular, the questionnaire would ask: "Have either of your parents ever had a heart attack? At what age?" "Did any of your grandparents have a heart attack? At what age?" Those children with positive family histories might automatically receive diet counseling, or they might be subjected to a cholesterol test to determine whether they should receive counseling.

In theory, one could reverse the order of the two "tests," first measuring cholesterol levels and then gathering data on family history from those with high levels. However, since the family history questionnaire is probably less expensive than cholesterol measurement, and since it more effectively narrows the pool of screenees for the second test, it is more advantageous to use the questionnaire first. In general, with dichotomous Sequential Screening tests, all of which must be positive to initiate treatment, it is more efficient to use first the test that yields the *most negative screenees* per test dollar (Cretin, 1977a). Even though the family history questionnaire and cholesterol measurements are not dichotomous, the same general principle applies.

While other factors besides cholesterol might help explain a positive family history, intervening in children in regard to smoking or high blood pressure might be premature. Nonetheless, because of the multiplicative action of risk factors, dietary intervention in the presence of a positive family history might be especially worthwhile, even for those children with average cholesterol values.

To evaluate the scope and efficiency of family history targeting, we must estimate some new descriptive parameters. Four new variables will be of special interest:

1. The expected yield of a family history questionnaire
2. The relative risk of disease in children with a positive family history
3. The expected cholesterol levels of children with a positive family history
4. The cost of gathering information on family history.

Details on the derivation of the first three of these variables are in Appendix J. Here we will only summarize the results of those calculations.

Yield of questions on family history of myocardial infarction

We have calculated the potential yield of accurately answered questionnaires asking 10-year-olds about family history of myocardial infarction by combining data on the age distribution of parents and grandparents with data on the age- and sex-related incidence of first myocardial infarction. Our computations yield the figures in Table 5-8.

About 0.85 percent of 10-year-olds would, in fact, have a positive history of myocardial infarction in a parent. The most restrictive ques-

Table 5–8. Yield of family history questionnaire (proportion of accurate respondents with a positive history)

			No parental history but		
*Most significant part of history**	*Father's MI <45 or Mother's MI*	*Father's MI ≥45*	*Grandfather's MI <45 or Grandmother's MI <55*	*GF <55 or GM <65*	*GF <65 or GM <70*
10-year-old children	.0055	.003	.067	.098	.118
15-year-old children	.010†	.010	.064	‡	‡

*Each child is placed in the left-most applicable column. Thus, asking about history of myocardial infarction in any parent has a potential accurate positive response rate from 10-year-olds of 0.85% (i.e., 0.55% + 0.30%).

†.008 father, .002 mother.

‡Never used in analysis.

tions (involving heart attack in a father under 45 years or in any mother) could be accurately answered "yes" by 0.55 percent of the 10-year-olds. Adding questions about grandparents raises the yield of the questionnaire nine fold even with the most restrictive inquiry (infarction in a grandfather under 45 or a grandmother under 55). All together, about 29 percent of 10-year-olds who answered accurately would give a positive history of myocardial infarction in at least one of the following: any parent, a grandfather under 65, or a grandmother under 70 years of age.

Relative risk of coronary heart disease in offspring of victims of myocardial infarction

Having estimated the yield of a family history questionnaire, our model next requires an assessment of the risk of coronary disease in positive respondents relative to the population as a whole. As explained in Appendix J, we have calculated these relative risks from studies of coronary disease among first-degree relatives of victims of myocardial infarction. We find the results of four of the major studies commensurable (Slack and Evans, 1966; Deutscher et al., 1970; Førde and Thelle, 1977; Sholtz et al., 1975). Table 5-9 shows the estimated relative risk in people who report a positive parental history of myocardial infarction.

Estimates of relative risk, given a positive history in *grandparents*, prove more difficult to make and require several tenuous assumptions about the transmissibility of risk through two generations. Our estimates, presented in Table 5-10, are based primarily on extrapolation from the risk estimates for positive parental histories.

Table 5–9. Risks of death from heart disease among people with a positive parental history relative to the population average

Age of CHD death in questionnaire respondent	*Age of parents' first MI*			
	Men <45 Women <55	*Men 45–54 Women 55–64*	*Men 55–64 Women 65–69*	*Other*
Men <45 Women <55	5.8	3.5	1.15	.58
Men 45–54 Women 55–64	3.8	3.8	1.25	.63
Men 55–64 Women 65–69	1.65	1.65	1.65	.83

Note. The earlier the disease appears in parents, the higher is the relative risk of premature coronary heart disease death in the offspring.

Table 5–10. Relative risk of death from heart disease in people with a positive history in a grandparent relative to the population average

Age of CHD death in questionnaire respondent	*Age of grandparents' first MI*			
	Men <45 Women <55	*Men 45–54 Women 55–64*	*Men 55–64 Women 65–69*	*Other*
Men <45 Women <55	1.75	1.5	1.0	.84
Men 45–54 Women 55–64	1.6	1.4	1.05	.88
Men 55–64 Women 65–69	1.2	1.15	1.05	.96

Note. The effect on risk among offspring is far less for a positive history in grandparents than in parents. We have no direct measurements of these relationships; these calculations are based on parent-child transmission of risk through two successive generations.

Cholesterol levels in offspring of victims of myocardial infarction

Since the victims of premature coronary disease have relatively high cholesterol levels, and since intrafamilial correlations of cholesterol level are positive, the children of victims of early heart disease can be expected to have higher cholesterol levels than normal. Knowledge of the expected cholesterol levels in the children who respond positively to a family history questionnaire is essential in predicting the yield of a Targeted Screening program.

We have shown earlier (Chapter 4, Appendix A) that the expected cholesterol level of a heart disease victim is β standard deviations above the population mean (where β is the coefficient of regression of risk on cholesterol in the logistic risk function). Since parent-child correlation coefficients are about .3, the child of a victim of early heart attack has an expected cholesterol level of $.3\beta$ standard deviation units above the mean.

The discussion in Appendix J shows that this prediction from our model is in good accord with most empirical data on offspring of survivors of myocardial infarction.

The cost of obtaining the family history

We would propose to use a family history questionnaire without follow-up. The costs thereby assumed would include printing, distributing, collecting, and processing the forms. We would expect this procedure to be quite inexpensive, and we estimate the cost to be about $0.25 per child. Since only a small fraction of children would then proceed to the cholesterol screen, the fixed costs of cholesterol screening may become proportionately quite important. We have assumed that those fixed costs are one-fifth the total costs of cholesterol screening. If fixed costs were too great a problem, children might conceivably be sent to a central site, or the family questionnaire program could be used in a longer cycle, screening a wider age range of children every 3 years, for example, instead of a smaller group every year.

Methods

In any period, the logistic risk model assumes that the risk of coronary disease is a function of $\alpha + \beta x$, where α and β are the regression coefficients from the Framingham study, and x is the cholesterol level. The two effects of a positive history, higher average cholesterol and increased risk at each cholesterol level, are represented by shifting x to $x + dx$ and changing α to α'. With these new estimates, the average risk is still approximated by the person at $\beta/2$ SD above the mean of the group. Hence, we can solve for α' by setting

$$\frac{\exp[\alpha' + \beta(\beta/2 + dx)]}{1 + \exp[\alpha' + \beta(\beta/2 + dx)]} = \frac{\mathrm{R}\exp[\alpha + \beta(\beta/2)]}{1 + \exp[\alpha + \beta(\beta/2)]}$$

where R is the risk of a positive history relative to average.

These α' can be used to generate life tables for different histories at each level of cholesterol, and we can then proceed with the methods of Chapter 4 to evaluate the benefits of a program. The optimal cutoff levels for treatment prescribed by our model will be different for people with different types of positive family histories. At the optimum, the lowest person treated in each type of family history category has the same expected benefits from treatment, and this benefit divided by the cost of intervention is equal to the benefit cost ratio of the program as a whole.

Results

Base case results

Returning to the base case estimates for relevant parameters, we can now use our new estimates for the yield of a family history questionnaire to predict the results of a Targeted Screening program. We assume a format in which cholesterol is measured in any child who reports a positive history in *any* parent or in a grandparent who meets the age and sex criteria specified in Table 5-11, which presents

Table 5–11. Scope and benefits of a targeted screening program

Intervention	*Sex*	*Cost/ YLS*	*Cost/ screenee*	*Change in cost/YLS of targeted screening compared with universal screening*	*Percentage of population whose cholesterol is measured*	*Percentage of population who are referred for treatment*	*Benefit per complying child (days of life saved)*	
							Undiscounted	*Discounted*
Intensive	M	$6730	$2.40	−37%	0.85%*	0.60%	478	43
Intensive	F	$7730	$1.90	−17%	0.85%*	0.46%	629	40
Minimal	M	$2520	$2.20	−19%	7.5%†	2.0%	374	32
Minimal	F	$2790	$2.80	− 1%	17.7%‡	2.6%	468	28

Note. A Targeted Screening program is most efficient if it uses only parental history, assuming that intervention costs are at the intensive level. For minimal intervention costs, the questionnaire should ask about parents *and* some grandparents.

Assumptions: Base case for all parameters.

*Those with a parent who had an MI.

†Those with MI in a parent or in a grandfather under 45 years of age or a grandmother under 55 years of age.

‡Those with MI in a parent or in a grandfather under 55 or a grandmother under 65.

the results for both minimal and intensive intervention strategies under base case assumptions. Our discussion will focus first on the results for intervention at the intensive level.

What strikes us first is that only a very few children (in the intensive program, only the 0.85 percent whose parents had a myocardial infarction) ever reach the second test, cholesterol screening. The questionnaire thus proves to be, as we expected, a powerful filter to narrow our population of interest. On the other hand, by so severely limiting the scope of our program, we have substantially limited its absolute potential social impact.

Of children whose cholesterol levels are measured, between 50 and 75 percent reach values high enough to merit intensive treatment. For this final group who "pass" both screening filters, the efficiency of our program is a good deal higher than in the Universal Screening program examined in Chapter 4. Targeted Screening incurs a cost per YLS of about $7700 for women (compared with $9300 under Universal Screening) and $6700 for men (compared with $10,600 under Universal Screening). The improvement in cost-effectiveness is thus about 17 percent for women and 37 percent for men.

The savings result primarily from the increase in benefits per complier. Compared with the results for Universal Screening in Table 4-7, Targeted Screening increases the gain in discounted days of life per complier by 87 percent for men and 48 percent for women. In *undiscounted* days of life, Targeted Screening yields benefits per complier that are 64 percent higher than those of Universal Screening for men and 33 percent higher than for women. The higher the discount rate used for health benefits, the greater will be the relative benefits of Targeted Screening for each treated person when compared with Universal Screening. In addition, although the average treated woman gains less added life than the average treated man at discount rates above 4 or 5 percent, the reverse is true at discount rates closer to zero. For example, at a discount rate of 5 percent, a treated woman expects to gain 7 percent fewer added days of life than a treated man, but at a discount rate of zero, the same woman's expected gain is almost one-third larger than the man's.

Unfortunately, we lack sufficiently detailed data on the relationship between nonfatal heart disease and a history of an early myocardial infarction in a parent to permit us to calculate the relative effectiveness of family history programs in reducing morbidity. Since nonfatal disease is much more common than fatal disease, we would expect a positive family history to have a smaller impact on disease than on death. In the Tecumseh study (Deutscher et al., 1970), the risk of any heart disease before age 60 was only two to three times higher for men with a parent who died of heart disease before age 65 than for those whose parents died of other causes, whereas their risk of *fatal* heart disease was eight times higher. From data like these, we draw the qualitative conclusion that the gain in discounted days free of disease per complier would probably be similar for people found by a positive family history to that for people with comparable cholesterol levels found through other forms of screening.

Why do men benefit differentially more from targeting than do women? The answer lies in the empirical finding that family history happens to be more important than cholesterol level as a predictive factor for early heart attack in males. For example, for a 30-year-old man whose father had a heart attack under the age of 45, the risk of early coronary disease death is about 5.8 times the average. In order to have a relative risk this great solely on the basis of high cholesterol, an individual would have to have a cholesterol level above the 99.9th percentile! With such high risk, given a positive family history, it is no wonder that an optimal Targeted Screening program treats a large percentage of those with a positive response to the questionnaire.

Turning attention to the results for the minimal intervention program, we notice that the advantage of Targeted over Universal Screening is far less impressive. Using the optimal strategy—which would require cholesterol testing in anyone with a positive parental history or a positive history in a grandfather under 45 or a grandmother under 55 years of age—the cost-effectiveness improves only 1 percent for girls and only 19 percent for boys as compared to Universal Screening. Our model specifies various cutoff levels for treatment of those children who reach cholesterol screening depending on the pattern of disease in the family. For example, among girls whose cholesterol is measured, the following proportions would be assigned to intervention: 75 percent of those with a positive history in a parent; 17 percent of those with a positive history of a heart attack in a grandmother under 55 or a grandfather under 45; and 9 percent of those with a positive history in a grandmother under 65 or a grandfather under 55.

The strategy of screening cholesterol in a child with *only* positive parental history is not necessarily the best. Perhaps we would gain in efficiency from discriminating among parental histories according to the *age* of the parent at the time of his or her heart attack. Such a modification in our approach seems reasonable on its face, since we already know that cholesterol level bears a stronger relationship to premature coronary heart disease than to disease in the elderly.

In fact, this refinement in strategy has a negligible impact on efficiency. For example, if we divided parental histories into two categories—one including young fathers (coronary disease under 45 years of age) and all mothers with ischemic heart disease, and one including all other parents with ischemic heart disease—the optimal strategy would treat 75 percent of the former group and 55 percent of the latter group. The gain in efficiency from this form of discrimination would be only about 0.3 percent, and the scope of the program would be practically identical to the case in which all positive parental histories are treated equally.

The problem of scope

Because family history is a filter of such great stringency, the potential scope of a Targeted Screening program is limited. The programs using the questionnaire achieve improvements in efficiency at the expense of narrowing their impact to a very small group of children. For example, a Universal Screening program (assuming intensive intervention) would recommend treatment for about 40 out of every 1000 boys tested, but a *Targeted* Screening program for the same 1000 boys using a family history questionnaire would conclude by treating only about 5 children. The latter program would be about 40 percent more cost-effective but would affect a group only one-eighth as large.

One way to increase the potential scope of a Targeted Screening program without much compromise in cost-effectiveness would be to relax the criteria for treatment. For example, since children with high cholesterol levels and an early positive history in a *grandparent* stand to gain only slightly less than do those with average cholesterol levels and a positive history in a parent, we might choose to regard *any* history of coronary heart disease in a parent *or* grandparent before age 65 as a signal to screen cholesterol levels, instead of preferentially screening children with positive parental histories. If we did so for females, for example, assuming intervention at the intensive level, we would nearly double the percentage of the population who reach treatment (from 0.46 to 0.85 percent) with a decay in efficiency of only 6 percent. Further laxity in criteria for screening or treatment would result in substantially more deterioration in cost-effectiveness.

Compared with cholesterol level, family history is such a powerful predictor of risk that it seems reasonable to consider intervening solely on the basis of a positive family history, without measuring cholesterol levels at all. Instead of treating those 10-year-olds with *both* a positive history in a parent *and* an elevated cholesterol level (amounting to 0.60 percent of boys and 0.46 percent of girls), we would treat all who met the first criterion (0.85 percent of both boys and girls).

We can calculate, however, that such a strategy is less efficient than Targeted Screening of cholesterol levels. Using history as the sole criterion for treatment increases cost per YLS in the base case by 15 percent for males (to $7700) and by 49 percent for females (to $11,500) over the optimal Targeted Screening programs. Interestingly, the cost-effectiveness of such a "questionnaire-only" program is greater than that of Universal Screening for men but less than that of Universal Screening for women. The difference is due to the relative ineffectiveness of treating any women with low or normal cholesterol levels, since such women reap benefits which, in our model, are both smaller and later than benefits to normocholesterolemic men.

Conditions under which targeted screening is relatively advantageous: sensitivity analysis

We have already noted that targeting by family history is a procedure of far more advantage to men than to women under base case assumptions and is more useful when the intervention is costly instead of cheap, that is, when we care a great deal about *not* wasting intervention on people whose benefit is not extraordinary.

Sensitivity to fixed costs of screening. Table 5-12 shows that the ratio of fixed to variable screening costs also affects the advantage of

Table 5-12. Sensitivity of cost-effectiveness and scope of targeted screening to the proportion of screening costs that are fixed costs

Proportion of screening costs that are fixed costs	*Sex*	*Cost/YLS*	*Change in cost/YLS of targeted screening compared with universal screening*	*Percentage of population whose cholesterol is measured*	*Percentage of population who are referred for treatment*
Fixed costs = 0	M	$5950	−44%	0.85%	0.44%
Fixed costs = 0.20 C_S	M	$6730	−37%	0.85%	0.60%
Fixed costs = 0	F	$6620	−29%	0.85%	0.33%
Fixed costs = 0.20 C_S	F	$7730	−17%	0.85%	0.46%

Note. The higher the fixed costs, the less efficient the program. This is true because so few children have their cholesterol levels measured.

Table 5-13. Sensitivity of cost-effectiveness and scope of targeted screening to B_{MHC}

B_{MHC}	*Sex*	*Cost/YLS*	*Change in cost/YLS of targeted screening compared with universal screening*	*Percentage of population whose cholesterol is measured*	*Percentage of population who are referred for treatment*
0.5	M	$ 9,180	−14%	0.85%	0.59%
1.0	M	$ 6,730	−37%	0.85%	0.60%
0.5	F	$10,580	+14%	7.5%*	0.62%
1.0	F	$ 7,730	−17%	0.85%	0.46%

Assumptions: base case, intensive intervention.
*If $B_{MHC} = 0.5$, then women with a positive history in a grandfather under 45 or a grandmother under 55 (in addition to those with a positive parental history) should have their cholesterol level measured.

Targeted over Universal Screening. If the fixed costs of cholesterol screening are low, Targeted Screening is abetted, since economies of scale do not apply. If fixed costs are high, then screening small groups of children becomes inefficient, and a program administrator might well consider assembling children with positive family histories in a central location for cholesterol measurement, attempting thereby to distribute fixed costs over large numbers of screenees. Indeed, if cholesterol screening is even moderately expensive, we might well look favorably on a program that intervenes on all 10-year-olds with a positive family history, dispensing entirely with lipid measurements.

Sensitivity to B_{MHC}. Just as in Case-finding, B_{MHC}, the relative benefit of intervening in a person with monogenic hypercholesterolemia compared with an average person at the same cholesterol level has a large impact on cost-effectiveness. We assume as our base case that $B_{MHC} = 1.0$ on the basis of epidemiological evidence that people in high-risk families incur heart disease at about the rate that would be predicted from their cholesterol levels, other risks factors begin held constant. Table 5-13 shows the impact on cost-effectiveness of Targeted Screening if that assumption is wrong, and if B_{MHC} is 0.5 instead of 1.0. For women, the effects are enormous, and it becomes more efficient, in fact, to *reverse* the order of the two-stage screen—first we should measure cholesterol levels and *then* ask about family history prior to choosing our targets for intervention. For men, reducing B_{MHC} to 0.5 does not invert the optimal order of tests—it is still better to use family history as the first screen—but efficiency deteriorates considerably, with costs per YLS more than 50 percent higher than when $B_{MHC} = 1.0$ ($9178/YLS vs. $6730/YLS).

Sensitivity to the discount rate. Family history is more strongly correlated with early than with late coronary heart disease, and thus Targeted Screening gains relatively more at early ages. Because of this shift in the *timing* of savings, we would expect that Targeted Screening fares better than Universal Screening under high rates of discount. Table 5-14 and Figure 5-13 show the sensitivity of cost-effectiveness to the discount rate. Under our stated assumptions, the Targeted Screening program yields its average benefits about 2 years earlier than does Universal Screening. At a discount rate of 10 percent, about *half* of the advantage of Targeted Screening is attributable to this earlier harvest of life-years. We should take note, however, that Targeted Screening dominates Universal Screening at all discount rates greater than or equal to zero, and thus its advantage is due not only to the earlier yield but also to its generally finer focus.

Sensitivity to age at intervention. The parents of 10-year-old children are relatively young, and as their children grow, some will experience premature coronary disease that would not be revealed in a history obtained from their children at age 10. If we were to wait, for example, 5 more years and administer family history questionnaires to 15-year-olds, the yield of positive parental histories would nearly double, as noted in Table 5-8. The effects of this postponement of our program are shown in Table 5-15, in which we make the tenuous assumption

Table 5–14. Sensitivity of Cost-Effectiveness and Scope of Targeted Screening to the Discount Rate

Discount rate	*Sex*	*Cost/ YLS*	*Change in cost/YLS of targeted screening compared with universal screening*	*Percentage of population whose cholesterol is measured*	*Percentage of population who are referred for treatment*
0	M	$ 680	−30%	0.85%	0.59%
5%	M	$ 6,730	−37%	0.85%	0.60%
10%	M	$47,700	−43%	0.85%	0.62%
0	F	$ 540	−12%	0.85%	0.44%
5%	F	$ 7,730	−17%	0.85%	0.46%
10%	F	$82,750	−21%	0.85%	0.48%

Note. As in Universal Screening, discounting profoundly affects cost-effectiveness. Assumptions: base case, intensive intervention.

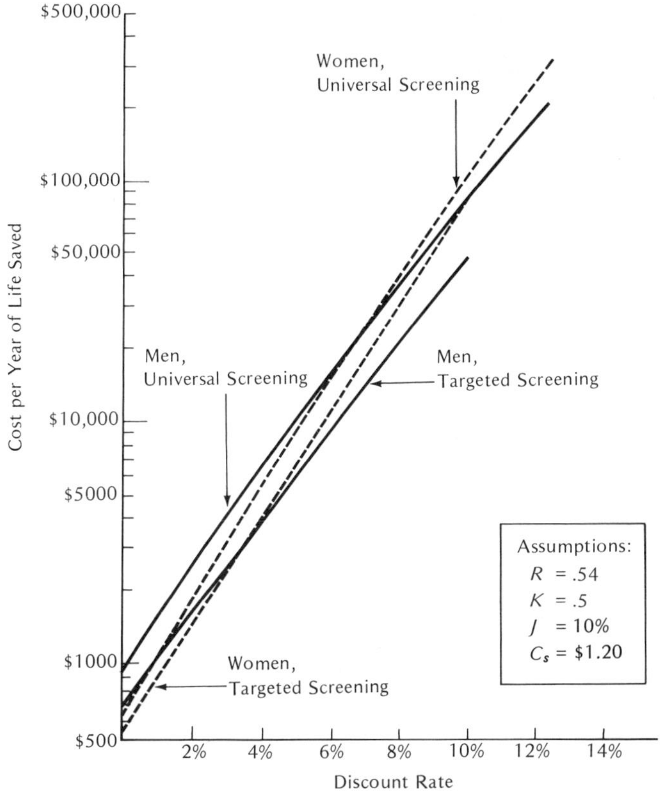

Figure 5-13. Sensitivity of Cost per Year of Life Saved to Discount Rate. Comparison of Universal and Targeted Screening (Intensive intervention program). Discounting profoundly affects cost-effectiveness but does not make Targeted Screening less efficient than Universal Screening.

that the decay in fraction of benefit and compliance from intervening in 15-year-olds instead of 10-year-olds exactly balances the gains in apparent efficiency from discounting benefits over 5 fewer years. The extra yield in positive parental history increases the scope of our treatment program by nearly 50 percent and improves efficiency by almost 15 percent for both men and women.

Confidence interval on cost-effectiveness of targeted screening. Two different perspectives are possible from which to explore the firmness of our base case estimate of the cost-effectiveness of Targeted Screening. On one hand, we can establish confidence intervals of specified width on the absolute magnitude of cost per YLS using much the same

Table 5–15. Sensitivity of Cost-Effectiveness and Scope of Targeted Screening to Age at Screening and Intervention

Age at time of family history questionnaire	*Sex*	*Cost/ YLS*	*Change in cost/YLS of targeted screening compared with universal screening*	*Percentage of population whose cholesterol is measured*	*Percentage of population who are referred for treatment*
10 years old	M	$6730	−37%	0.85%	0.60%
15 years old	M	$5880	−45%	2.0%	0.88%
10 years old	F	$7730	−17%	0.85%	0.46%
15 years old	F	$6540	−30%	2.0%	0.66%

Note. If we can delay the age at which we take the family history, the questionnaire yield rises and cost-effectiveness improves.
Assumptions: Base case, intensive intervention.

analysis as we did for Universal Screening. On the other hand, we can confine our attention to the parameters that affect the efficiency of Targeted Screening but that do *not* have an impact on Universal Screening, thus testing our confidence in our estimate of the *relative* performance of the two programs.

Calculations of the first sort lead to the entries in Table 5-16. There, much the same parameter intervals are tested as in the Universal Screening program, but in addition, we have added variation in estimates of parameters that affect Targeted but not Universal Screening—parameters including the relative benefits of intervention in a monogenic as opposed to a polygenic hypercholesterolemic person (B_{MHC}) and the relative proneness to disease among close relatives of victims of early myocardial infarction. Combining the variances appropriately, we conclude that the cost per YLS for Targeted Screening has as its ±1 SD confidence limits $2960 and $12,500 for men and $3400 and $14,200 for women, a statement equivalent to the conclusion that the chances are two out of three that the true values lie within those limits.

If we confine our view to those parameters that could affect Targeted Screening differently from Universal Screening, we arrive at the entries of Table 5-17. In this table, only four parameters are allowed to vary: the relative risk of disease in close relations of victims of premature myocardial infarction, the relative reduction in cholesterol achievable in people with positive family histories, the relative compliance of those people with dietary therapy, and the relative benefits to monogenic hypercholesterolemics (B_{MHC}). We believe that the presence of a positive family history may increase the motivation

Table 5–16. Contributions to Variance of Cost-Effectiveness of Targeted Screening

Parameter	Base case estimate	Range	Contribution to variance of log (cost/YLS) M	F
Cost of screening (C_S)	\$1.20	\$0.70–\$2.25		
Stability of level (R)	.54	.40–.60	.232	.203
Cost per visit	\$10	\$7–\$14		
Logistic coefficients	(as in Table 4–12)			
Reduction in cholesterol (J)	10%	8–14%	.11	.11
Compliance (K)	.5	.38–.78	.13	.13
Relative benefit to monogenic hypercholesterolemic (B_{MHC})	1.0	0.7–1.0	.006	.006
Relative risk of disease in relatives of victims of early myocardial infarction	(See Appendix J)	±40%	.05	.07
Total variance			.528	.519
±1 SD (as percentage of base case)			44–186%	44–184%

Note. Dollar values for confidence intervals can be calculated by multiplying the appropriate base case estimate by the stated percentages.

Table 5–17. Contributions to Variance of Relative Cost-Effectiveness of Targeted Screening Compared with Universal Screening

Parameter	Base case estimate	Range	Contribution variance of log (cost/YLS)	
			M	*F*
Relative risk of disease in relatives of victims of early myocardial infarction	(See Appendix J)	±40%	.05	.07
Relative reduction in cholesterol level	1.0	1.0–1.25*	.015	.015
Relative compliance	1.0	1.0–1.2†	.008	.008
Relative benefit to monogenic hypercholesterolemic (B_{MHC})	1.0	0.7–1.0	.006	.006
Total relative variance			.079	.099
±1 SD as percentage of base case			68–119%	66–123%
±1 SD of cost/YLS of Targeted Screening as percentage of cost/YLS of Universal Screening			43–75%	50–102%

*Interval equal to K = .5–.6.

†Interval equal to J = 10–12.5%.

Note. In these calculations, the only parameters that are allowed to vary are those on which the cost-effectiveness of Universal Screening does not depend.

to comply with a therapeutic diet, and we have therefore assumed that both J and K *may* be higher for those treated under Targeted Screening than under Universal Screening. Using these estimates, we find ±1 SD confidence limits, which imply that Targeted Screening has a cost per YLS of between 43 and 75 percent of that for Universal Screening for men and between 55 and 102 percent of that for Universal Screening for women.

Summary and discussion of targeted screening

A Targeted Screening program, using in sequence a family history questionnaire and a cholesterol measurement in 10-year-old children, is a promising strategy when compared with Universal Screening. Its improvement in cost-effectiveness—nearly one-third less in cost per YLS—is substantially larger than the improvements we can predict from the modifications or supplements to Universal Screening that we have considered so far, such as Case-finding, Universal Rescreening, and Sequential Rescreening.

The major deficiency of Targeted Screening is its limited potential scope, although a public health administrator with a tightly constrained budget might welcome an effective preventive program of smaller total scope than Universal Screening.

One more remote advantage of Targeted over Universal Screening is its testability. Proving the effectiveness of a Targeted program would be costly and time-consuming, but much less so than a similar effort for a Universal program. Some calculations will illustrate.

Suppose that we followed for 25 years a cohort of people initially aged 25 to 30 with a positive history of myocardial infarction in a parent. Such a group has a risk of heart attack before age 55 of about 25 percent as compared with 7 percent for the average man. For a given chance of observing a real difference (a feature known as "experimental power"), a study of such a group need be only $(0.07/0.25)^2 = 8$ percent as large as a study of the general population.

Using the base case assumptions of Chapter 4, and assuming that we seek an 80 percent chance of detecting an effect at a significance level of 5 percent (one-sided), we would need about 7500 subjects at the end of our study. Our model predicts that our program would achieve a reduction in heart attacks in males aged 55 from 25 percent to 22.5 percent, and if we have treatment and control groups of equal size, we require $2(0.25)(0.75)(6.2)/0.025^2 = 3720$ people in each group. Stratification or matching by other risk factors could reduce this requirement somewhat. An experiment of the same power in the general population of people without regard to family history would require experimental and control groups numbering nearly 50,000 people *each*.

The attractiveness of an experiment on Targeted Screening is diminished by uncertainty about its generalizability, given our ignorance of the correct value for B_{MHC}. Extrapolation from Targeted to Universal Screening would be unduly pessimistic if B_{MHC} is less than 1.0 and unduly optimistic if B_{MHC} is greater than 1.0.

TRIGGERED SCREENING

Description of a program

Obtaining a family history is not the only possible road to profiting from the tendency of heart disease to run in families. Another plan, which we call Triggered Screening, would use not *history* but rather the *morbid events, themselves* to initiate screening or treatment of relatives of victims of coronary heart disease. We can, with little difficulty, imagine a surveillance program watching over hospital coronary care units or physicians' offices and awaiting the arrival of a new victim of premature atherosclerosis. That victim's family members—children and grandchildren—become immediate candidates for preventive intervention or at least measurement of risk factors, including cholesterol level, and our hypothetical surveillance program can thereby target its efforts in an ongoing fashion on a group of people whose risks, and therefore whose benefits, may be especially high.

We will not engage in an elaborate quantitative analysis of such a Triggered Screening program but instead will attempt some rough comparisons with the Targeted Screening program discussed above. The cost of Triggered Screening would likely be very high compared with mass screening efforts based in public schools, since Triggered Screening requires an ongoing surveillance apparatus for the detection of relatively rare events. On the other hand, since Targeted Screening for 10-year-olds (assuming intensive intervention) results in cholesterol measurements in only 0.85 percent of all questionnaire respondents, and since Triggered Screening "finds" a positive family history in 100 percent of the people it identifies, we can tolerate a surveillance cost almost $100\%/0.85\% = 118$ times as high as the cost of our family history questionnaire. Thus, even if surveillance is very expensive, it may nonetheless prove more efficient than a family history questionnaire.

A surveillance program for Triggered Screening has a potential scope limited by the incidence of morbid events. Extrapolating from Framingham study data (Table 5-18), we would have expected about 71,000 myocardial infarctions in men under 50 years of age and women under 60 years in the United States in 1977, or an incidence of about one heart attack per 3000 people. Making the rough assumptions that the appropriate follow-up of a single index case requires about one working day and that there are 250 working days in a year, a surveillance program would require a population base of 250 × 3000 = 750,000 people to support a single surveillance officer. By comparison, the venereal disease control program in Massachusetts employs about one public health nurse for every 170,000 people in the state.

Results of triggered screening

Although every myocardial infarction is a relatively rare event, the potential scope of a Triggered Screening program is larger than that of Targeted Screening. A family history questionnaire for 10-year-olds would involve about one-sixtieth of the U.S. population each year. Each child questioned would have, on the average, 2.3 siblings, and about 0.85 percent of the respondents would report a positive history of heart attack in a parent. Overall, then, a Targeted program based on family history would pinpoint about 100,000 children each year for treatment or further screening. By comparison, the 71,000 young victims of myocardial infarction each year who are investigated by a

Table 5–18. Estimated Number of First Myocardial Infarctions in the U.S. Population, by Age of Onset

Age (years)	*Incidence of first myocardial infarction before the stated age*	
	Men	*Women*
39	14,000	†
44	28,000	2,000
49	50,000	7,000
54	*	12,000
59	*	21,000

Source. 1977 U.S. population data combined with Framingham study incidence figures.
*Not used in this analysis.
†Less than 500.
Note. These early infarctions could act as the "trigger" for cholesterol measurement in relatives.

surveillance program would have slightly over two children each on the average, and depending on how easily these children can be located, from 100,000 to 150,000 would thereby be identified as being at high risk. Adding grandparents' histories to a questionnaire program increases its yield by a factor of 9, whereas extending surveillance to grandchildren only doubles the yield of Triggered Screening.

The real advantage of Triggered over Targeted Screening depends on the rate of decay of potential benefits from intervention with the passing of years—the so-called fraction of benefit. The average age of an index patient in a Triggered Screening program would be about 46 years, and the average age of the *children* of these heart disease victims would be about 20 years. If, as we have assumed without proof, the fraction of benefit decays completely between age 10 and age 20, then Triggered Screening can have little to offer. If, on the other hand, a 20-year-old can reduce his or her risk through cholesterol alteration no less than a 10-year-old can, then the older ages of the children identified by Triggered Screening are no handicap.

The event initiating screening or treatment in a program of triggered intervention is far more dramatic than in a targeted program—a sudden serious illness in a close family member instead of a remembered tragedy in the more or less distant past. We find it reasonable to speculate that the impact of such drama may alter both compliance with recommendations for dietary change and the psychological costs and benefits of intervention. If compliance is greater and if the psychological costs are favorably altered, then Triggered Screening may reap some gains to counteract its possible loss from decay in the fraction of benefit.

The most critical factor needed to permit comparisons of Triggered Screening with its alternatives is the relationship between the age at intervention and the level of benefit achievable from dietary lowering of cholesterol. If dietary intervention at an early age holds little advantage over later efforts, then Triggered Screening may indeed be a very cost-effective program. We will return once more to this central issue in our final chapter.

6. Population-wide interventions

INTRODUCTION

Reasons for a population-wide perspective

Coronary heart disease has reached epidemic levels in our culture, and the risk factors that predispose to it, including hypercholesterolemia, are so prevalent as to make us doubt that the average American is in any useful sense "normal." As we have seen, even those of us in the developed world with cholesterol levels below average are hypercholesterolemic in comparison to people in more primitive societies, where the burden of coronary heart disease is also lower.

If most of us are "abnormal" in our lipid levels, then the screening efforts described in Chapters 4 and 5 may be misguided from the outset. Those who hold this view—including the American Heart Association (1973a) and the Inter-Society Commission for Heart Disease Resources (1970)—view hypercholesterolemia, not as a personal health problem to be detected and treated in a few of us, but rather as a cultural health problem to be corrected in us all.* If high cholesterol is a population-wide problem instead of an individual one, then its solution may require population-wide efforts instead of expanded per-

*Recommendations with respect to universal childhood intervention have been more cautious, but an ad hoc committee of the American Heart Association's Steering Committee for Medical and Community Programs recently took a step in this direction in a statement for physicians, which included these words: "Although the evidence does not yet support the recommendation that cholesterol and saturated fat should be reduced in the diet of all children, the public should be advised that such modification appears to be safe and very likely to be beneficial" (Glueck et al., 1978b).

sonal health services. This logic directs our attention away from the doctor's office or the nutritionist's counseling room and toward activities that permit access to a larger proportion of the populace—toward the mass media, government regulatory authorities, and the production and sale of food, for example.

In this chapter, we explore some of the avenues that might lead to community-wide alterations in dietary habits and thereby favorably affect the cholesterol levels of entire populations without any attempt at screening individuals. Although many uncertainties still exist about the effects of community-wide programs on diet and heart disease risk, a few well-designed social experiments are beginning to yield valuable information on our ability to change health-related behaviors in communities. Such data permit rough comparisons between population-wide efforts and programs using screening and focused intervention.

Two strategies for community-wide change

Technical interventions

Intervention on whole populations can take one of two forms: technical or behavioral. By *technical* interventions, we mean those that alter food production and consumption in ways that do not require conscious or motivated changes in the behavior of consumers. The fat composition of beef, for example, can be influenced through the animals' diet and age at slaughter. Cattle fed on grass produce meat that is lower in saturated fat content than meat from grain-fed cattle. Cattle that are fed capsules containing polyunsaturated oils yield meat and dairy products that are substantially higher in polyunsaturated/saturated fat ratio than are the products from cattle fed normal diets (Hoover, 1973). The cholesterol content of eggs, the major source of exogenous cholesterol in American diets, can be reduced by 35 percent by adding a plant sterol, sitosterol, to chicken feed (Clarenberg) et al., 1971). Government regulatory policies could be constructed to encourage such innovations as these in the production and sale of farm products, thereby favorably altering the saturated fat intake of the meat- and dairy-eating population.

Food labeling laws provide a second example of technical interventions that require little voluntary consumer compliance to achieve healthful changes in diet. Podell (1974) has pointed out that numerous trade regulations have long existed that tend to discourage the marketing and consumption of cholesterol-lowering foods. Until 1972, for example, the Food and Drug Administration explicitly forbade listing the cholesterol content of a food on a package label, nor could a product be advertised as appropriate for a cholesterol-lowering diet. Ice cream in which vegetable oil replaces some saturated fat (Mellorine) is illegal in many states, and until 1972, when the federal Filled Milk Act was ruled unconstitutional, the transportation of filled milk (in which butter fats are replaced by vegetable oils) in interstate commerce was illegal. The federal Filled Cheese Act, repealed in 1974, imposed a tax on the sale of filled cheese at wholesale and retail levels. Some states still restrict the sale of such "altered fat" products, even though they are a major component in most cholesterol-reducing diets (Hoover, 1973).

Regulations that now exist have substantial effects on the types of meat products that reach the marketplace. For example, the tenderness of beef is determined by the age of the animal at slaughter and by the fat content of the meat. Labeling laws now permit only older, fattier beef to be called "USDA Choice," a desirable designation in food marketing. Changing these laws would allow younger beef, with less fat (but equally as tender), to be sold as "Choice."

Not all writers agree that technical modifications in food production, regulation, and marketing are effective and economically feasible ways to change the American diet. Heywood (1977) concludes that the health impact of new meats from cattle with fat-modified diets would be minimal. Moreover, Meyer (1973) warns of "chaos . . . in the whole agricultural economy" should we attempt sudden and marked changes in fat-consumption patterns. Nonetheless, major secular trends in diet are already under way without undesirable economic consequences, and innovative products exploiting texturized vegetable protein substitutions for high-fat meats have met with considerable success in the marketplace (Altschul, 1973). More such advances are well within the reach of the food industry (Stare, 1973; Robertson, 1973); what they require is an appropriate regulatory and economic environment for food manufacturers. More work is needed to draw together and analyze technical modifications in food production and regulation that would lead to more healthful American diets, but this is not our field.

Behavioral interventions

Ultimately, the selection of foods for consumption rests with the American shopper (or restaurant-goer), and the shaping of consumption choices is the goal of most proposals for dietary interventions.

Strategies that alter choice—we call them *behavioral* strategies—are in some ways less attractive than technical changes. They are, for instance, more likely to require ongoing intervention instead of "one-time-only" efforts and thus are more demanding in personnel training and time. On the other hand, if a behavioral strategy can alter consumer demand, it may thereby generate just those incentives needed for industry to adopt technical changes in food production without government intervention.

Modern advertising media, especially television, have acquired enormous power to influence consumer choices. Their success offers hope that healthful, population-wide dietary change can be facilitated through many of the same devices that now boost our consumption of cosmetics, beer, and packaged soups. The *potential* reach of mass media messages on health behavior is difficult to imagine for those of us used to viewing health care as a "one-to-one" enterprise. The average American television set is turned on 5¾ hours every day; from the second to the sixty-fifth year of life, the average television viewer will watch over 3000 entire days of programming—over 8 *years* of continuous viewing (Manoff, 1973). Upon graduation from high school, the average American child has spent an estimated 12,000 hours in formal education and about 22,000 hours in front of a TV set. That television exposure has included 350,000 commercial messages, totaling 5000 hours (Looney, 1971).

Despite its power, however, even television is limited in its ability to change behavior. Commercial advertisers are pleased when a campaign increases a sponsor's share of the market by 1 or 2 percent (Bauer, 1964). Furthermore, efforts to change beliefs and behaviors generally meet with more resistance than efforts to change knowledge or to influence consumers' choices among very similar products, and unfortunately, health-related campaigns usually must seek to change behavior. Evidence suggests that offering healthy substitutes for current behaviors may be more effective than seeking to abolish old behaviors or create new ones. Warner (1977) notes, for example, that a major impact of antismoking campaigns may have been to cause consumers to change to brands with less tar and nicotine instead of giving up smoking entirely.

Methodologically rigorous measurements of the impact of medical health campaigns are rare. A recent review of 25 published studies of televised health campaigns found that nearly half used inadequate correlational designs that did not permit inferences about cause and effect (Lau et al., 1978). Of the remaining 13 studies with at least semiadequate design, only 6 demonstrated any discrete effect of media campaigns on behavior, belief, or knowledge, and in several cases, the effect was only transient.

Among the better-designed studies was Warner's analysis of correlations between the major events in the "antismoking crusade" in the United States and the price-adjusted annual per capita cigarette consumption between 1947 and 1975. He concluded that the impact of the antismoking efforts was substantial and that in the absence of those health education and media efforts, cigarette consumption in 1975 would have been 20 to 30 percent higher than it actually was. Furthermore, he suggested, antismoking campaigns resulted in relative increases in the consumption of low-tar and nicotine cigarettes, an effect overlooked by simple measurement of total consumption.

O'Keefe (1971) studied the impact of televised antismoking messages, which appeared at the rate of 80 to 100 per week in parts of Florida. One percent of ex-smokers and nonsmokers said that the campaign had influenced their behavior. The greatest effect was on those who smoked least, and the commercials seemed to influence attitudes more strongly among those who had a prior inclination to quit smoking than among those with no such inclination, observations consistent with the thesis that persuasion is more powerful in *confirming* beliefs than in *changing* beliefs.

From their review of the published studies, Lau et al. (1978) concluded that although the data in general are deficient and unimpressive, those few studies that have used adequate experimental design and have also achieved a high level of exposure of the target population to the message have found "reasonably major effects of health campaigns."

Not all forms of community-wide behavioral interventions must rely on mass media. An alternative approach might use the public school system as the point of contact with the community. Such a school education program is "community-wide" in the sense that it does not attempt to limit intervention to those at especially high risk, and furthermore, if the program is a continuing one, it will eventually reach nearly everyone in the community.

While we have some information on the effects of mass media campaigns on community cholesterol levels (we will review this information below), we have no information on the possible effects of school education programs on children's cholesterol levels. It is conceivable that dietary education in schools would be more effective than mass media campaigns, since schoolchildren may be more impressionable than adults, and since peer group pressures may reinforce a well-planned educational message. On the other hand, school programs could be far *less* effective than mass media, since parents may fail to reinforce or respond to the lessons taught their children in school, and since peer group pressure may be as likely to invalidate an educational message as to endorse it. Programs in the school system to combat teenage smoking, pregnancy, and venereal disease have not met with dramatic success, and we must remain skeptical about whether dietary education programs would do any better.

EXPERIENCE WITH POPULATION-WIDE INTERVENTIONS

The North Karelia Project

Our knowledge of the costs and effectiveness of community-wide intervention to prevent coronary disease comes almost exclusively from two studies completed in the late 1970s—the North Karelia Project in Finland, and the Stanford University Heart Disease Prevention Program in northern California. The latter has bred a third major effort—the Five Cites Study, results of which are expected in the mid-1980s.

North Karelia, a rural county in east-central Finland with about 180,000 inhabitants, suffers from one of the highest ischemic heart disease burdens in the world. Finns are subject to cardiovascular death rates more than twice as high as those of their other Scandinavian neighbors, and the risk among North Karelians in 1972 was 50 percent higher than Finland's already extraordinary average.

Under these near-emergency conditions, the Finnish government and the University of Kuopio initiated the North Karelia Project in 1972, designed to be a community-wide, systematic, comprehensive assault on cardiovascular risk factors, with the intermediate objectives of reducing hypertension, smoking, and cholesterol levels in the target population and with the ultimate objectives of reducing cardiovascular morbidity and mortality, especially in middle-aged males.

The North Karelia Project used five sorts of community-wide intervention. First, it sought to *distribute information to the public.* Primarily a rural area, North Karelia lacked significant television service, and so information was distributed through other routes such as radio, newspaper, leaflets, and health education meetings in a variety of settings.

Second, the North Karelia Project attempted to assist in modifying the *organization of services* in the community, reorienting elements of the existing health system toward prevention, and providing new basic health services where needed.

Third, *supplementary training for health industry and other community personnel* was provided to improve their contributions to prevention services.

Fourth, the North Karelia *health environment* was improved wherever possible. The project enlisted, for example, the cooperation of the local dairy industry to produce and market low-fat dairy products in greater variety and higher volume. Restrictions on smoking in public places were increased and enforced.

Finally, the North Karelia Project created a new configuration of *internal information services,* including patient registers and surveying mechanisms to identify areas of need for services and to monitor the impact of interventions.

The project seems to have been successful. In the initial 5-year period, 1972 to 1977, the net reduction in the calculated cardiovascular risk compared to a control region was 17 percent among men and 12 percent among women. The net reduction in the prevalence of smoking was 2.5 percent for males and 6.1 percent for females. North Karelia men achieved a net reduction in diastolic blood pressure of 2.6 mm Hg and a 4.1 percent net reduction in cholesterol. For women, the net reduction in diastolic blood pressure was 3.4 mm Hg while the net reduction in cholesterol level was 1.2 percent (Puska et al., 1979).

During the period of the program, mortality from cardiovascular disease decreased by 13 percent among men and 31 percent among women. This decrease seems to be, in part, a continuation of a declining trend which began in 1970, since similar decreases were observed in the control region. Because cardiovascular disease develops over decades, it is premature to expect a statistically significant decrease in cardiovascular mortality in North Karelia, so continued monitoring is planned (Salonen et al., 1979).

During the study period, women in the control region experienced a decline of 1.5 percent in cholesterol level, while levels for men in the control region increased slightly, as would have been expected due to aging. For this reason, the *net* reduction in cholesterol level for North Karelia women compared to the control region was only about 1 percent, although the *absolute* reduction was over twice that. We do not know why the women in the control region experienced declines in cholesterol levels, while their scores on the other risk factors remained relatively stable. When we later review the results of our model in light of the North Karelia findings, we will usually refer to the *net* reductions, rather than the absolute reductions, although this may underestimate the effectiveness of the campaign for women.

Despite these successes, the North Karelia experience holds lessons of only limited value for the American policymaker. The Finnish investigators worked in a health care system that differs in organization, philosophy, and financial structure from that of the United States. One of the most effective information services in the North Karelia Project, a strong Housewives' Association (with over 300 chapters), has no clear analogue in the American consumer scene. On the other hand, the major potential media vehicle for disseminating information in the United States, television, was not available in North Karelia. Because of such differences, conclusions about costs and effectiveness of media are especially difficult to generalize from the North Karelia Project to our country.

The North Karelia Project had a budget of approximately $200,000 per year in its 5 initial years, of which about 40 percent was spent on actual program costs (as distinguished from costs related to its experimental nature). To this figure should be added the value of donated services that otherwise would have had alternative uses. It seems reasonable to estimate the total annual program costs of the North Karelia Project at between $0.50 and $0.75 per person in the target communities. We will compare this rough estimate with other data on the likely costs of community-wide campaigns.

The Stanford Heart Disease Prevention Program

The Stanford Heart Disease Prevention Program, begun in 1972, was similar to the North Karelia Project in undertaking multifactorial risk factor interventions aimed at cigarette smoking, hypertension, and cholesterol. Unlike the Finnish study, however, the Stanford group relied heavily on mass media strategies, which were developed only after preliminary research on the knowledge gaps and media use patterns of the target populations. The ultimate media campaign in the two experimental communities (with populations of slightly less than 15,000 people each) used two 9-month exposure periods with radio and television spot commercials, several hours of both television and radio programming, newspaper columns and advertisements, billboards, posters, and direct mail literature. Special materials were developed for Spanish-speaking consumers (Farquhar et al., 1975; Maccoby and Farquhar, 1975).

In one of the experimental communities, some people at especially high risk were assigned to intensive face-to-face interventions involving personal instruction and counseling. In these cases, the results of the Stanford study represent a hybrid program of mass media and altered personal health services.

Within 2 years of the start of the Stanford program, the two target communities experienced significant alterations in risk factors as compared with the control community, alterations that were similar in magnitude to those seen in North Karelia (see Table 6-1). Compared to the control community, plasma cholesterol values in the two experimental communities fell by 3.2 percent and 2.0 percent overall and by 3.8 percent in those high-risk subjects who received intensive intervention in addition to the media campaigns. Systolic blood pressure fell by 7.5 percent and 5.0 percent and cigarette smoking by 5 percent and 23 percent in the same 2-year period. The Stanford study's multiple logistic risk equation projected a net reduction of 23 to 28 percent in the experimental population's risk of coronary events as compared with the control community. Interestingly, although the high-risk subjects receiving individualized instruction achieved a more *rapid* reduction in risk than did the general population, the *ultimate* risk reduction in the overall population was virtually the same as in the intensively treated group by the end of the second year of the experiment. Cost data on the Stanford study are not yet available.

The similarity of impact of these two major studies on cholesterol levels (see Table 6-1), though possibly fortuitous, may offer us some confidence in our ability to predict the likely effects of media and community-wide campaigns in other settings: We would expect that reasonably intensive community-wide campaigns can achieve a reduction of 1 to 5 percent in a population's average cholesterol level over a period of several years.

Two hypothetical programs

In exploring the potential efficiency of Community-wide Intervention without screening, we will focus discussion on two hypothetical programs, which we denote as School Education and Mass Media. For each of these, we will attempt to generate estimates of costs and benefits and to compare our results with those for screening programs.

We contemplate a School Eduation program that would provide health education instruction in public schools for grades five through nine (children aged approximately 10 through 14 years), the intent of

Table 6–1. Effects of community-wide interventions on cholesterol levels

Study	*Initial mean cholesterol level (mg/dl)*	*Change in cholesterol level**
Stanford Heart Disease Prevention Program		
Gilroy (experimental)	212	0.0%
Watsonville (experimental)	213	+1.1%
Tracy (control)	209	+3.8%
North Karelia Project		
North Karelia (experimental)		
Men (25–59)	269	−3.7%
Women (25–59)	265	−2.5%
Reference county (control)		
Men (25–59)	260	+0.3%
Women (25–59)	259	−1.5%

Sources. Farquhar et al., 1975, 1977; Puska et al., 1978, 1979; Salonen et al., 1979.
*Changes are those reported in the Stanford study after 2 years and in the North Karelia Project after 5 years.

which would be to encourage use of the "prudent diet." As described below, the program would provide each class of children with twice-yearly instruction throughout the five designated school years. Such a program tacitly assumes some advantage to early intervention, just as in the Universal Screening programs examined in Chapter 4. This advantage could take many forms; for example, heightened biologic susceptibility to plaque prevention in preadolescent children, psychologic susceptibility to modification of diet, or reduced intervention costs because of the accessibility of children in large groups in school. Since a School Education program does not distinguish its clients according to risk but rather according to age, it can be viewed as an age-targeted form of Population-wide Intervention.

A Mass Media program such as we imagine would have even a broader clientele than School Education. Our hypothetical Mass Media efforts would use television, radio, the press, and other forms of advertising and public relations to create community-wide awareness of dietary risk factors and to encourage the adoption of a more prudent diet. We do not postulate a "one-time-only" media campaign in our model but rather imagine a need for continued or at least repeated exposure to the message in order to maintain useful behavioral changes.

The sophistication of the modern advertising industry would, in reality, permit media efforts to be targeted at groups for whom behavioral change or change in risk can be realized most easily. Aiming messages at such selected markets is one of the primary principles of efficient advertising. Our model of a Mass Media program uses a parameter that represents the cost per person to the *entire* population of interest, even though we recognize that an actual budget should reflect rationally focused efforts for certain susceptible subpopulations. When we calculate the *total* program costs, we take care to assign those costs only to the appropriate target group.

A MODEL OF POPULATION-WIDE INTERVENTION

As in previous chapters, our evaluative models for School Education and Mass Media programs require several new parameter estimates. Three are of particular interest: the cost of a School Education program, the cost of a Mass Media program, and the expected change in cholesterol level that results from each program. In addition, we must examine carefully the assumptions in our benefits model before applying that model directly to the population-wide programs.

Costs of school education—C_E

We require an estimate of the cost per child of providing a nutrition education program in school during grades five through nine. Only crude estimates are feasible.

One half-time health educator plus support staff and supplies would cost approximately $25,000 per year, and we assume that funding at this level could provide a reasonable instructional program for a school system that has about 5000 children in the 10- to 14-year age group (roughly the size of that group in the Santa Monica, California, School District). Assuming a school year 180 days long, a half-time educator could meet twice yearly with each class of 25 children and still have 6 hours or more a week left over for program development and administration.

The cost of such a program would be about $5 per child per year. This is our best guess for the parameter C_E, and we further estimate that the true cost would lie between $1 and $10 per child per year.

As in evaluating previous programs, we wish here to discount costs using the age of 10 (or fifth grade) as the index year. Table 6-2 gives the total discounted cost per child for a School Education program under the conditions listed, and it can be compared with C_I (the cost of intervention) in previous chapters.

Table 6–2. Total discounted cost of a school education program per person (adjusted to age 10)

C_E *(Cost per child per year of program exposure)*	*Discount rate*		
	0%	*5%*	*10%*
$1.00	$5.00	$4.55	$4.16
$5.00	$25.00	$22.75	$20.85
$10.00	$50.00	$45.50	$41.70

Note. Program costs are spread over five years in our School Education intervention model.

Costs of mass media programs—C_M

In an effort to estimate the probable costs of effective media campaigns, we enlisted the advice of a number of professionals from the advertising industry and encountered a trade community of enormous sophistication, able to engineer highly targeted media efforts in response to particular goals. Those we consulted, however, seemed far more equipped to respond to requests for the design of campaigns of certain intent subject to specific budgetary guidelines than to questions about the budget that would be needed to achieve specific goals, such as a 20 percent increase in the substitution of filled milk for whole milk in a given geographical area.

We remain convinced that the enormous capacities of the advertising industry ought increasingly to be brought to bear specifically on programs for health-related behavioral change, but we are forced by the limitations in our experience to use cruder estimates of media costs, based on the benchmarks of current expenditures of the food industry on advertising. Table 6-3 shows the total expenditures on major media advertising in 1977 by the American food industry for some selected products.

The data in Table 6-3 convey a subjective sense of the relationship between media exposure and the amount of money the food industry spends on advertising some representative food types. On the average, in 1977, each American was exposed to about $1.13 worth of messages about beer and wine, about $0.50 worth of advertisements about coffee, tea, and cocoa, and about $0.16 worth of soup advertising. Since some of these products were advertised to highly targeted subgroups, the average figures may be misleading (whether they are misleadingly low or misleadingly high depends on whether or not the reader happens to have been in a targeted group). Nevertheless, these

Table 6–3. United States food and beverage advertising expenditures, 1977 (some sample figures)

Type of product	*Total media expenditures* (1000s of dollars)*	*Expenditures per person in U.S. population†*
Citrus fruits	$ 7,380	3.3¢
Ice cream and sherbet	$ 9,814	4.4¢
Cheese	$ 23,349	10.5¢
Fruit juices	$ 27,167	12.2¢
Soups	$ 36,101	16.2¢
Pastas	$ 42,185	18.9¢
Milk, eggs, and butter	$ 52,425	23.5¢
Shortenings and oils	$ 66,308	29.7¢
Coffee, tea, cocoa, and derivatives	$109,883	49.3¢
Candy and gum	$148,028	66.4¢
Cereals	$185,822	83.3¢
Beer	$196,515	88.1¢
Beer and wine	$252,000	113.0¢

Source. LNA Multi-Media Report Service. Class/Brand YTDS, vol. 4, no. 3. New York: Leading National Advertisers, Inc., Jan.-Dec. 1977.

*Estimates include six measured media, excluding spot radio and newspaper advertising.

†Assumes 1977 U.S. population of 223 million.

figures are helpful in generating rough subjective estimates of media costs.

The spread of advertising costs between heavily marketed foodstuffs and lightly advertised ones goes from more than $1.00 per American to less than $0.05. Most products fall between $0.10 and $1.00 per capita, and it is within this range that we have proceeded to explore the cost-effectiveness of a hypothetical media campaign to change diets in healthful directions. More precise estimates of cost must await appropriate data from the critical Community-wide Intervention experiments.

In summary, the analysis we will present of the impact of community-wide dietary intervention assumes a possible reduction of average cholesterol level of about 2 percent at an annual cost per person somewhere between what was spent in 1977 in advertising cheese (10.5¢) and what was spent in advertising beer and wine ($1.13). For the base case analysis of Mass Media programs, we select a yearly per-person expense (C_M) of $0.50, or about what was spent in 1977 for advertising coffee, tea, cocoa, and their derivatives (see Table 6-3). In comparing community-wide programs with screening, sensitivity analysis on C_M will be critically important. We will be particularly interested in identifying the levels of media expenditure and efficacy at which population-wide efforts begin to appear more cost-effective than the Universal and Targeted Screening programs examined in Chapters 4 and 5.

The shift in cholesterol from population-wide intervention—J_E and J_M

Population-wide efforts to change diets are more dilute than the personalized interventions that would follow Universal or Targeted Screening. Assuming a conventional dose-response relationship between dietary change and expenditures on intervention, we would expect that the average changes in cholesterol level harvested from School Education or Mass Media programs (J_E or J_M) would be lower than the changes postulated in Chapters 4 and 5 (J). The exact magnitudes of J_E and J_M, on which we have few empirical data, are much more uncertain at any given level of educational or media expenditure than is the magnitude of J, on which we have copious experimental data.

As discussed above, the Stanford Heart Disease Prevention Program and the North Karelia Project observed differences in cholesterol levels between experimental and reference communities of 1 to 4 percent of initial values, with the drop in North Karelia compared to the reference county being greater for men than for women. Given the relevant initial levels, this corresponds to an absolute drop in cholesterol of between 3 and 10 mg/dl.

We have chosen to express the change in cholesterol from population-wide programs (J_E and J_M) as percentage changes.† We will explore the cost-effectiveness of Mass Media intervention over a range of values of J_M from 0.2 percent (0.4 mg/dl) to 6.0 percent (12 mg/dl), choosing as our base case $J = 2.0$ percent (4 mg/dl), a value at the low end of the range observed in the Stanford and North Karelia studies. Since the North Karelia Project, in particular, involved some interventions that went beyond a simple media campaign, we feel that this is an appropriately low estimate.

†In our technical developments in Appendix K, we will measure the change in cholesterol in terms of Δ, the number of standard deviations from the mean log cholesterol level. In these units, the base case J (10 percent) used in Chapters 4 and 5 would be 0.5 SD units. In general,

$$J_E(\text{or } J_M) = \frac{\Delta}{5}$$

For School Education campaigns, we will allow J_E to vary over the same range, but we will choose a somewhat less ambitious base case value than for Mass Media, namely $J = 1.0$ percent (2 mg/dl). This low value reflects skepticism about the effects of school education, a result in part of the lackluster results of antismoking and other health-oriented campaigns in schools and, in part, of our feeling that because school-based programs are dependent on the competence of individual educators in each district, there may be more variability in the content and quality of school education programs than of Mass Media programs.

The actual effects of a Mass Media or School Education campaign are not likely to be distributed evenly across the target populations. It may be more realistic to expect a "lumpier" distribution of dietary responses, with some people changing behavior dramatically and some people totally ignoring the campaign. This unevenness of response poses a problem in associating health benefits with a particular average J_E or J_M if the relationship between degree of cholesterol change and degree of risk reduction is nonlinear. Fortunately, within the rather narrow range of applicable values, a linear model relating cholesterol change and risk change is an excellent approximation of the more complex relationship implied by the logistic function, and therefore J_M (or J_E) is a useful average parameter even if, for example, the true cholesterol change were $2J_M$ (or $2J_E$) for one-half of the population and zero for the rest.

The benefits model

Cohort analysis: the general approach

When we evaluated the potential impact of the screening programs described in Chapters 4 and 5, we relied heavily on the assumption that our efforts were targeted at discrete cohorts of children. For the most part, screening occurred at age 10, and treated children were followed for specific periods of time beginning at that age. Each child in the population could be considered a member of a cohort, and calculations of costs and benefits were carried out from the perspective of a 10-year-old entering the cohort. We refer to this method of accounting for costs and benefits as "cohort analysis."

For a School Education program, cohort analysis is easy to apply. Intervention costs are incurred at particular ages beginning with 10-year-olds, and the assumptions about fraction of benefit that we made in Chapters 4 and 5 seem equally applicable to the children in the "treated" grades. In fact, a School Education program can be thought of as a Universal Screening program in which C_S equals zero, all 10-year-olds are treated, and C_I equals the (discounted) program cost per member of the cohort.

The community-wide advertising program presents special problems in cost and benefit assessment that did not arise in looking at the screening or School Education programs, and the applicability of cohort analysis is no longer obvious. Two factors made the screening programs easy to analyze: First, it was possible to identify a complete, discrete program package. Second, it was possible to identify a particular group—a cohort of children—that would receive the complete program of screening and intervention. We did not need to consider cases where the program stopped prior to the completion of the interventions, or where children entered midway through the intervention program. These things might happen, of course, but it seemed reasonable to analyze a base case in which they did *not* occur.

A Mass Media campaign is different. When such a campaign begins, everyone is exposed to the intervention, including people who have already adopted a prudent diet, those who never will, and those who are too old or too young to benefit from a change in diet. Although some targeting of a media message is possible, the intervention is, by its nature, indiscriminant and is most appropriate if a majority of the population will (potentially, at least) benefit from the exposure.

With most programs, when we reduce the scope, we reduce the costs. It is not clear, however, that a media campaign is any less expensive when the real targets are only a subset of the population. Whether the campaign is aimed at 60 percent of the population or at 100 percent, the same overall budget may be necessary to ensure that each person in the target group will be sufficiently exposed to the campaign. In determining the cost-effectiveness of the program, however, it is critically important whether the total costs in a given year are attributed to everyone in a community or just to those in a certain age range, for example 10 to 50.

The problem is most obvious during the start-up phase of a Mass Media campaign. Media costs are typically calculated on a per-person or a per-household basis. If there are many people for whom the proposed diet changes come too late in life to do any good, then perhaps the costs of a media program ought not be attributed to them but rather to the younger people in the population who can still benefit from dietary change. While it may not be as obvious, if this is true in the start-up phase, then it is also true in any given year of an ongoing program.

These considerations of who really benefits from a media campaign also influence what the "ideal" campaign strategy would be. A continuous campaign would be indicated if individuals must receive the diet message throughout their lives or throughout some broad critical span of their lives (e.g., ages 10 through 40). In either of these cases, any interruption in the campaign would presumably reduce its effectiveness. If, on the other hand, people only need periodic reminders about their diet or if exposure during a short period within some critical age category (e.g., a 2-year exposure any time between ages 10 and 30) is sufficient, then a pulsed or periodic media campaign may be much more efficient than a continuous one.

To assess the cost-effectiveness of a media campaign properly, we must therefore make some assumptions about whom the program seeks to affect, who should bear the costs, who will reap the benefits, and how long the campaign will last. Unless there is a clearly defined group at whom the campaign is aimed, it is not possible to define a "completed" campaign. Unlike the screening programs, it would matter a great deal if a Mass Media program were terminated after a few years or months of operation. Our expectations about the benefits of an aborted program would be very different from our expectations about an ongoing program.

The assumptions we must make—about how long the campaign will last, who will benefit, and how to allocate the costs—may seem far more arbitrary than those we needed to make to evaluate the screening programs. Our goal in establishing the framework of assumptions within which to analyze the Mass Media program will be to construct a "reasonable worst case"; that is, whenever possible we will seek to overestimate costs and underestimate benefits, in effect placing Mass Media programs at the maximum reasonable disadvantage as we estimate their cost-effectiveness. We do this because, in the face of so much uncertainty, it seems more useful to establish a relatively firm lower limit on efficiency than a fuzzy best guess of the cost-effectiveness. As we will see, however, even in a "worst case," media campaigns perform considerably better than the childhood screening strategies.

The framework for analysis of a mass media program

Since the media campaign affects all age groups simultaneously, it may seem unlikely that cohort analysis, a method of evaluation based, for example, on a cohort of 10-year-olds, could apply. However, if a program continues for several "completed cohorts," the cohort analysis will provide a good estimate of the cost-effectiveness. The longer the program continues, the less important are start-up effects. The question is: How does our calculation of the cost-effectiveness of the campaign for the completed cohort compare with the cost-effectiveness for individuals who only were exposed to the media message for part of their lives, and who therefore receive only part of the benefits possible? If a "complete" campaign has an optimal design, then these "incomplete" groups must incur a higher cost per year of life saved than the "completed" cohort. (Otherwise, the campaign is not optimal but instead should be pulsed or shortened.) The specific campaign we are analyzing may not be optimal, however this is consistent with our effort to provide a "reasonable worst case."

Our estimates of the cost-effectiveness of a media campaign are most appropriate if the campaign is assumed to continue indefinitely, always incurring yearly costs of C_M to maintain a cholesterol shift of J_M. If such a campaign were terminated before at least one cohort experienced a completed campaign, benefits reaped might be small or nonexistent.

Allocating the costs of mass media

As discussed above, we estimate that a reasonable media campaign might cost from \$0.10 per person per year to \$1 per person per year, with a median guess of about \$0.50 per person per year—the amount now spent to advertise coffee, tea, and cocoa products. While it is convenient to think in terms of costs on a per-person-per-year basis, we must be careful when calculating the cost-effectiveness to allocate costs only to targeted individuals in the population. It may not seem reasonable, for example, to allocate costs to very young or to very old individuals. If we hold the overall budget constant as we reduce the size of the target population, the yearly cost per targeted individual rises. However, depending on whether we exclude young or old individuals from the targeted group, the present value of the discounted costs may rise or fall. (When the discount rate is zero, the total cost per person is not affected by the age of the target population.)

When costs are not attributed to individuals *above* a certain age, the present value of the discounted costs rises. Two forces, with opposite effects, are at work to change the present value. Since total costs are allocated over a smaller number of years of an individual's life, the undiscounted cost per year increases. On the other hand, the years in

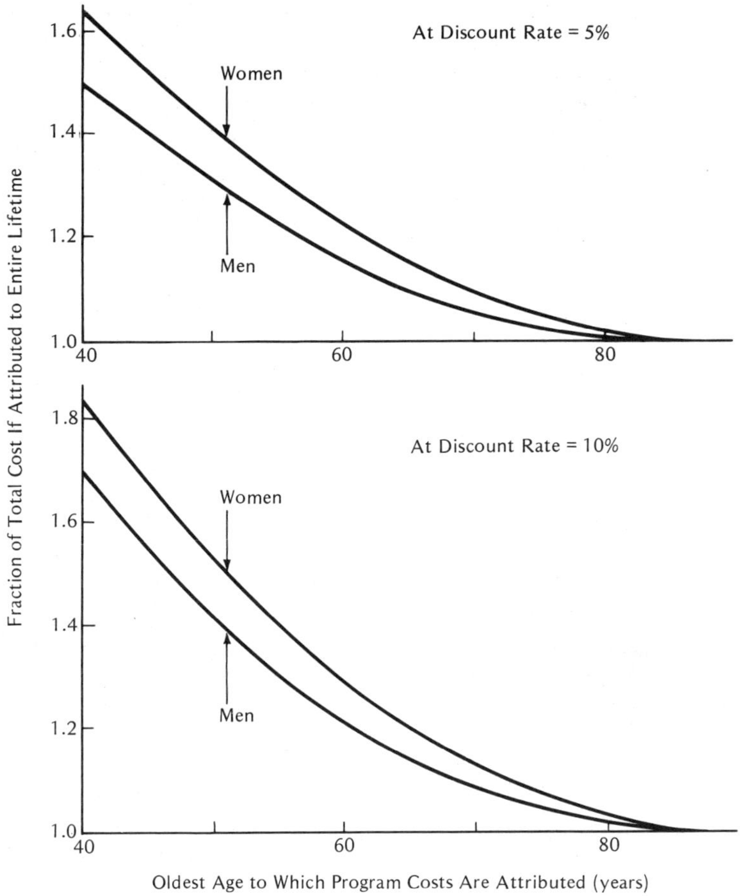

Figure 6-1. Total Media Program Cost per Person vs. Oldest Age to Which Costs Are Attributed. Discounted cost per person rises if we do not attribute media costs to older people.

which no costs are incurred come late in life, and because of the discount factor, the contribution to total costs from these later years is quite low. It turns out that the highly discounted savings from late in life do not offset the increased cost per year incurred early in life. Figure 6-1 shows the effects on costs of excluding individuals over a certain age from the target population. At a zero discount rate, the timing of costs exerts no effect on total costs.

For our base case in examining the Mass Media program, it seems reasonable and consistent with "worst case" analysis not to attribute costs to older individuals. The statistical risk model we use assumes

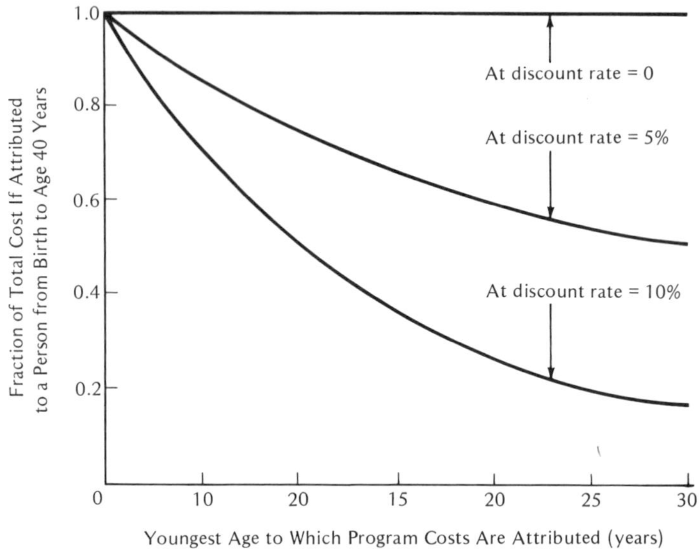

Figure 6-2. Total Media Program Cost per Person vs. Youngest Age to Which Costs Are Attributed. Discounted costs fall as we exclude younger people from the population to which costs are attributed. Costs are shown here as a fraction of the costs that would be assigned per person if costs were attributed from birth to age 40.

that cholesterol has no appreciable effect on heart disease morbidity and mortality for men after age 65 and for women after age 75. Although it could be true that individuals who have artificially lowered their cholesterol through diet ought to stay on that diet even in old age, we have chosen not to attribute costs to men or women after age 40. This will provide a reasonable upper bound on total costs. It is true that excluding people below 40 years of age would result in even higher costs, but if this were desirable, it is likely that School Education or some other program aimed just at young people would be preferred in the first place.

When costs are not attributed to individuals *below* a certain age, the present value of the discounted costs *falls*. As Figure 6-2 shows, starting from a base case in which costs are attributed to everyone in the population from birth to age 40, excluding infants and young children from the target population reduces the overall discounted present value of the costs. It is true that the cost per year (for those years in which costs are incurred) will be higher. Now, however (as opposed to when older people are excluded), the decrease obtained from discounting more than offsets the increase obtained from a smaller target group, since the included years occur later in life. Figure 6-2 shows the net effect of excluding young children from the target group for discount rates of 5 and 10 percent. Since *including* young children results in higher costs, we will include children from birth in attributing costs to a cohort. This may or may not be realistic, but it is consistent with our construction of a "reasonable worst case."

Using the assumptions we have made about cost allocation, we can now calculate the discounted present value of the costs to a 10-year-old of Mass Media campaigns of varying intensity, attributing costs from birth to age 40. Table 6-4 shows the results for programs of varying intensity at varying discount rates. Because we have adjusted all cost figures to age 10, the entries in Table 6-4 are directly comparable with the costs discussed in Chapters 4 and 5, as well as those for School Education.

Cohort analysis may create a problem of interpretation when we speak of the total costs of a Mass Media program. Confusion arises because there are two different perspectives from which total costs can be viewed: first, from the perspective of the cohort and, second, from the perspective of an annual operating budget. From the viewpoint of the *cohort,* "total costs" will refer to the present value of the lifetime expenditures expected by someone at age 10. Since this present value is affected by both discounting and attrition in the size of the cohort through death, the cohort's "total cost" will be less than the annual operating budget.

For a budget director, this year's actual program budget is simply $C_M \cdot N$, where N is the number of people in the target population. We will return to these two different estimates of total yearly cost later in this chapter.

Table 6–4. Total Discounted Cost of a Mass Media Program Per Person (Adjusted to Age 10)

*Cost per person per year of program exposure** *(C_M)*	*Sex*	*Cost per targeted person per year†*	*Discount rate*		
			0%	*5%*	*10%*
$0.10	M	$0.17	$ 6.80	$ 4.90	$ 4.80
	F	$0.19	$ 7.50	$ 5.50	$ 5.30
$0.50	M	$0.86	$34.20	$24.60	$24.10
	F	$0.95	$37.50	$27.30	$26.40
$1.00	M	$1.72	$68.40	$49.10	$48.20
	F	$1.89	$75.00	$54.60	$52.90

*Costs allocated from birth to death. This figure multiplied by the total population equals the annual program budget.

†Costs allocated only to men and women under the age of 40.

A review of assumptions

Before presenting the results of our model for Population-wide Interventions and comparing them with results for Universal and Targeted Screening, let us briefly review some of the important assumptions we have made that could, if wrong, result in too favorable a view of media programs as compared with screening programs.

First, we assume that mass media (or school health education) can be effective in altering dietary habits. The Stanford and North Karelia programs suggest that they can, but results of comparable efforts aimed at smoking and automobile safety in the United States are not so consistent or so certain.

Second, our benefits model assumes that even people with low cholesterol levels experience a reduction in risk from further lowering. Cross-cultural comparisons support this thesis, which is consistent with the Framingham logistic risk model. This assumption does not greatly affect the calculations on Universal and Targeted Screening, because those programs do not treat people with low cholesterol. In the Mass Media and School Education programs, however, benefits are attributed to a population of people half of whom have initial cholesterol levels below the median. If benefits from diet do not accrue to those at the lower levels, then the model of Population-wide Intervention overestimates efficiency.

Third, we have evaluated Mass Media efforts as if the programs lasted a long time, an assumption that is necessary, since we also postulate that continuous media pressure is required to maintain behavioral change. If a Mass Media program were terminated abruptly a few years after its inception, its efforts would be wasted if people reverted quickly to their old habits and their old risks. By comparison, if the School Education or screening programs evaluated in Chapters 4 and 5 terminated suddenly, the treated cohorts of positive screenees would still go on to reap their benefits later in life, since their behavior, we assume, would have been permanently changed for the better. Thus, given the vagaries of public financing, the assumption that media efforts must be continuous to be effective makes Mass Media programs look riskier than screening and short-term intervention. If, on the other hand, Mass Media campaigns, like personal interventions, can effect enduring behavioral changes, then they may not differ so much in riskiness from the other programs.

Some of our assumptions have the effect of making Mass Media programs look *less* effective than they may be. For example, if fraction of benefit does not decay with age, Mass Media programs would turn out to be far more efficient (and realize benefits earlier) than our analysis suggests. It may also be the case that continuous media effort is not necessary to change a population's behavior for good. If, for example, an intensive 10-year Mass Media program could produce permanent healthy changes in the American diet and life-style, costs would thereafter fall to zero, benefits would continue to accrue, and the true cost-effectiveness ratio of the whole program would be far lower than predicted by the cohort analysis model of a continuous Mass Media program.

We should note, finally, that the efficiency of Mass Media programs might well improve over time as susceptible target audiences are identified, more effective media devices are developed, and psychological barriers fall as "prudent diets" become more the cultural norm. How rapidly such processes could evolve, if at all, is a question beyond our competence to explore.

RESULTS OF THE MODEL OF POPULATION-WIDE INTERVENTION

Base case results

For our base case analysis, we choose, as in previous chapters, a discount rate of 5 percent and assign values to the relevant new parameters as follows:

J_M, the change in average cholesterol from a Mass Media program = 2 percent.

J_E, the change in average cholesterol from a School Education program = 1 percent.

C_E, the cost per person per year of a School Education program = \$5.00.

C_M, the cost per person per year of a Mass Media program = \$0.50.

Benefits assessed include days of life saved and days free of coronary heart disease added.

The health benefits of community-wide intervention are assumed to come from achieving a shift in the population's distribution of cholesterol. The details of this calculation and the results in terms of absolute benefits are included in Appendix K. The estimated cost per year of life saved for the School Education and Mass Media programs are found by dividing the appropriately discounted costs from Tables 6-2 and 6-4, respectively, by the appropriate benefits from Table K-2 of Appendix K. The results are shown in Table 6-5, which presents the base case performance of the two programs.

For men, Mass Media is only one-fourth as costly per YLS as Universal Screening, and only 40 percent as costly as Targeted Screening, assuming intensive intervention in the screening programs. Indeed, Mass Media appears substantially more efficient than the screening programs even if C_I is \$80, the minimal intervention estimate.

School Education, although less cost-effective than Mass Media, is still better than either Targeted Screening or Universal Screening (with intensive intervention). If we assume the minimal intervention cost (C_I = \$80 instead of \$308), the screening programs look more efficient than School Education.

For the expected benefits shown in Table 6-5, each cohort member pays a discounted total of \$25 to \$27 under the Mass Media program and about \$23 under the School Education program. It may be instructive to compare these results to those for Universal Screening in Tables 4-5 and 4-7, where we find that screenees pay about half as much as under a Mass Media program but can expect benefits in extended life only one-seventh as large. More extensive comparisons appear later in this chapter , but the overall conclusion is clear: under base case assumptions, the Mass Media program is more cost-effective than any screening program that we have examined.

Sensitivity analysis

Sensitivity to cholesterol shift—J_E and J_M—and to cost per cohort member—C_E and C_M

Our estimates of both cholesterol shift and program costs for population-wide interventions are tenuous, and sensitivity analysis is therefore especially important. Figures 6-3 and 6-4 show the relationship between cost per YLS and these variables for the School Education program for men and women, respectively. Figures 6-5 and 6-6 present the same analyses for the Mass Media program. Each of these figures represents, in fact, sensitivity analysis of two variables simultaneously, J_E and C_E, or J_M and C_M.

Within the limits of our ranges of estimates for J_E, J_M, C_E, and C_M, cost-effectiveness of the Population-wide Intervention program varies enormously. At the worst combination of cost and cholesterol shift for Mass Media programs for men ($J_M = 0.2\%$, $C_M = \$1$), cost per YLS is

Table 6–5. Results of Base Case Analysis of School Education and Mass Media Programs

Program	*Sex*	*Cost YLS*	*Change in cost/YLS compared with universal screening* *	*Change in cost/YLS compared with targeted screening* *	*Cost per cohort member (adjusted to age 10)*	*Days of life saved per cohort member (at age 10)*	*CHD-free days added per cohort member (at age 10)*	*Stroke-free days added per cohort member† (at age 10)*
Mass media	M	\$2720	−74%	−59%	\$24.60	40.9	70.8	4.3
	F	\$3830	−59%	−50%	\$27.30	47.5	61.5	5.8
School education	M	\$5060	−53%	−24%	\$22.75	20.8	35.8	2.2
	F	\$6500	−30%	−16%	\$22.75	24.1	31.0	2.9

Assumptions: Base case, $J_E = 1\%$, $J_M = 2\%$, $C_E = \$5$, $C_M = \$0.50$, $D = 5\%$.

*With intensive intervention ($C_I = \$308$).

†Benefits are stated in *undiscounted days*.

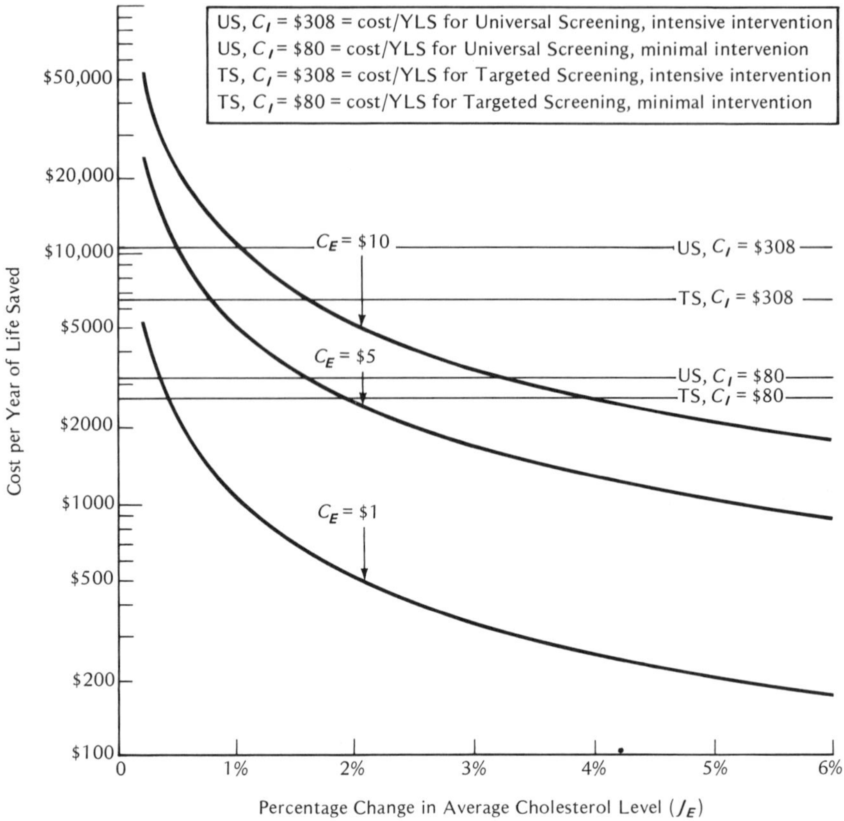

Figure 6-3. Cost per Year of Life Saved, for Men, School Education Program, at $D = 5$ Percent. Cost-effectiveness is shown for three different values of C_E. The cost-effectiveness of the Universal Screening and Targeted Screening programs for both minimal and intensive intervention are indicated for comparison.

nearly 300 times as great as at the most favorable combination ($J_M = 6\%$, $C_M = \$0.10$). Examining these extreme cases, however, is less instructive than testing combinations of J_M and C_M that are more consistent with the data that we do have. If we assume that the cholesterol shift observed in the Stanford Heart Disease Prevention Program, for example, is unlikely to underestimate or overestimate by more than a factor of 2 the shift achieved by our hypothetical Mass Media program, then we may look at cost-effectiveness in the range between $J_M = 1\%$ and $J_M = 4\%$, again letting C_M vary from $0.10 to $1.00. In this more limited region, cost per YLS for men goes from $290 to $10,910, a 40-fold variation. Only combinations of J_M and C_M

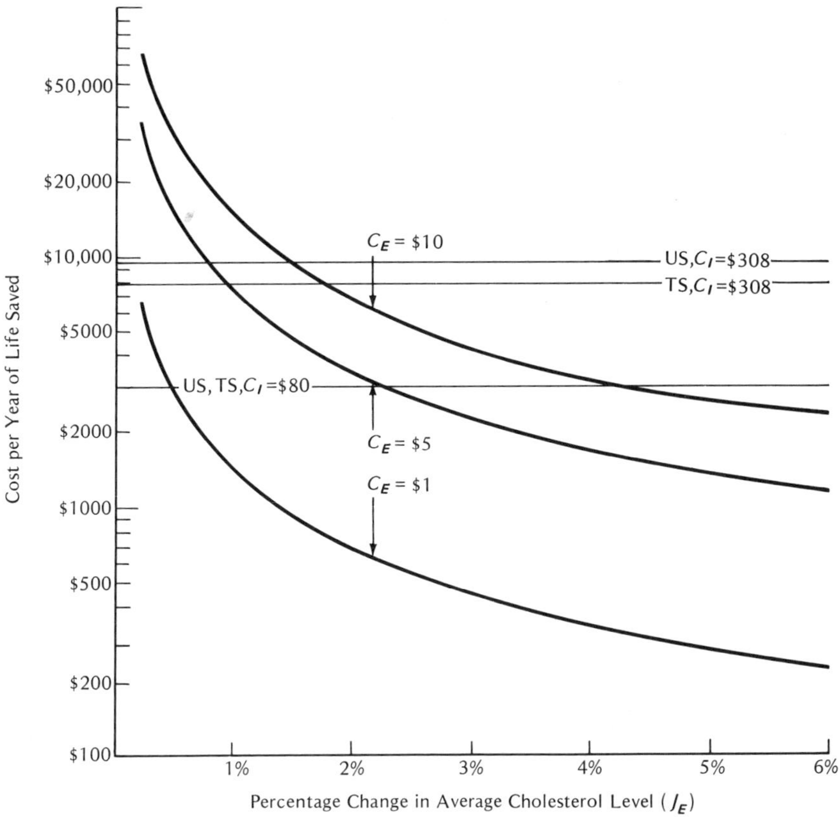

Figure 6-4. Cost per Year of Life Saved, for Women, School Education Program, at D = 5 Percent.

within this range that are near the worst case ($J_M = 1\%$ and $C_M = \$1.00$) result in cost-effectiveness with which Targeted and Universal Screening are competitive.

Even for a tiny shift in average cholesterol level ($J_M = 0.2\%$, or about 0.5 mg/dl), at the cheapest cost we explore ($C_M = \$0.10$), Mass Media interventions are more cost-effective for men than the best screening programs analyzed in the preceding chapters. For women, the Mass Media campaign under these conditions is superior to Universal Screening and about equal to Targeted Screening.

School Education fares less well in the same type of comparison. If J_E is as low as 0.6 percent (and $C_E = \$5$), or if C_E is as high as $10 (and $J_E = 1\%$), then the School Education program is worse than Targeted Screening for either sex and worse than Universal Screening for women.

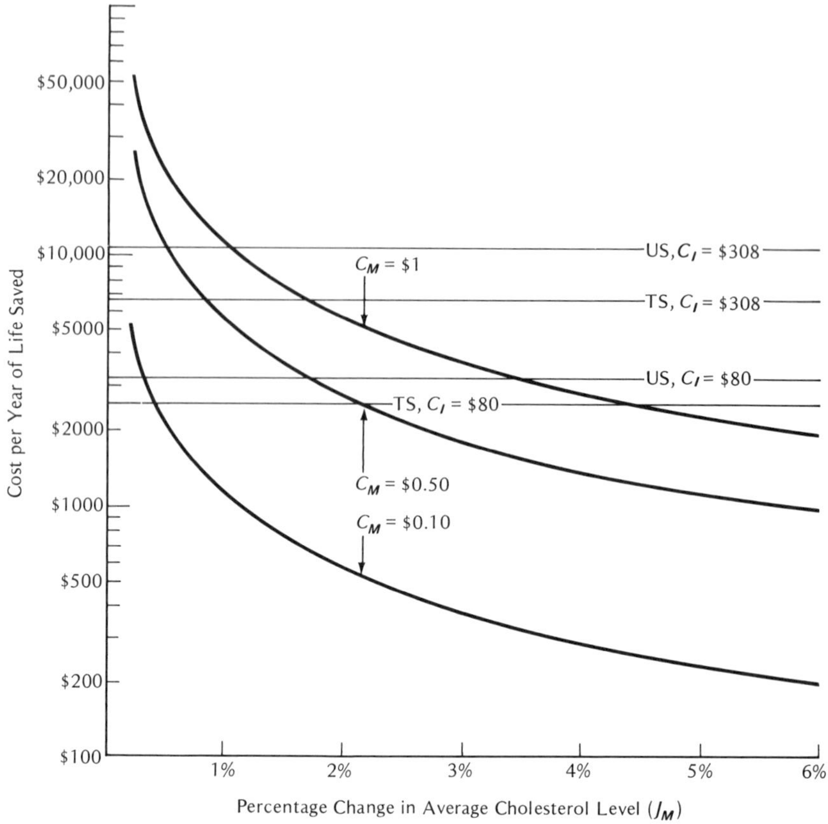

Figure 6-5. Cost per Year of Life Saved, for Men, Mass Media Program, at $D = 5$ Percent. Cost-effectiveness is shown for three different values of C_M. The cost-effectiveness of the Universal Screening and Targeted Screening programs for both minimal and intensive interventions are indicated for comparison.

Both population-wide programs in the base case achieve costs per YLS that are lower for men than for women, whereas the opposite was true for the screening programs in Chapters 4 and 5. At a discount rate of 5 percent, the cost per YLS for men in a Mass Media program is 30 percent lower than that for women.

As in the screening programs, the cost per YLS is less for women than for men at a discount rate of zero, and, as in the screening programs, higher discount rates favor programs for men. In the Universal Screening program, the crossover point (the discount rate at which programs for the two sexes have equal cost-effectiveness) occurred between 5 and 10 percent. In the population-wide interventions, the

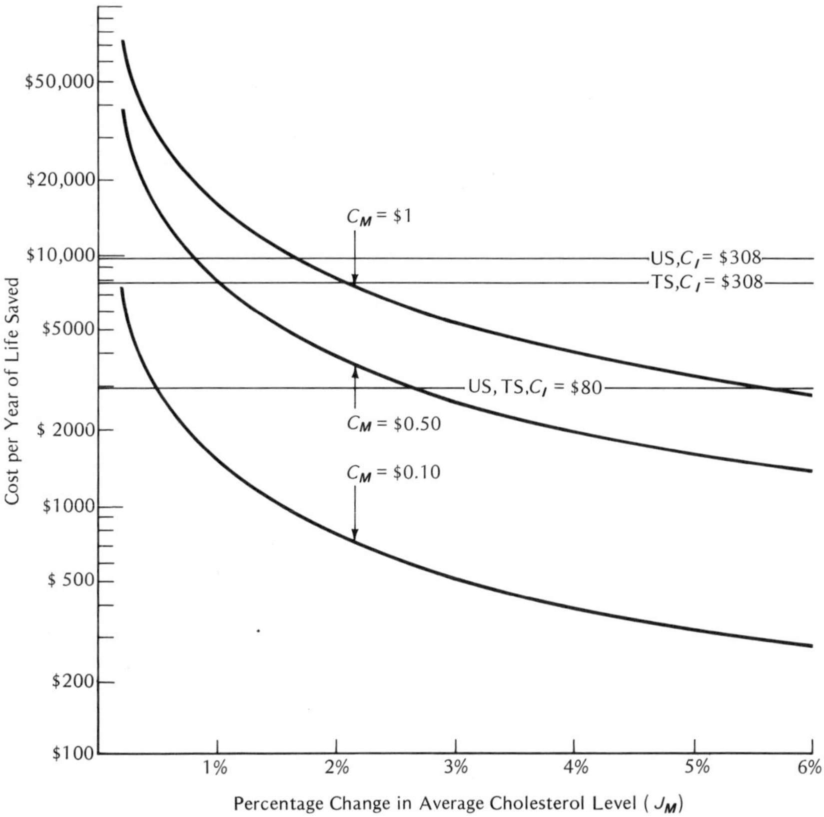

Figure 6-6. Cost per Year of Life Saved, for Women, Mass Media Program, at $D = 5$ Percent.

relative advantage of discounting for men is more dramatic, and the crossover occurs at a lower discount rate—between 0 and 5 percent.

In both cases, screening and population-wide programs, the stronger influence of discounting on the cost-effectiveness of programs for women results from the tendency of women to have their fatal cardiovascular events at later ages than men. It is also true, however, that young women who die of heart disease are even more likely than men who die at the same ages to have elevated cholesterol levels. This factor tends to offset the lateness of most heart disease in women in the Universal Screening program, which treats hypercholesterolemic women and thus selects women who are more likely to experience premature death.

No such selectivity occurs in the School Education or Mass Media program. These programs are assumed to alter behavior without re-

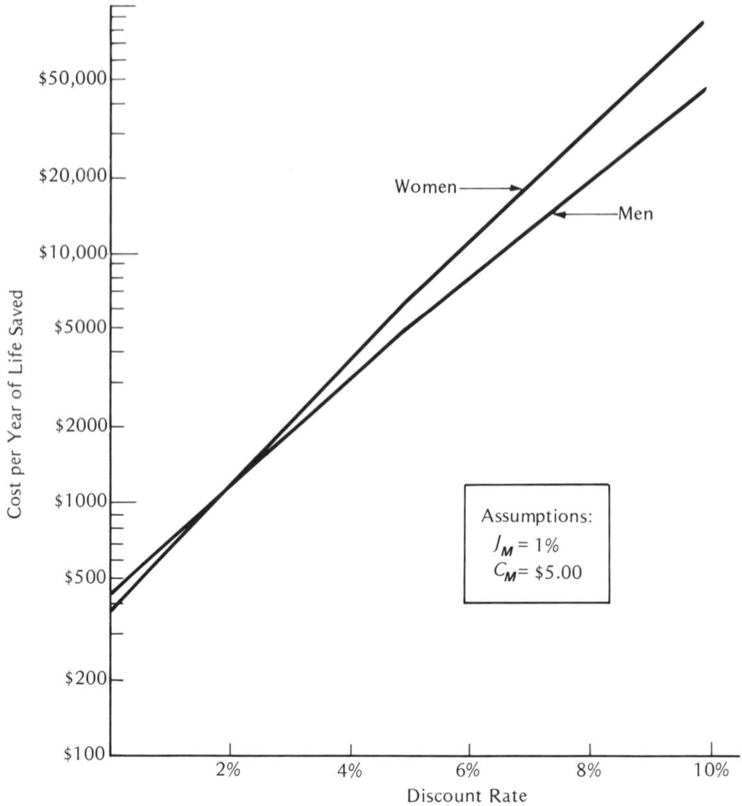

Figure 6-7. Sensitivity of Cost per Year of Life Saved to Discount Rate, School Education Program. At discount rates above 2 percent, programs are more efficient for men than for women.

gard to cholesterol level, and to predict the timing of benefits, we must look to the average individual, not the hypercholesterolemic one. The *average* women experiences coronary disease later than the *average* man, and so average benefits to women are attributed to a later age. Under Mass Media programs, then, discounting more strongly attenuates benefits to women than to men.

Sensitivity to the discount rate—D

As is true of the screening program, the cost-effectiveness of population-wide interventions changes more dramatically with the discount rate than with any other parameter within the ranges tested. Figures 6-7 and 6-8 show this relationship for School Education (at

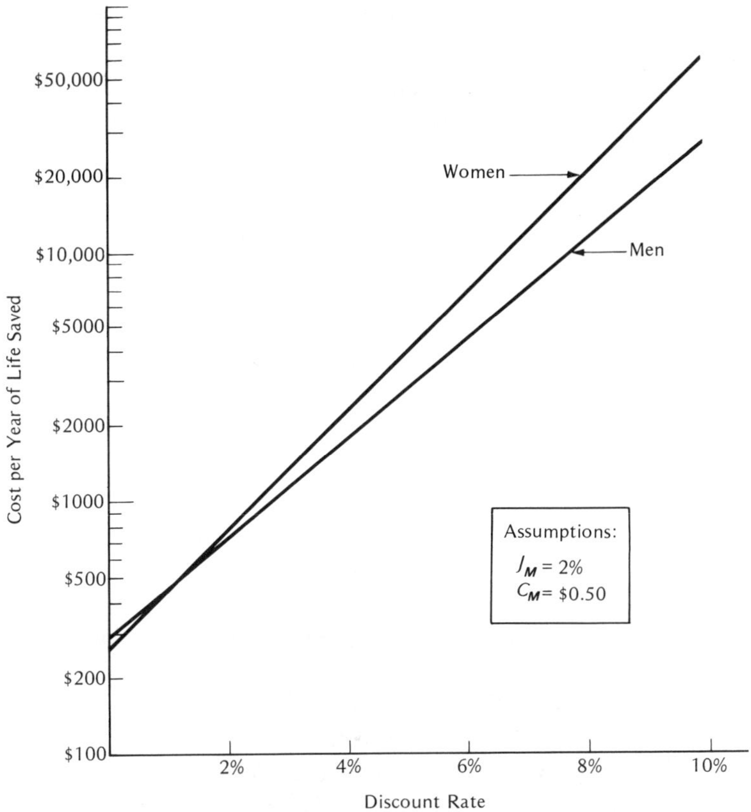

Figure 6-8. Sensitivity of Cost per Year of Life Saved to Discount Rate, Mass Media Program. The difference in cost-effectiveness for the two sexes is more exaggerated at higher discount rates.

$J_E = 1\%$, $C_E = \$5$) and Mass Media (at $J_M = 2\%$, $C_M = \$0.50$), respectively, for both sexes.

From a discount rate of zero to one of 10 percent, the change in cost-effectiveness is enormous—approaching two orders of magnitude for many comparisons. The effect is somewhat greater on the School Education program than on the Mass Media program; for men, cost-effectiveness between $D = 0$ and $D = 10$ percent increases 105 fold for the former program and 90 fold for the latter. This difference in sensitivity occurs because the time streams of cost for the two programs have different durations. For the Mass Media program, both costs and benefits are discounted over several decades, and a rising discount rate acts on both, with effects that tend to cancel each other—discounted benefits fall as the discount rate rises but so do discounted costs. In contrast, the School Education program incurs its costs early in the cohort's lives (ages 10 to 14), and so benefits fall as the rate of discount rises but without as dramatic a compensatory fall in costs.

To dramatize the differential effect of discounting on the two types of programs, let us select values of J_M, J_E, C_E, and C_M that, at a discount rate of zero, are approximately equal in efficiency. At $J_E = 3\%$ and $C_E = \$1$, School Education costs \$30 per YLS for men, equal to the cost-effectiveness of Mass Media for men at $J_M = 4\%$ and $C_M = \$0.10$. At the same parameter values but with a discount rate of 5 or 10 percent, the School Education program costs 20 percent more per YLS than does Mass Media.

A summary expression for sensitivity—G

In Chapter 4 we explored the usefulness of expressions for elasticity as summary measures of the sensitivity of Universal Screening programs to changes in important parameters. With a single number, an estimate of elasticity could summarize very complex relationships. It would be equally useful to develop a simple way of expressing the complex relationships between the cost-effectiveness of population-wide programs and the critical parameters C_E, C_M, J_E, and J_M.

For both Mass Media and School Education programs, the cost per year of life saved can be expressed in a fairly simple algebraic form‡

$$\text{Cost/YLS} = \frac{(C_M)\ (\text{discount factor})}{-(L + 3C)\ (5J_M) + Q(5J_M)^2 - C(5J_M)^3}$$

where L, Q, and C are parameters relating the shift in cholesterol to years of life saves (see Appendix K). Given the small values of J_E and J_M that we explore (i.e., less than 6 percent), and small values of Q and C in our model (see Table K-1, Appendix K), the above expression can be approximated well by simply ignoring the quadratic and cubic terms in J_M, giving us the following simplified equation:

$$\text{Cost/YLS} \simeq \frac{(C_M)\ (\text{discount factor})}{-(L + 3C)\ (5J_M)}$$

‡In the development of this formula as presented in Appendix K, the change in cholesterol level is expressed in terms of standard deviation units from the mean level of log cholesterol, Δ. The percentage change in level (J_E or J_M) is approximately one-fifth as large as Δ. For example, a J_M of 6 percent (0.06) corresponds to a $\Delta = J_M \times 5 = 0.06 \times 5 = 0.30$.

Table 6–6. The Value of Factor G to be Used for Estimating Cost Per Year of Life Saved in Population-Wide Programs

		Factor G		
Program	*Sex*	*D = 0%*	*D = 5%*	*D = 10%*
Mass media*	M	12.36	109.10	1069.90
	F	11.52	156.00	2116.30
School	M	0.91	10.12	92.60
Education†	F	0.77	13.00	166.80

*Cost per YLS≅ $(C_M/J_M)\,G$.

†Cost per YLS≅ $(C_E/J_E)\,G$.

Note. To find cost per YLS in the range of values tested, multiply G times the ratio of C_M to J_M or C_E to J_E, as shown below.

In both of these equations, C_M is the cost per person per year of the program. Put another way, the cost per YLS for this population-wide intervention can be expressed as a simple linear function of the ratio of C_M to J_M:

$$\text{Cost/YLS} \simeq \left[\frac{C_M}{J_M}\right] G$$

in which we have defined a new factor, G, which depends on the program, the sex of the target group, and the discount rate, and which provides a simple estimate of the sensitivity of cost per YLS to the ratio of C_M to J_M for Mass Media and of C_E to J_E for School Education. This factor, G, is *not* equivalent to elasticity, but it serves somewhat the same function of simplifying some very complex relationships. Table 6-6 gives the values of G that apply for different programs, sexes, and discount rates. From Table 6-6, one can calculate the cost per YLS for any estimate of C_M, C_E, J_M, and J_E within the ranges we have defined.

Confidence interval on cost-effectiveness of population-wide interventions

As in previous chapters, we are interested in knowing how our uncertainties about individual parameters combine to produce uncertainty in our estimate of cost-effectiveness. Our goal will again be to estimate the variance of the logarithm of cost per year of life saved. For population-wide interventions, the calculations are somewhat simpler than for the screening programs because the number of parameters is smaller. In this case, we can partition the parameters into two independent groups as follows:

1. The Intervention Groups—including the cost (C_M or C_E) and reduction in cholesterol (J_M or J_E).
2. The Risk Group—including the effects of cholesterol on risk, summarized in this model by the parameters L, Q, and C.

Within the Intervention Group, we would expect the scope of a program to be linked with the effectiveness of that program in reducing cholesterol levels. As in the screening programs, we will deal with this correlation by holding constant the scope of intervention and then estimating our uncertainty in the cost and cholesterol reduction *relative to* this fixed scope. In the cases at hand, this means that we will estimate a confidence interval on cost-effectiveness of a Mass Media program with the same scope as U.S. advertising of coffee, tea, and cocoa, and of a School Education program that involves two sessions per year for 5 years.

The Risk Group for population-wide interventions is dealt with exactly as in the screening programs by allowing the logistic parameters to vary from 1 SD below the Framingham estimates to 1 SD above.

Table 6-7 summarizes these results for School Education and for Mass Media at a discount rate of 5 percent. For School Education, the interval on cost-effectiveness comprising ±1 SD lies between $2070 and $12,220 per YLS for men and between $2800 and $15,300 per YLS for women. For the Mass Media program, the comparable limits are $1280 and $5820 for men and $1840 and $7930 for women. Uncertainty in the risk coefficients has less effect on the population-wide programs than on the screening programs because the former do not depend on a special distribution of risk for their results.

When we compare the *relative* cost-effectiveness of population-wide and screening programs, it would be misleading to regard the uncertainties in the estimated cost-effectiveness of two types of program as independent. The cost and cholesterol reduction parameters may or may not operate independently in the population-wide and screening programs, but the Risk Group reflects the same underlying parameters—the Framingham logistic risk coefficients—no matter what the program. To test our uncertainty in evaluating the efficiency of population-wide programs *relative to* screening programs, we must confine our attention to variables that affect the two *differently*. Table 6-8 shows the relative variance in cost per YLS of School Education and of Mass Media compared with Universal Screening. From that table, we estimate that the true cost per YLS of Mass Media for men is between 11 percent and 33 percent of the cost per YLS for Universal

Table 6–7. Contributions to variance of cost-effectiveness of population-wide programs from individual parameters

Parameter	Base case estimate	Range (±1 SD)	Contribution to variance of log (cost/YLS)	
			M	*F*
For mass media				
Cost per person (C_M)	$0.50	$0.40–$0.60	.04	.04
Reduction in average cholesterol (J_M)	2%	1.0–3.8%	.45	.45
Logistic coefficients	(As in Table 4–12)	(As in Table 4–12)	.09	.04
Total variance of log (cost/YLS)			.58	.53
±1 SD as a percentage of base case			47–214%	48–207%
For school education				
Cost per person (C_E)	$5.00	$4–$6	.04	.04
Reduction in average cholesterol (J_E)	1%	0.4–2.0%	.65	.65
Logistic coefficient	(As in Table 4–12)	(As in Table 4–12)	.09	.04
Total variance of log (cost/YLS)			.78	.73
±1 SD as a percentage of base case			41–242%	43–235%

Note. Dollar values for confidence intervals can be calculated by multiplying the appropriate base case estimate by the stated percentages.

Table 6–8. Contributions to variance of relative cost-effectiveness of population-wide programs compared with universal screening

Parameter	*Base case estimate*	*Range (±1 SD)*	*Contribution to variance*
For mass media			
Cost per person (C_M)	\$0.50	\$0.40–\$0.60	.04
Reduction in cholesterol (J_M)	2%	1.2–3.3%	.26
Total relative variance of log (cost/YLS)			.30
±1 SD as percentage of base case			58–173%
±1 SD as percentage of base case for universal screening (men)			11–33%
For school education			
Cost per person (C_E)	\$5	\$4–\$6	.04
Reduction in cholesterol (J_E)	1%	0.6–1.7%	.30
Total relative variance of log (cost/YLS)			.34
±1 SD as a percentage of base case			55–179%
±1 SD as percentage of base case for universal screening (men)			26–85%

Note. In these calculations, the only parameters that are allowed to vary are those which do not affect the cost-effectiveness of Universal Screening.

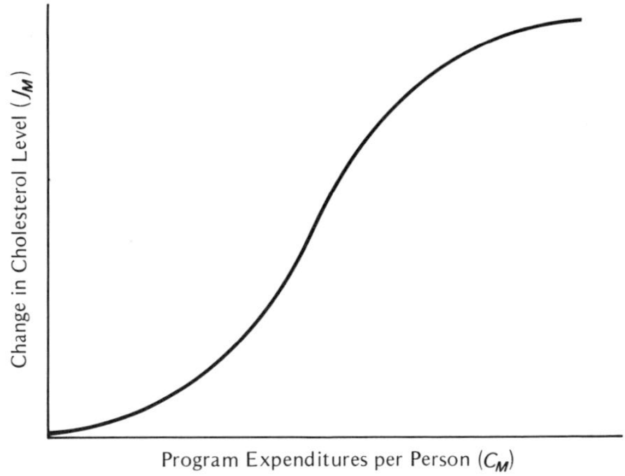

Figure 6-9. Hypothetical "Dose-Response" Curve, Mass Media Expenditure vs. Resulting Change in Cholesterol Level. We have little information on the true shape of this curve.

Screening in the base case. Similarly, we believe that the chances are two out of three that School Education for men costs between 26 percent and 85 percent of the cost per YLS for Universal Screening.

SELECTING OPTIMAL LEVELS OF EXPENDITURES: A THEORETICAL DISCUSSION

Although we have treated C_E and C_M as if they were fixed amounts, they are, in fact, subject to choice. We might reasonably expect a dose-response relationship between the chosen level of expenditure per person and the average cholesterol shift achieved by a Population-wide Intervention program. Such dose-response relationships are usually characterized by a sigmoidal, or S-shaped dependence of effect on treatment. In pharmacological models, at least, sensitivity to a drug is a normally distributed attribute in a population. At a low dosage, only a few highly susceptible individuals respond fully; in the mid-range, most potential responders show the effects of the drug; and at very high dosage, only those few who are inordinately resistant to its effects begin to respond.

An analogous dose-response curve relating J_M to C_M (or J_E to C_E) is shown in Figure 6-9. Data do not exist on the true functional relationship, and so we have left the "cost" axis unlabeled, merely wishing to suggest the *shape* of the function. This sigmoidal shape suggests to our eye what may not be immediately apparent to our mind—that the

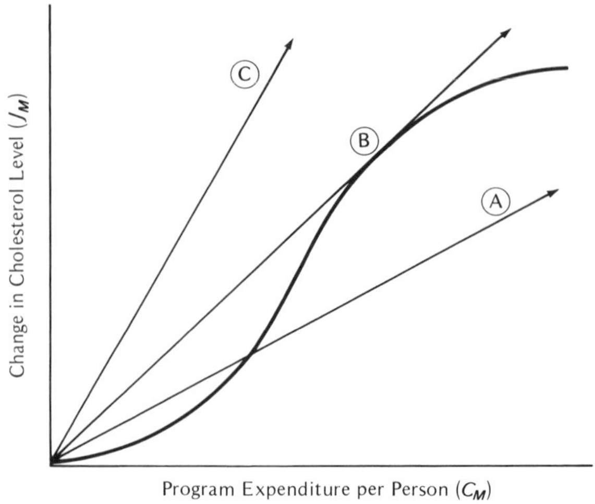

Figure 6-10. Lines of Constant Cost-effectiveness and Hypothetical "Dose-Response" Curve. Programs on line A are feasible but are less efficient than the program on line B at the point of tangency, which is also feasible. Programs on line C are more efficient than either A or B, but they cannot be achieved.

optimal expenditure per person for Mass Media or School Education may *not* be that which achieves the maximum cholesterol shift, J_M or J_E. As the dose-response curve begins to flatten, we get smaller and smaller increments in J_M or J_E for each additional dollar spent, and at some point, it probably is not wise to spend more money. Where is that point, or, in other words, what are rational criteria for selecting the optimal C_M or C_E?

The preceding discussion of the linear approximation of cost per YLS, in which we estimate cost per YLS to be a function of the ratio C_M/J_M or C_E/J_E, suggests a way of finding the optimal expenditures. For any given program, cost-effectiveness remains approximately constant as long as the ratio of C_M/J_M or C_E/J_E remains constant. The graph of those constant ratios superimposed on Figure 6-9 would be a straight line, and the more cost-effective the program, the greater will be the slope of that line.

In Figure 6-10, we have chosen a hypothetical set of such lines of constant cost-effectiveness, superimposed on the dose-response graph from Figure 6-9. In that figure, line A represents a less efficient program than line B, and line C represents a more efficient program than either line A or B.

The dose-response curve represents the frontier of achievable cholesterol shifts for all levels of expenditure, and this curve of possible programs intersects many, but not all, lines of constant cost-effectiveness, such as lines A, B, and C. It is apparent from Figure 6-10 that the parameters of the most efficient feasible program lie at the point at which the dose-response curve touches the most nearly vertical cost-effectiveness line. In Figure 6-10, the program on line B at the point of tangency with the dose-response curve is more efficient than (and just as achievable as) programs on line A which lie under the dose-response curve. Programs on line C are even more attractive than B but are not achievable. The optimal program achievable spends the amount C_M (or C_E) and harvests the cholesterol shift J_M (or J_E), which are defined at the point of tangency between the sigmoidal dose-response curve and the cost-effectiveness lines. Although this method of optimization works in theory, its application would require data that we do not have on both cost-effectiveness and dose-response relationships for media and educational programs.

COMPARISONS OF UNIVERSAL SCREENING, TARGETED SCREENING, AND POPULATION-WIDE INTERVENTION

In the remainder of this chapter, we will draw together some of the results of our models of Universal Screening, Targeted Screening, and Population-wide Intervention in order to compare their merits. This comparison will continue in Chapter 7, where we will explore more general conclusions. Since Mass Media programs in the base case are more efficient than School Education, we will tend to use the former as the better representatives of population-wide intervention.

Comparisons under varying combinations of J_M *and* C_M

In Figures 6-3 through 6-6, we have sketched in as horizontal lines the base case estimates for cost-effectiveness of Universal Screening and Targeted Screening programs. The points of intersection between these horizontal lines and the graphs of cost-effectiveness for the Mass Media program constitute a set of *points of equivalency*. At these points, the designated combinations of J_M and C_M would result in a cost-effectiveness estimate for the Population-wide program that is just equal to the cost-effectiveness of the relevant screening program. It is instructive to graph these points of equivalency as lines indicat-

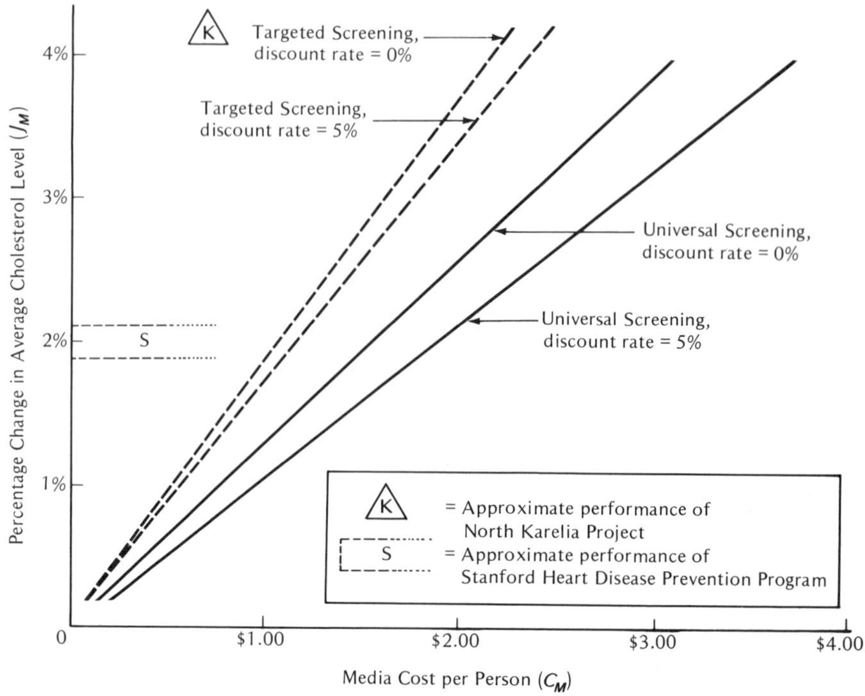

Figure 6-11. Lines of Equivalency for Screening Programs and Mass Media Programs for Men. For combinations of J_M and C_M that lie above and to the left of any line, Mass Media performs more efficiently than the program indicated by that line. Mass Media is less efficient for combinations of J_M and C_M that lie below and to the right of any line.

ing combinations of J_M and C_M, as we have done in Figure 6-11 for men and Figure 6-12 for women.

In Figures 6-11 and 6-12 each *line of equivalency* bisects the plane into two regions. Above the line are found combinations of J_M and C_M at which Mass Media is a more cost-effective strategy than the screening program to which that line pertains. Below the line, Mass Media programs are less efficient in cost per YLS than the screening program.

The estimated combinations of J_M and C_M experienced in the North Karelia Project are also indicated in Figures 6-11, and 6-12, and for men this point lies deep within the regions of dominance of the Mass Media programs. For North Karelia women, the modest cholesterol lowering achieved in comparison with the control region would result in a cost per YLS comparable to that of Targeted Screening and only slightly better than Universal Screening. We have no cost data on the

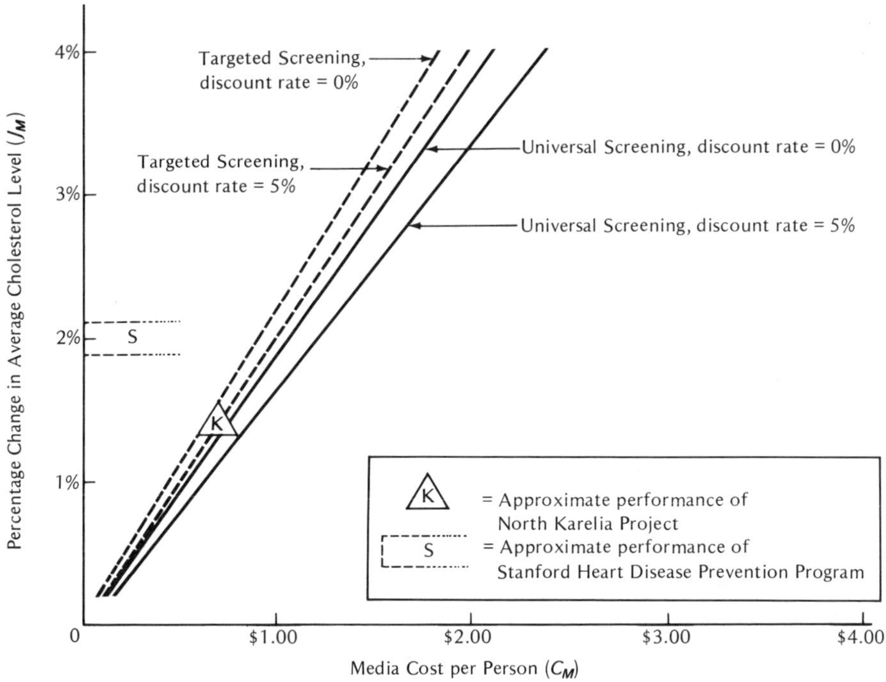

Figure 6-12. Lines of Equivalency for Screening Programs and Mass Media Programs for Women. For combinations of J_M and C_M that lie above and to the left of any line, Mass Media performs more efficiently than the program indicated by that line. Mass Media is less efficient for combinations of J_M and C_M that lie below and to the right of any line.

Stanford study, but we observe that at any C_M less than about $1.50 for men or $1.00 for women, its J_M of 2 percent would make it more cost-effective than any of the base case screening programs at a discount rate of 5 percent.

Interestingly, substantial portions of the area portrayed in Figures 6-11 and 6-12 lie between the Targeted and Universal Screening lines, in which cases, Mass Media would be less efficient than the former and more efficient than the latter. There are sex differences as well, with some combinations of J_M and C_M dictating a preference for one program for men and a different one for women. As previously noted, a Mass Media program seems to hold more consistent advantages over screening programs for men than for women.

Figures 6-11 and 6-12 show the relationships at a discount rate of zero as well as at 5 percent. We note in comparing the two discount rates that fewer combinations of J_M and C_M lie above any given equivalency line at the discount rate of zero, indicating that discounting tends to put the Mass Media program at an advantage relative to the screening efforts. This advantage results primarily from the impact of discounting on program costs. For Mass Media, program costs are discounted over a longer period (40 years) than for screening programs (8 years in the intensive intervention program), and therefore, the costs of Mass Media decrease more rapidly in response to discount rates. Even if the discount rate is zero, the combinations of J_M and C_M that we ascribe to the North Karelia Project still result in a more efficient program than any of the screening programs for men. Without any discounting, the average J_M in the Stanford study would indicate a preference for Mass Media over screening if C_M is less than about $1.

Fraction of benefit and comparative efficiency

Underlying most of our calculations is the assumption that the potential fraction of benefit—the reduction of risk achievable through lowering cholesterol levels—is a rapidly decreasing function of age. Cretin (1977b) has analyzed in some detail the simultaneous effects of diminishing costs and decaying fraction of benefit with advancing age. Figure 6-13 shows a schematic version of these two effects. The line labeled $f_c(x)$ represents the cost of a program as a function of the age at which those costs are incurred. Costs are expressed as the fraction of the total costs to a 10-year-old cohort, and the present value of those costs falls to the fraction $f_c(x) = [1/(1 + D)]^x$ for any age x at a discount rate of D. The line labeled $f_b(x)$ represents a hypothetical decay curve for fraction of benefit, assuming that the fraction is 1.0 at age 10. In fact, we have very little information at present on the actual shape of this function $f_b(x)$.

As Cretin shows, the optimal age at which to operate a program with the characteristics shown in Figure 6-13 is *not* the age at which both fractional costs and fractional benefits are 1.0. Instead, the cost/benefit ratio is at a minimum where the following equation holds:

$$f'_c(x)/f_c(x) = f'_b(x)/f_b(x)$$

Solving the above equation for x would yield the age at which the ratio of $f_c(x)$ to $f_b(x)$ is at a minimum, and which is therefore the most efficient target age for a program.

In the screening program analysis, we assume that fraction of benefit decays quickly enough after age 10 to outweigh the burden of a

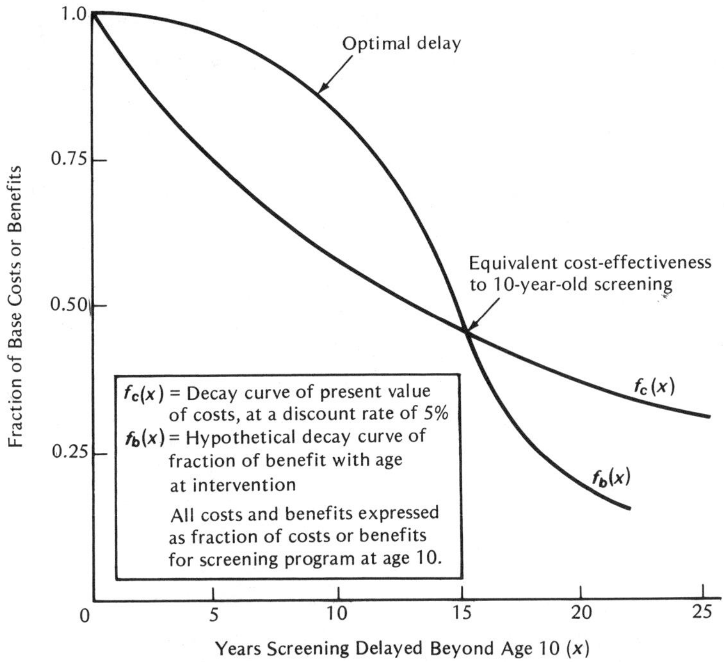

Figure 6-13. Effect on Discounted Costs and Benefits of Delaying Screening for *X* Years Beyond Age 10. (Reproduced with permission from S. Cretin, Cost/benefit analysis of treatment and prevention of myocardial infarction. Health Serv Res 12:174–189, 1977.)

positive discount rate; that is, we assume that if we waited until a later age to screen and treat, we would lose more in potential fraction of benefit than we would gain by not having to discount future benefits over quite so many years. In the Mass Media program cohort analysis, we assume that fraction of benefit falls quickly enough over a lifetime that cohort analysis provides an estimate of the maximum achievable benefits and thus of the minimum cost per YLS.

Suppose for a moment that we have been wrong in these assumptions—that, for example, potential fraction of benefit remains at 1.0 right up until the age of 30. How would this new assumption affect the performance of each of the three major programs: Universal Screening, Targeted Screening, and Mass Media?

Universal Screening would clearly benefit. Instead of screening 10-year-olds, we could now afford to wait until age 30 to screen and intervene, reducing by 20 years the period over which the benefits must be discounted. If we assume that 30-year-olds could be screened and treated as efficiently as 10-year-olds, then the 20-year reduction in discounting would increase benefits by a factor of $(1 + D)^{20}$, which at $D = 5$ percent amounts to 2.65. Costs remain the same as in the program for 10-year-olds, so cost per YLS is only $1/2.65 = 38$ percent as high for 30-year-olds as for 10-year-olds.

The effect on Targeted Screening is even more favorable. If fraction of benefit remained 1.0 until age 30, we could, once again, wait until that age to screen and so avoid 20 years worth of discounting benefits. In addition, the delay increases the yield of a family history questionnaire, since the parents and grandparents of 30-year-olds have had a longer opportunity to display coronary disease than the parents of 10-year-olds. At age 30, for example, 6.9 percent of people responding accurately would report a history of myocardial infarction in a father under 55 or a mother under 65, which is nearly ten times the yield of the same question asked of 10-year-olds. Because a higher proportion of family histories are positive, the cost per positive screenee falls. At a discount rate of 5 percent, the net effect of preservation of full benefits and delaying the screening program until age 30 is that cost per YLS falls to 28 percent of that for 10-year-old boys and 26 percent of that for 10-year-old girls.

Changing this assumption about the efficacy of intervention later in life has complex effects on the Mass Media program. The cohort analysis as we report it attributes both costs and benefits to a cohort member at age 10. If fraction of benefit remains at 1.0 until age 30, we can ascribe benefits instead to people at age 30, raising them from benefits at age 10 by a factor of $(1 + D)^{20}$. Total costs, on the other hand, are divided among the members of a smaller segment of the population. Instead of attributing them to all men from birth to age 40, for example, we choose the age range 30 to 40. The net effect is a relative increase in the discounted total costs per member of the cohort.

Figure 6-14 shows how four programs, Universal Screening, Targeted Screening, Mass Media, and School Education, fare as we increase our estimate of the maximum age at which fraction of benefit equals 1.0. If we can implement a Universal Screening program as late as age 25 with full benefits, then it becomes more cost-effective than School Education. Targeted Screening performs more efficiently than School Education if the former can be deferred to age 15 or later with no loss in benefits. At no point in this comparison does any program exceed the efficiency of Mass Media.

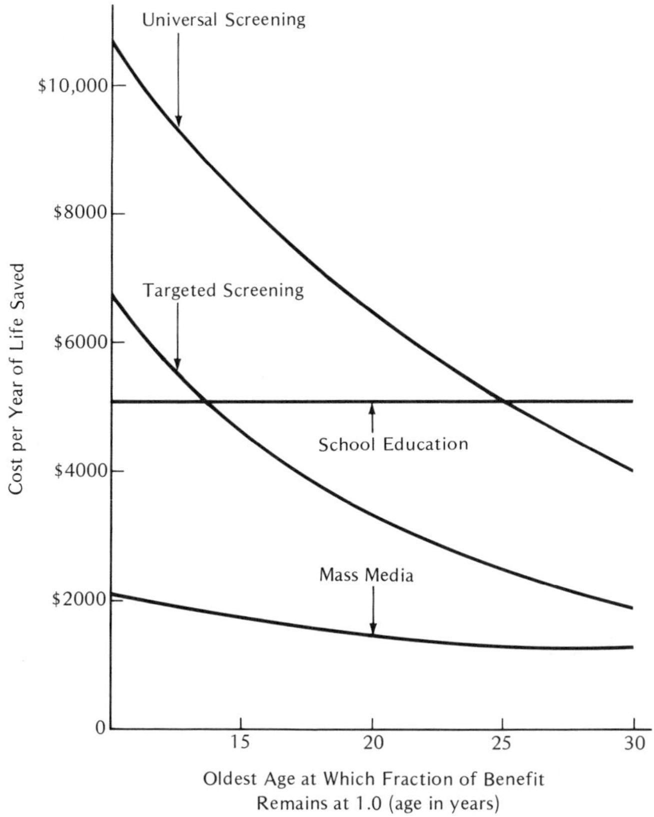

Figure 6-14. Dependency of Cost per Year of Life Saved on the Oldest Age at Which Full Fraction of Benefit Is Obtainable, for Men, at Discount Rate = 5 Percent. The longer we can delay screening without loss of benefits, the more cost-effective screening becomes. There is no equivalent effect on the School Education program, and the effect on Mass Media is small.

Comparisons of efficiency, scope, and total budget

No single number can capture all the attributes by which we would wish to compare alternative programs. The simplest in many ways is our primary cost-effectiveness yardstick—cost per year of life saved—but this measure does not reveal such other important features as total cost, evenness of distribution of benefits in a population, or total benefits. In Tables 6-9, 6-10, and 6-11, we summarize a wide variety of performance features of the six major programs we have analyzed: Universal Screening, Sequential Rescreening, Case-finding

Table 6–9. Comparison of programs: cost effectiveness*

Program	Sex	*Base case cost per YLS†*	*Probable range of cost per YLS†,‡*	*Cost per cohort member*	*Benefits per cohort member (undiscounted)*		*Benefits per treated cohort member (undiscounted)*	
					Days of life added	*Heart disease-free days added*	*Days of life added*	*Heart disease-free days added*
Universal screening	M	$10,660	$5,540–$20,680	$13.30	5.8	8.4	145	210
	F	$ 9,300	$4,930–$17,670	$10.10	7.0	5.5	241	190
Sequential rescreening	M	$10,500	—	$13.40	5.8	8.5	147	215
	F	$ 9,120	—	$10.45	7.4	5.7	246	189
Case-finding (on sib-	M	$10,600	—	$14.20	6.0	8.9	158	234
lings)	F	$ 9,240	—	$10.60	7.4	5.8	274	215
Targeted screening	M	$ 6,730	$2,960–$12,500	$ 2.40	1.4	§	239	§
(family history)	F	$ 7,730	$3,400–$14,200	$ 1.90	1.5	§	315	§
School	M	$ 5,050	$2,070–$12,220	$22.80	20.8	35.8	21	36
education	F	$ 6,500	$2,800–$15,300	$22.80	24.1	31.0	24	31
Mass media	M	$ 2,720	$1,280–$ 5,820	$24.60	40.9	70.8	41	71
	F	$ 3,830	$1,840–$ 7,930	$27.30	47.5	61.5	48	62

Note. Comparisons shown are for the screening programs with intensive intervention. Benefits are expressed in undiscounted figures. If discounted at 5 percent, most benefits would be only one-tenth to one-fifteenth as large.

The two right-most columns show expected benefits per *treated* cohort member. The expected benefits per *complier* are twice as large, since we assume that only half of treated members of the cohort actually comply with a therapeutic diet. (This applies to all the screening programs but not to the population-wide programs.)

*Adjusted to age 10.

†Cost per YLS calculated based on benefits discounted at 5 percent.

‡Range expressed as mean estimate ±1 SD; i.e., the odds are approximately 2:1 that the true value lies within this range (see text, p. 158).

§Insufficient data to estimate.

Table 6–10. Comparison of programs: scope and reach*

Program	*Sex*	*Percentage of cohort "treated" (%)*	*Percentage of cohort with cholesterol measured (%)*	*Number of 10-year-olds in U.S. "treated" per year†*	*Total years of life saved by 10-year-old cohort in U.S.*	
					Undiscounted	*Discounted at 5%*
Universal screening	M	4.01	100	60,100	23,810	1,890
	F	2.90	100	43,500	28,770	1,640
Sequential rescreening	M	3.96	100	49,400	19,830	1,910
	F	3.01	100	45,150	30,410	1,730
Case-finding (on siblings)	M	3.8	100	57,000‡	24,660	2,010
	F	2.7	100	40,500§	30,410	1,730
Targeted screening (family history)	M	0.60	0.85	9,000	5,750	530
	F	0.46	0.85	6,900	6,160	370
School education	M	100	0	1,500,000	85,480	6,750
	F	100	0	1,500,000	99,040	5,250
Mass media	M	100	0	1,500,000	168,080	13,500
	F	100	0	1,500,000	195,210	10,500

Note. Number of children treated and total years saved are calculated for these programs applied to the entire United States, which includes 3 million 10-year-olds each year.

*Calculations for base case.

†Assumes 3×10^6 ten-year-olds per year.

‡Plus 6600 siblings of different ages.

§Plus 6150 siblings of different ages.

on Siblings (a modification of Universal Screening), Targeted Screening using a family history questionnaire, School Education, and Mass Media. We have omitted two other programs—Universal Rescreening and Triggered Screening—the former because it is dominated in all respects by Single Screening, and the latter because our analysis of it was limited to qualitative observations.

Table 6-9 reviews the major features related to cost-effectiveness. The population-wide programs are far more efficient than the others but at a substantially higher expected dollar price per participant. Targeted Screening is the least expensive per participant and produces the highest expected benefit to each *treated* individual, but its overall scope is comparatively small, and the average discounted benefit per screenee is so tiny that it is best expressed in *hours* of life saved.

Issues of scope are more fully explored in Table 6-10. There we see that Targeted Screening, though more efficient than other screening programs, reaches barely one-seventh as many individuals and attains only one-fourth the total benefits as the Universal Screening programs. In this table, as well, the massive scope of the population-wide programs is evident. In total years of life saved, Mass Media surpasses Universal Screening and its variants by a factor of 6 or 7.

For a policymaker, ultimate choices may depend as much on total costs as on efficiency. Although the completely rational policymaker should spend budget dollars first on programs of maximum cost-effectiveness, it may be important to know the cost of a program as applied to a population of predetermined size. These are the figures presented in Table 6-11, representing two ways of calculating total cost for each of the programs if extended to the entire U.S. population (220 million people). The total discounted cost to a cohort of 10-year-olds represents total costs as seen from the point of view of beneficiaries, with remote costs being discounted appropriately. Of somewhat more political interest is the total budgetary cost per year, the actual amount that would appear in any given year's budget as the price of the program that year. Here, the small scope of the Targeted Screening program again surfaces, with total costs only one-twelfth as large as those of the Mass Media program. Applied to a uniform population base, the most efficient program—Mass Media—is also the most costly.

Although population-wide programs are by far the most cost-effective under our base case assumptions, no single program dominates the others under all political circumstances or under all sets of

Table 6–11. Comparison of programs: total budget

Program	*Total discounted cost to national cohort at age 10**	*Total yearly budget in U.S. in "steady state"†*
Universal screening	$35,100,000	$40,192,400
Sequential rescreening	$35,775,000	$40,743,450
Case-finding (on siblings)	$37,200,000	$39,639,750
Targeted screening (family history)	$ 6,427,000	$ 6,483,600
School education	$68,400,000	$75,000,000
Mass media	$77,850,000	$110,000,000

*Assuming discount rate of 5 percent.
†Assuming U.S. population = 220 million, with 3 million 10-year-olds.

objectives. With a strictly limited budget to cover a large population, Targeted Screening may be the best compromise. If efficiency is prized above all else, then the Mass Media program seems best.

Because of the uncertainty in the parameter estimates that affect the performance of each of these programs, we cannot express great confidence in our best guesses about the actual cost-effectiveness figures displayed in Table 6-9. We have far more confidence, though, in the rank ordering of the programs, which remains relatively stable within the range of our uncertainty. In the concluding chapter we will deal further with the impact of uncertainty on the rank ordering of our program preferences.

7. Conclusions and recommendations

INTRODUCTION

In this final chapter, we will develop some general conclusions from the specific results of the preceding chapters. As a first step, we will place our analysis in context by comparing our cost-effectiveness results with those for other health programs that have been similarly evaluated. Second, we will discuss some of the critical determinants of the efficiency of the hypothetical cholesterol-reducing programs discussed in Chapters 4 through 6. Third, we will examine the potential impact of factors that we have *omitted* from our formal analysis, paying particular attention to features other than cost-effectiveness that might lead us to prefer one strategy over another. Finally, we will try to generalize some of our conclusions to the field of preventive medicine as a whole and to highlight the strengths and weaknesses of biomedical research, especially research on lipids and heart disease, in generating the kind of information needed for formulating sound public policy.

THE TERRAIN OF COST-EFFECTIVENESS IN PUBLIC HEALTH

Before a health program is adopted, it should meet two economic tests: first, the program should yield an adequate return for its costs (just like any investment), and second, it should be attractive when compared with its alternatives. The cost-effectiveness numbers generated in the last three chapters allow us to subject cholesterol programs to both of these tests, the absolute and the relative.

Absolute cost-effectiveness

How do the costs per year of life saved for the programs we have evaluated compare with the value that our society places on one year of human life? The question is difficult, for it requires us to struggle with assessing the value of human life, an issue that we can sidestep by simply comparing the cost-effectiveness of our programs with the cost-effectiveness of other health care programs. We will proceed here to examine our results briefly in absolute terms, but we believe that the relative comparisons in the end provide more useful information.

Philosophers may hold that human life is priceless, but societies, including our own, seldom act as if this were the case. Under the pressure of inflation in the health care sector of our economy, there have been increasing demands that even lifesaving programs must somehow prove their worth. Some examples will illustrate the pressure.

Both the Occupational Safety and Health Administration (OSHA) and the Environmental Protection Agency (EPA), which have traditionally tried to minimize hazards to health whenever technologically feasible, must now be concerned with cost as well as with hazards to health. Negotiations between the Council of Economic Advisors and OSHA, for example, have resulted in a standard for acrylonitrile exposure that implies a value of about $3.5 million per life saved, instead of choosing a stricter but technologically feasible standard that would have implied a value of about $16 million per life saved. We can infer that, in this instance at least, each human life is implicitly valued at more than $3.5 million and less than $16 million. Unfortunately, such inferences about the implicit value of life drawn from other societal decisions yield highly disparate estimates. The decisions made in one state highway program, for example, imply a tacit value of $3000 per life, less than one-tenth of 1 percent of the value inferred from the OSHA acrylonitrile standard (Carlson, 1963).

Part of the variation in these estimates of the value of life results from the imprecision of the underlying risk estimates. If we were setting standards for saccharin exposure, for example, we would have to deal not only with the valuation of life but also with the estimate that saccharin may cause between 0.0007 and 3640 cases of bladder cancer per year! Even when the magnitude of the risks is known, other factors, such as the *type* of risk, influence policy decisions. It seems, for example, that society is far more willing to spend public money to reduce involuntary risks than to reduce voluntary risks.

Because of these complexities, inferential estimates of the value we place on life are necessarily crude, but the fact remains that our governmental policies do recognize limits on our willingness to pay to preserve health and life. Most serious attempts to estimate a "dollar value" for a year of life have proposed figures that are from $10,000 to $50,000 per year *higher* than the cost of the cholesterol-reducing programs analyzed in this book. It does seem unlikely that a nation as wealthy as the United States would regard $5000 as too much to spend for an extra year of life, and therefore, without applying the first economic test strictly, we may still conclude with some confidence that although saving life-years through cholesterol-lowering programs is expensive under most assumptions, it is by no means *prohibitively* expensive. Lowering cholesterol probably represents a productive use of our resources in absolute terms. With this in mind, it makes sense to compare the cost-effectiveness of our hypothetical cholesterol programs with the cost-effectiveness of other preventive medical programs.

Relative cost-effectiveness

From a number of recent studies of the cost-effectiveness of prevention, we have chosen those shown in Table 7-1 as being both careful and representative. To facilitate comparison with the cholesterol-lowering programs, whenever possible we have restated the results of other studies in terms of 1975 dollars and years of life saved discounted at 5 percent. In some cases, these recalculations have required us to make assumptions about when the life-years saved would occur. As a result, our adjusted figures are both different from and somewhat less reliable than the estimates in the original sources.

Among the most interesting comparisons are those with the cost-effectiveness of renal dialysis. Since 1972, the U.S. government has assumed the full cost of treatment for more than 90 percent of Americans suffering from end-stage renal disease. In underwriting this program, our government implies that the years of life saved are worth the cost. From the work of Stange and Sumner (1978), we estimate that the cost per year of life saved (in 1975 dollars) is $22,000 for facility dialysis, $14,000 for home dialysis, and between $12,500 and $18,000 for kidney transplantations. Since the costs per year of life of all the cholesterol-reducing programs we examined are lower than the cost of extending life through renal dialysis and transplantation, the cholesterol programs lie within the range of cost-effectiveness in which the federal government sometimes acts.

A number of studies of preventive medical practices, including screening, have produced cost-effectiveness estimates that compare favorably with those for renal dialysis. It is easy to overestimate the value of screening and prevention programs by neglecting to take account of false-positive screenees, spontaneous cures, iatrogenic complications, and cases that would have been detected without a screening program. Nevertheless, even taking these limitations into account, some preventive practices seem extremely attractive. Axnick et al. (1969), for example, studied the decline in incidence of measles following the immunization campaigns of the 1960s and calculated reductions in death and retardation from measles encephalitis alone costing only $2100 per discounted year saved. (For assumptions in our recalculations, see Table 7-1.) Rubella vaccination may be even more cost-effective, but vaccination for mumps, from which severe complications are rarer, is probably much less efficient (Witte, 1974).

A study of the cost-effectiveness of neonatal screening for phenylketonuria (PKU) (Bush et al., 1973) produced estimates of about $5000 per year of severe retardation averted. Routine *follow-up* rescreening for PKU, on the other hand, has an unattractively low yield (only four new cases in 2.3 million children tested, compared with 290 cases found on the initial screening [Sepe et al., 1979]).

Tuberculosis screening in children is apparently very expensive, costing between $25,000 and $90,000 per year of life saved (depending on the value assigned to years of life compromised by nonfatal complications). Tuberculosis today is too rare, too indolent, and too treatable in symptomatic stages for screening for asymptomatic disease to have a great impact.

In the field of adult screening for asymptomatic disease, Weinstein and Stason (1976) analyzed the efficiency of public programs for screening and treating hypertension. Outcomes are measured in terms of "quality-adjusted" life-years, in which years of life compromised by the side effects of disease or treatment are assigned a slightly lower value than years entirely free of ill health. The authors conclude that a screening and intervention program for hypertension would cost between $7000 and $15,000 per discounted, quality-adjusted life-year saved. Without adjusting for the quality of life, the cost per life-year would be 10 to 20 percent lower. The adult screening programs analyzed by these authors are much less affected by discounting than are the childhood programs that we have analyzed.

Cancer screening has also been subjected to this form of analysis. The cost per year of life saved for programs such as biennial Pap smears for cervical cancer, physical examination for breast cancer, and

Table 7–1. Cost-Effectiveness of Health Programs; Some Representative Studies

Author	*Medical condition*	*Program evaluated*	*Cost per year of life added (1975 dollars, discounted at 5%)*
Treatment and Prevention			
Stange and Sumner (1978)	End-stage renal disease	Facility dialysis	$22,000
		Home dialysis	$14,000
		Transplantation (with facility dialysis of failures)	$12,000–$18,000
Cretin (1977b)	Coronary disease	Coronary care units	$3,000
		Mobile coronary care units	$4,300
Axnick et al. (1969)	Measles	Immunization	$2,100[b,d]
Screening			
Bush et al. (1973)	Phenylketonuria	Screening neonates and dietary treatment	$5,000[b,c]
Sepe et al. (1978)	Phenylketonuria	Follow-up screening of initially negative screenees	$30,000[b,c]
Bush et al. (1972)	Tuberculosis	Screening children	$25,000–$90,000[e]
Weinstein & Stason (1976)	Hypertension	Screening and treatment	$7,000–$15,000[a]
Berwick et al., (this volume)	Hypercholesterolemia	Changing diets	$2,800–$10,000
Kisch & Keeler (1977)	Breast cancer	Screening with physical exam by trained lay people	$4,000

		Screening with mammogram (marginal effect)	\$33,000
Eddy (1978)	Breast cancer	Screening 50-year-old women with annual physical exam	\$983[f]
		Annual physical exam and biennial mammograms	\$2,778[f]
	Cervical cancer	Screening 25-year-old "average-risk" women with:	
		Annual Pap smear	\$1,716[f]
		Pap smear every 5 years	\$368[f]
	Bladder cancer	Screening 45-year-old men with:	
		Annual urinalysis	\$6,260[f]
		Annual urinalysis and cytology	\$6,555[f]
	Colon cancer	Screening 50-year-old women with:	
		Annual occult blood test and sigmoidoscopy every 5 years	\$367[f]

Note. The cholesterol programs analyzed here have cost-effectiveness levels within the range of current active public health intervention.

[a]Life-years are quality adjusted for discomfort resulting from side effects and morbidity of disease. In "pure" life-years saved, these numbers would be 10 to 20% lower.

[b]Assumes that years of severe retardation have no value (are equivalent to death).

[c]Assumes that treatment is harmless and effective and that all cases would be severely retarded without the screening program.

[d]Only the effects of measles encephalitis are considered.

[e]The different values reflect different methods of quality adjustment of life-years. Costs are higher here than in the original paper because of the estimated effects of discounting and inflation.

[f]Costs discounted at 3% per year, benefits undiscounted.

stool guaiac tests for colon cancer ranges from just under $400 per year (without discounting benefits) to $50,000 per year.

Cretin (1977b) used many of the same methods employed in this book to estimate the efficiency of coronary care units (CCU) and mobile coronary care units (MCCU). Using a 5 percent discount rate, Cretin estimated the cost per year of added life (without quality adjustment) to be about $3000 for CCUs and about $4300 for MCCUs.

In summary, our analysis of cholesterol-reducing programs shows them to be comparable in cost-effectiveness to a number of other preventive medical programs. Such a comparison is helpful in choosing among programs that are all acceptable on an absolute cost-benefit scale. Choices must frequently be made, since limitations on budget and management capabilities usually prohibit us from investing in all productive enterprises at once. The observation that cholesterol-reducing programs are comparable in performance to many other health programs has at least three important implications for policy. First, it suggests that implementation of cholesterol control programs, at least on a trial basis, is reasonable. Since alternative programs are expected to yield about the same benefit per unit of cost, mistakes in choosing among programs are not likely to be very expensive (assuming that estimates of efficiency are comparably sound).

Second, since cost per year of life saved (our primary measure of effectiveness) is similar among alternative preventative programs, other measures of performance, such as the quality of the years added, the scope of the undertaking, the distribution of benefits, and political and administrative constraints, acquire more significance. These secondary measures may prescribe action more fully than they would if the primary ratings of efficiency were less ambiguous.

Third, when alternative programs have the same expected efficiency, the potential degree of error in the estimates of efficiency becomes more important. Particularly for large programs, whose true effectiveness will not be known for several years, we may prefer to implement programs with tighter intervals in estimates of cost-effectiveness, even if those programs have a slightly inferior *average* expected performance.

KEY FACTORS IN RELATIVE COST-EFFECTIVENESS

From the analysis of the previous chapters, three factors stand out as the most critical in determining both the relative and absolute cost-effectiveness of the programs we have evaluated: the discount rate, the malleability of dietary behavior, and the effect of cholesterol reduction on risk.

Discount rate

The most powerful determinant of the efficiency of pediatric screening programs is the degree to which we discount future costs and benefits. This conclusion turns our attention away from a search for more accurate factual information and toward a search for societal values. We have characterized the different values placed on the present and the future by incorporating a constant rate of discount into our models. Although the discounting model is convenient and ubiquitous, it is not necessarily the only or the most accurate way to characterize society's preferences over time. We accept the discounting model as reasonably consistent with the observed behaviors of people. Furthermore, the use of more complex models of time preferences might change our quantitative results but would have little effect on our qualitative conclusions. Formal methods exist for inferring discount rates from the observed behaviors and choices of people. For any society, however, the choice of the discount rate remains a value-based decision, under human control.

Whether or not atherosclerotic lesions regress, or cholesterol levels change with diet, or media advertisements alter tastes are questions with factual answers, not matters of value and opinion. In contrast, whether we so value the present against the future that we express this preference through a discount rate of 10 percent or 5 percent or 0 percent is a choice very much up to us, subject to debate, to disagreement, and ultimately to decision by consensus. The discount rate chosen should reflect societal values.

It is not surprising that policymaking requires such judgments of value. Judgments are to be expected in weighing one type of benefit against another or in translating different sorts of costs into comparable units. The surprise lies in the potency of discounting as a determinant of choice. The formulation of consistent policy on the pediatric prevention of adult disease requires the prior selection of an appropriate rate of discount for costs and benefits.

Choosing a discount rate above zero does *not* imply that pediatric programs to prevent adult diseases ought never to be implemented. We will still want programs of pediatric prevention, even when benefits are long delayed, as long as the benefits are very large compared with the costs. Discounting, however, does lead us to favor programs with both immediate and long-term benefits, and we will especially prefer preventive programs that can be implemented at later ages without much decline in benefit. Pediatric prevention will seem desirable only when achievable benefits fall with advancing age at a rate faster than the rate of discount (Cretin, 1977b).

The choice of discount rate affects not only the absolute performance of the programs studied—important in deciding whether any preventive program is warranted—but also the relative efficiency of the programs with respect to each other. At low rates of discount, for example, programs for men cost more per year of life saved than for women, but the situation is reversed at higher rates. Furthermore, the crossover point lies within the region of current debate about applicable discount rates for public programs.

Despite the burden that discounting places on preventive programs with delayed benefits, we are convinced that costs and benefits should be discounted at the same rate and, furthermore, that the same rate of discount should be used in evaluating the cost-effectiveness of all social programs. On the other hand, valid reasons do exist for investing in programs for children even when those programs are *less* cost-effective than other alternatives according to economic measures. Our society may feel, for example, a special obligation to provide for the health and welfare of its young, especially the disadvantaged young.

Public investment in programs for children is also a way to encourage savings without favoring the rich. Some economists feel that people in the United States at present consume too much and save too little for our economic well-being, and one implication of this argument is that the government ought to adopt policies that encourage savings. Unfortunately, most such policies tend to benefit the wealthy at the expense of the poor. Programs that invest resources in the future welfare of children avoid this maldistribution of benefit.

Just as society may favor programs for children, so may it favor programs that encourage people to preserve their health through changes in life-style and the use of preventive medical services. Our current system of medical insurance, because it covers acute care more completely than preventive medical services, tends to shift consumption toward acute care services and consequently to increase medical care costs. Coverage of preventive services, such as immunization programs or specific disease screening programs, may help to restore some balance to the orientation of our health services, but there is still an incentive to rely on medical services rather than to try to prevent illness through appropriate self-care and healthful life-styles. All the programs we have analyzed encourage individuals to reduce their risk of disease by adopting good health habits. A government like ours, which is heavily involved in financing medical care, may save resources by underwriting programs that encourage individuals to take responsibility for their own health through appropriate self-care and improved life-styles (Phelps, 1978).

Strong reasons exist, therefore, to prefer programs for children and programs that encourage healthful behaviors even when those programs are not as cost-effective as alternatives, but these countervailing reasons do not support the conclusion that the attenuating effects of discounting on the cost-effectiveness of some preventive programs are unimportant or ought to be ignored. When choosing *among* programs in pediatric prevention, for example, discounting will still lead us to favor programs with immediate payoffs over those with remote payoffs. Furthermore, when intervention can be delayed—that is, undertaken at a time closer to the time at which benefits are realized—with little or no decrease in benefits, discounting will lead us to take advantage of that delay instead of shouldering intervention costs at an unnecessarily early time.

The malleability of taste and behavior

In preparing our estimates of cost-effectiveness, we have had an especially difficult time with those variables that relate to the determinants of people's behavior. Predicting compliance with diet, estimating program expenses, designing and "costing out" media campaigns, and selecting the most acceptable dietary adjustments—each of these tasks calls upon a level of understanding of the determinants of life-style that has not yet been achieved.

The efficiency of the interventions examined in this work is highly dependent on these issues of compliance and behavioral change. Despite some scattered pieces of evidence, we still have only an imprecise notion about how malleable dietary choices are, about how to get receptive people to change what they eat, and about the proportion of people who are essentially immune to efforts to alter diet. We are encouraged to note that the changes in behavior required to reduce American cholesterol levels are mainly substitutions, not eliminations, more like switching from high-tar to low-tar cigarettes, which many have done, than like giving up smoking altogether. The results of the North Karelia Project and the Stanford study, as well as significant secular trends in the American dietary pattern, tell us that change can occur, but the exact dose-response relationship between counseling or media on the one hand, and alteration in diet, on the other, remains undefined.

The importance of this dose-response relationship was introduced in Chapter 6. If most of the returns from efforts to modify dietary behavior occur early in those efforts—if each additional dollar spent produces much less response than the first dollars spent—then the screening programs, which spend large amounts of money trying to influence a few people to change their habits a lot, are at a distinct disadvantage compared with population-wide programs. However, programs of intensive, targeted intervention are favored over media efforts if dietary behavior is very refractory to change with small investments of effort. In this case, the dilute exposure achieved by Mass Media could be completely ineffective and a total waste of money. To make sound policies, we need to know much more than we do about the relationship between the amount of resources expended and the degree of behavioral change that can result.

The effect of cholesterol reduction on risk

As we have seen, prospective longitudinal studies reach a consistent conclusion: low cholesterol levels are associated with better cardiovascular health than are high cholesterol levels. Even though the reported range of the observed connections between cholesterol and risk is fairly broad, these uncertainties turn out to have only a relatively small effect on our estimates of cost-effectiveness. A much more serious concern for us than the exact functional relationship between lipid levels and risk is the question of how late in life dietary modifications can begin and still be effective in reducing risk. What fraction of the full benefit of a low cholesterol level can be achieved by diets introduced in adulthood?

When we use our benefit curves, computed by "inverting" the Framingham study data, to predict the results of the dietary intervention studies in Finland (Turpeinen, 1979) and Los Angeles (Dayton et al., 1969), we find a disconcerting result: our model would have predicted these intervention programs to be less effective then they were. In the study of Finnish mental hospitals, for example, our benefits model would have predicted a reduction in cardiovascular disease only four-fifths as large as that observed, *even if* there were no decay in benefits with age (i.e., if fraction of benefit remained at 1.0 for the middle-aged population in that study). We have no convincing single argument to explain this discrepancy. It is possible that these studies achieved simultaneous alteration in weight, exercise, or smoking that confounded and exaggerated the apparent effects of dietary change or that the populations studied represented, for some reason, a particularly high-risk group in whom particularly high benefits were attainable.

If, as this discrepancy between observed and predicted results may suggest, we have systematically underestimated the benefits achievable from reduction of cholesterol level, then obviously we have underestimated cost-effectiveness. As we saw in Figure 6-14, if the fraction of benefit that can be achieved with a diet starting late in life is equal to that achieved with a diet started in childhood, then this implies a substantial relative advantage for a Targeted Screening program. More generally, this preservation of fraction of benefit would make all the programs that we have evaluated (except School Education) seem like better buys.

CONSIDERATIONS OTHER THAN COST-EFFECTIVENESS

As we built our models, we chose to omit some considerations that, however important to the evaluation of a program, seemed particularly resistant to quantification or formal expression. It is useful now to review some of those omissions and to ask how their inclusion might affect the design and relative attractiveness of the different programs.

Psychological costs and benefits

Nowhere woven into our numbers are the mental costs and benefits of the various programs. Some such effects seem clearly negative, among them the foregone pleasure in forbidden foods, the pain of taking blood samples, the discomfort of worrying about illness and risk, and the invasion of privacy involved in any public program intervening on individual health. Other effects seem positive and desirable, such as the sense of control over one's body that may accompany personal efforts to change risk, the pride of added knowledge about how one's body works, or the reassurance (even if unwarranted) to someone whose cholesterol level is found to be low.

In fact, these omissions are probably more important in the ideal design of each program than in determining one program's attractiveness relative to that of another. Ideally, screening programs should try to avoid the negative effects of labeling people and families, and interventions should be designed to minimize the disability of "nondisease" such as has been reported in screenees positive for hypertension (Haynes et al., 1978) or sickle cell trait (Hampton et al., 1974). Labeling is a smaller problem for population-wide intervention programs, but these also should seek to promote healthful change in behavior without inducing anxiety in noncompliers. It is likely that interventions that alter tastes at young ages avoid many of the psychological costs of giving up harmful foods.

"Preferences" about ways of dying constitute another psychological factor. The reduction of cardiovascular deaths would result in a slightly older population and a small increase in the chances of dying from other causes. Whether death from cancer is viewed as better or worse than death from heart disease depends on one's preference for a particular mode of dying, a gloomy thought but one that nonetheless may alter the apparent cost-effectiveness of a preventive program that shifts mortality patterns.

At what age lives are saved may also be important. The screening programs, by focusing on hypercholesterolemic people, would save life-years at earlier ages than the population-wide programs, an effect that places the screening programs at an advantage if we regard, for example, the fourth decade of life as more valuable than the sixth.

Psychological costs and benefits that are tied to an individual's knowledge of his or her *own* personal risk would have more impact (positive or negative) on the screening programs than on the population-wide programs. The effects of changing mortality and morbidity patterns would be felt more under the population-wide programs, since their scope is so much larger than the screening programs. Even the population-wide programs, however, would have very little effect on the age distribution of our population or on the causes of death.

Multiple risk factor interventions

By confining our attention to interventions on a single cardiovascular risk factor, cholesterol, we have perhaps underrated the preventive programs we examined. The risk factors for heart disease are, in fact, multiple, and as explained in Chapter 2, they interact multiplicatively with each other. Interventions confined to a single risk factor sacrifice the opportunity to capitalize on this interaction, and an analysis of single factor intervention may thereby underestimate the potential efficiency of prevention.

The opportunity to capitalize on multiple risk factors takes several forms.

First, simultaneous reduction of several risk factors may multiply benefits just as the factors together multiply risk. A hypercholesterolemic person who smokes can achieve perhaps three times as much reduction in risk as a person who has one, but not both, risk factors. A screening and intervention program that focuses on "multiple risk" individuals, then, can aim for a greater improvement per patient than can a single program.

Second, interventions to alter risk may echo from factor to factor, and therefore the cost of reducing two risk variables may be far less than twice the cost of reducing one. We know, for example, that some of the costs of screening, such as recruiting screenees, would be no larger for a multiple risk factor intervention program than for a cholesterol program alone.

Furthermore, psychological and sociological theories would predict that some of the goals and facilitators of behavioral change—perceived susceptibility to disease, for example, or motivation to change—remain constant across risk factors. The same program dollar that buys dietary adherence may simultaneously purchase smoking cessation or compliance with antihypertensive medication regimens. Compliance in changing one risk factor may trigger or reinforce compliance with other changes.

Third, even if we ignore the opportunity to intervene on several factors, our calculations have not estimated the secondary effects of a cholesterol-lowering diet on risk. For instance, calorie restriction, which is a feature of a prudent cholesterol diet, would for many patients reduce body weight, which would not only lower cholesterol further but also might help lower blood pressure. The less obese one is, furthermore, the more she or he may exercise, helping once again to lower both cholesterol and blood pressure levels.

Data permitting calculations of the efficiency of multiple risk factor intervention will emerge in the next few years, as the results of several large studies take shape. We anticipate that such data will be more favorable to multifactor screening programs than our constrained investigation of single factor screening.

The potential for multiple risk factor intervention has more positive implications for the screening programs than for the Population-wide programs and probably offers more advantage to Targeted Screening than to Universal Screening. The reason is that any factor that increases potential benefit to high-risk individuals more than it increases benefit to low-risk individuals would improve the cost-effectiveness of screening. Being able to aim efforts at multiple risk factors has the same impact on efficiency as does an increase in the curvature of a risk factor/risk relationship, making the identification of high-risk individuals a more productive enterprise.

Secular trends and spontaneous change

We have tacitly compared each of the programs investigated with an unchanging status quo, assigning that status quo a reference value of zero. As any reader of the lay press knows, however, the status quo in cardiovascular disease is hardly unchanging. Between 1968 and 1975 the coronary heart disease mortality rate in people aged 35 to 74 fell 19 percent for white males and 24 percent for white females in the United States, for reasons that remain unclear (Stamler, 1978). It is difficult to predict whether this trend will continue, but if it does, our models will have overestimated the benefits of intervention; after all, we cannot take credit for preventing disease that would not have occurred in the first place.

Such uncertainties about the future increase the relative desirability of programs with small front-end costs, which realize benefits early and which can be discontinued abruptly without serious loss. In this light, Mass Media programs, which may involve the development and amortization of expensive program materials and which may require long-term operation to produce effects, are perhaps the most precarious of all, and the screening programs are perhaps the least threatened by secular improvements in risk. For these and other reasons, it will be important to discover if the results of the media campaigns in the Stanford and North Karelia studies are sustained after the discontinuation of those campaigns or if repeated or continuous public education is required to maintain healthful changes in life-styles in a community.

Program interactions

Although we have treated Universal Screening, Targeted Screening, Mass Media compaigns and their relatives as if they were mutually exclusive options, they are not. The combination of Mass Media and Targeted Screening, for example, is easy to imagine, and their benefits may be nearly additive. Other combinations seem less logical. Targeted Screening and Universal Screening, for instance, make little sense as joint programs, since the whole point of the family history questionnaire is to use an inexpensive means of *avoiding* measuring everyone's cholesterol level. In general, any of the population-wide programs could be used in conjunction with any of the screening programs with only slight decrements in the cost-effectiveness of each. One must wonder, however, whether the impact of a Universal Screening program might be to reassure a negative screenee falsely that he or she need pay no attention to a media campaign and thereby render the population-wide effort less effective.

Alternatives to early prevention

Concentrating on pediatric prevention, we have not evaluated other worthwhile ways to deal with our burden of coronary heart disease. For one, we have not dealt fully with prevention in adulthood, specifically with the possiblity that early atherosclerotic lesions may be capable of regression.

If the established lesions of atherosclerosis are reversible through dietary interventions, then a program of early prevention obviously has no substantial advantage over a "curative" program. Given the same ultimate health outcome, it would be far more efficient to reverse disease in a 40-year-old than to prevent disease in a 10-year-old. Determining the degree of reversibility of atherosclerotic lesions should be a research enterprise of high priority.

Another alternative not examined here is an assault on coronary-disease-related death through emergency medical interventions. Stress test screening for silent coronary disease and expansion of emergency medical capabilities are both being explored actively as alternatives or supplements to primary prevention. Although the potential savings from active coronary resuscitation training programs are not enormous, they are far from negligible, and because benefits are immediate, discounting is much less an issue than in pediatric prevention. Cretin's (1977b) comparison analyses of primary prevention and emergency medical services find the latter to have substantial advantages when discount rates are high.

Scope and equity

In a simplified world, we may wish to choose public programs solely in ascending order of cost-effectiveness. If we wish to "save life-years" with a limited budget, we would simply instruct a computer to begin buying life-years through the most efficient program until potential clients for that program were exhausted, then to move to the next most efficient program, and so on until the budget has been used up. Of course, some programs may appear as "take-it-or-leave-it" packages, and although the program may be efficient, the package price may exceed the budget available. Mass Media campaigns, for example, may require a minimum threshold expenditure to begin to produce effects in the target audience, and that threshold may exceed available funds. In that case, second-best programs must be purchased, with some sacrifice in cost-effectiveness.

In reality, however, rarely can we rely only on considerations of cost-effectiveness and budget to select from among possible programs. At least two other constraints frequently apply: requirements of scope and requirements of equity.

Constraints on scope depend on both the resources and the jurisdiction of the decision maker. The public health officer for a small town may accept our estimate of Mass Media as nearly five times more cost-effective than Universal Screening but may nonetheless find the observation irrelevant. A small town is unlikely to be able to mount a media campaign, at least one using primarily television and radio, without enormous waste in the population reached, and so the public health officer may choose to consider seriously only the screening programs, since they can be scaled down easily to a small population. Similarly, a public health commissioner may notice that Targeted Screening, although more efficient than Universal Screening, has a much smaller potential aggregate impact. Lacking the administrative resources to mount the programs in sequence (using the most efficient first), the commissioner may reasonably decide to use only the program of wider scope, getting a higher total benefit, albeit at a higher cost per unit of benefit.

For decision makers at a community or regional level, some of the figures in the summary tables at the end of Chapter 6 are too global to be useful, being calculated on a nationwide scale. Trade-offs come into sharper focus if we describe the performance of the three major programs as they would apply to a smaller population, say a city of 100,000 inhabitants. The public health commissioner of such a city would have in his or her charge some 1400 ten-year-old children, spread through 15 to 20 elementary schools. The health department's annual budget would typically include between $1 million and $1.5 million for surveillance, health code enforcement, school health, and administration, excluding the budget of city hospitals and other major municipally owned facilities.

Table 7–2. Three Options for a City of 100,000

	Universal screening	*Targeted screening*	*Mass media*
Reach of program			
Number of people screened yearly	1,400	1400—Questionnaire 12—Cholesterol	0
Number of people "treated" yearly	49*	7	100,000 (1400 ten-year-olds)
Optimal annual budget†			
Screening costs	$ 1,400	$360	0
Treatment costs	$17,600	$2,500	$50,000
Total costs	$19,000	$2,860	$50,000
Cost-effectiveness			
Total life-years added per year (undiscounted)	25.0	5.2	169.5
Cost per year of life saved‡	$10,000	$7,100	$3,200

*Calculated at a discount rate of 5%. If the discount rate is 0%, then 45 people are treated at the optimum.

†Optimal budget is calculated assuming a discount rate of 5%. At a discount rate of 0%, $1400 less is spent for treatment under Universal Screening. The other figures remain unchanged.

‡Cost per year of life saved for males and females weighted by the number of years saved in each sex. Costs and benefits discounted at 5%.

Table 7-2 shows how Universal Screening, Targeted Screening, and Mass Media programs to control cholesterol look to the commissioner of our hypothetical city. In actual fact, a city of 100,000 people may be too small a base for a well-designed media campaign, and so it may be more realistic to consider that possibility as if it were an option to buy shares in a consortium of neighboring municipalities to design and operate a Mass Media program jointly.

The differences in scope are striking. Targeted Screening appears as a tiny program—a potential afterthought to a million dollar budget—with comparably small returns. The Universal Screening and Mass Media programs appear more ambitious, with budgets comparable to the salaries of one or two full-time departmental employees.

If the health department's program budget were $1 million overall, then Targeted Screening would consume less than 0.3 percent of it, Universal Screening would use nearly 2 percent, and Mass Media efforts would use 5 percent.

By assumption, the cost-effectiveness of the program is the same as previously calculated, but the commissioner may also be interested in the total health gains for the community. Universal Screening without discounting adds about 25 life-years per year of program operation, Targeted Screening adds almost 6 life-years, and Mass Media adds over 169 life-years. At a discount rate of 5 percent the gains are less than one-tenth as large.

Even given programs of similar scope, considerations of equity and distributional imperatives may limit choice. Whether to mount programs for men, for women, or for both is clearly a matter for decision, but the decision maker may go well beyond mere cost-effectiveness in making that choice. A purist would recommend directing programs first at the sex with the greater cost-effectiveness and treating the other sex only after all of the first had been dealt with. A pragmatist, however, may notice political hazard in offering services only to men or only to women for a disease that both can get and so may sacrifice efficiency in the interest of an equitable distribution of services. Similarly, the rights of today's elderly may be insisted upon in selecting between a program for children and a less efficient program for older adults.

In a rigorous cost-effectiveness analysis, these political and administrative constraints could be represented formally as benefits sought (improved equity or wider scope) or costs incurred (maldistribution of benefits or limitation of impact). Such quantitative translations are difficult to make, however, and we prefer to regard these as superimposed considerations to be used in interpreting the narrower cost-effectiveness ratios that we do supply.

Flexibility

One program feature that is difficult to represent numerically but is important in rating alternatives is the adaptability of a program to changing circumstances. We have already noted that Mass Media programs that require sustained efforts may be undesirable in politically unstable contexts. A screening program aborted by an administration with an extraordinarily low priority on health care may nonetheless reap the benefits expected in our model for the cohorts already treated. An aborted Mass Media program, on the other hand, could conceivably represent wasted money—incurring high cost and no substantial effect. Alternative strategies must be reviewed with an eye toward those relevant circumstances that seem likely to change in the future, and it may be better in the end to select programs of higher durability even if they are less cost-effective.

One element of flexibility that is of special importance is the "testability" of programs on a small scale. Given uncertainties in actual performance, one may desire to see a program function on a small scale before buying the full-scale version. Pilot programs permit confirmation of guesses about performance and also allow modifications that improve efficiency in ways not anticipated in the planning stages. Indeed, the perfectability of a program—the chance that ways will be found to improve it—can itself be a desirable component of flexibility. To be testable, a cholesterol-reducing program must be capable of expansion from small to large versions without important distortions in performance and must have measurable intermediate outcomes that bear a close relationship to the actually desired ultimate outcomes. Screening programs, whose effects are expected to be more discernible than population-wide program effects, may therefore be easier to improve as time goes by.

We regard Targeted Screening as one of the most testable and flexible of the programs we have examined. It is relatively adaptable to a small scale (a single community, for example); its performance may be measured in terms of questionnaire yield, screening and intervention costs, and cholesterol reduction; and one would expect its performance on a small scale to be similar to that on a large scale, at least for the first few years of operation. Furthermore, since it treats mainly cohorts of individuals, its achievements at each stage do not depend on its own future.

Prolonging life and preserving health

The health outcomes of preventive programs have been expressed here in two categories: the prolongation of life (years of life saved) and the postponement of nonfatal disease (heart-disease-free and stroke-free years added). We have not even tried to express these in common units. How to trade off such different benefits against each other is an important value decision that deserves public discussion.

The relative weight assigned to these different outcomes, as we have seen, directly affects the relative attractiveness of the different programs. Programs for women fare better than programs for men in preserving life, but they fare worse in postponing disease. Even within sexes, anomalous rank orders exist, although the effects are small. For example, for women, Sequential Rescreening gives slightly more expected days of life per complier than does Universal Screening but slightly fewer added days free of heart disease. We have not estimated stroke-free days for many of the programs, since the magnitude of that benefit seems so small in comparison with others, but even the delay of stroke could affect rank ordering if it were for some reason valued extremely highly. For example, Universal Screening delays heart attack more efficiently for men but delays strokes more efficiently for women.

The conversion of years of life *with* a stroke or *with* a nonfatal infarction into equivalent years of fully healthy life, a conversion attempted by Weinstein and Stason (1976) and by Bush et al. (1972) among others, is one way to deal with this problem of multiple outcomes. This approach, has several serious problems, however. It generally imposes a simple linear trade-off between years of life with disability and years of life without disability, whereas the real preferences of people are probably far more complex. More importantly, such conversions tend to impose the analyst's values on the results in a way that makes it difficult for people with different values to use those results.

WHICH PROGRAMS ARE BEST?

Given the warnings, the omissions, and the uncertainties, what conclusions about the programs can our results support? How do cholesterol-reducing programs compare with other health-enhancing programs, and how do they compare with each other?

Compared with the health programs we reviewed earlier in this chapter, every cholesterol-lowering programs we analyzed—Univeral Screening, Targeted Screening, School Education, and Mass Media—is at least competitive with existing health programs on the grounds of cost-effectiveness. Universal Screening, at a cost of roughly $10,000 per year of life saved, is certainly at the high end of the spectrum, but it is still better than screening children for tuberculosis or treating end-stage kidney disease with dialysis programs. Targeted Screening (at about $7000 per year of life saved) and School Education (at $5000 per year of life saved) have a yield typical of many other health programs, including hypertension screening, phenylketonuria screening, and the most efficient forms of cancer screening. Mass Media, at a cost of a little over $2000 per year of life saved, is as good as any other health program for which we have found comparable evaluations.

We are admittedly uncomfortable with reporting only point estimates of the cost-effectiveness of the programs we have analyzed. We feel it important to ask, therefore, how our cholesterol programs fare when we look at the *ranges* of estimates of cost per year of life as projected in our composite sensitivity analysis. We are especially interested in how the cholesterol programs compare with others when their cost-effectiveness is at the *high end* of the estimated range.

As detailed in Chapter 6, we have attempted to construct ranges that have a 2:1 chance of including the true value of the cost-effectiveness for each program. In other words, there is roughly one chance in three that the true value lies outside the range, or one chance in six that it lies above and one chance in six that it lies below the stated range.

To review, our range estimates for cost per year of life saved at a discount rate of 5 percent are as follows:

For Universal Screening:
From $5500 to $20,700 for men
and from $4900 to $17,700 for women
For Targeted Screening:
From $3000 to $12,500 for men
and from $3400 to $14,200 for women
For School Education:
From $2100 to $12,300 for men
and from $2800 to $15,300 for women
For Mass Media:
From $1000 to $4300 for men
and from $1800 to $7900 for women

Although we do not have comparable range estimates for the other health programs reviewed in Table 7-1, it seems that in comparison with efforts in other health fields, Universal Screening, in particular, may well be too costly a program to implement. Targeted Screening and School Education still seem to be worth considering, and Mass Media looks promising indeed despite our uncertainties.

We have, in general, been comparing these programs using a discount rate of 5 percent. Those readers who would choose discount rates other than 5 percent can use our results by recalculating range estimates using as the base case the cost-effectiveness that corresponds to another discount rate. A lower rate would make all the cholesterol programs look much more cost-effective. On the other hand, at a rate as high as 10 percent, these programs would have much higher costs per year of life saved—on the order of $100,000 or more.

It is also true that many of the other health programs listed in Table 7-1 would have very different costs at different discount rates. Some are relatively insensitive to discount rate, however; mobile coronary care units or dialysis, for example, incur costs and yield benefits almost simultaneously.

In terms of efficiency, Mass Media seems by far the best program to implement. However, it is also the program to which we have attached the most caveats. Therefore, before making any summary recommendations, it is important to review the relative advantages and disadvantages of the programs we have analyzed, focusing on the three archetypal programs: Universal Screening, Targeted Screening, and Mass Media. We have summarized some of these considerations in Table 7-3.

Mass Media programs are almost certainly the most cost-effective. They distribute benefits widely through a population, produce the highest absolute benefit per cohort member, and purchase the largest number of added years of life and health in a population of given size at the lowest price per year. On the other hand, as we describe them, the total cost of Mass Media programs is high; they require the largest expenditure per member of the population and cost nearly twice as much as the next most costly program when applied to a population of given size. Furthermore, Mass Media programs in our model are the most dependent on a stable future and run the highest risk of waste if terminated prematurely.

Targeted Screening, through a family history questionnaire, is less cost-effective than Mass Media. On the other hand, it avoids many of the problems of the population-wide program. The yield in added health per cohort member is tiny with Targeted Screening because so few are treated, but the gains per *treated* person are higher than in any other program. Targeted Screening delivers personal services to a group with an extraordinarily high expected benefit in our model. In addition, if Targeted Screening can be implemented in young adulthood with full effect, it looks *better* than School Education, although Mass Media is still the most cost-effective program. The potential scope of a Targeted Screening program is small—an advantage because its total cost for a given population is low, but a disadvantage because its ultimate total impact is so limited. We may reasonably designate Targeted Screening as the best "low-budget" program, when population-wide efforts are not possible.

Universal Screening has few advantages. It is neither as cost-effective as Mass Media nor as limited in total cost as Targeted

Table 7–3. Advantages and Disadvantages: Three Programs

Universal screening
- Advantages
  1. Treats many of the high-risk people
  2. Informs everyone of his or her own level, facilitating individual decisions
  3. Loses little effect through abrupt termination
- Disadvantages
  1. Falsely reassures "negative" screenees and creates anxiety among positive screenees
  2. Incurs high cost per year of life saved
  3. Incurs high total cost per cohort member (or given population)
  4. Invades privacy

Targeted screening
- Advantages
  1. Reaps very large benefits per treated individual
  2. Incurs lower cost per year of life saved than Universal Screening
  3. Incurs low cost per cohort member (or given population)
  4. Loses little effect through abrupt termination
  5. May achieve higher compliance in high-risk families
- Disadvantages
  1. Has small overall scope
  2. Misses many high-risk people
  3. Stigmatizes families
  4. Requires more elaborate administrative structure than Universal Screening
  5. Invades privacy

Mass media
- Advantages
  1. Incurs lowest cost per year of life saved
  2. Addresses the high-risk status of most Americans
  3. Minimizes invasion of privacy
  4. Reaps highest total yield and highest yield per cohort member
- Disadvantages
  1. Incurs highest cost per cohort member (or given population)
  2. May lose a large proportion of benefits through abrupt termination
  3. Incurs high "front-end" costs

Screening. Universal Screening seems a wise purchase only when population-wide programs cannot be mounted and when Targeted Screening seems too small an undertaking. Even under those circumstances, the more rational strategy would be to run a Targeted Screening program first and then to use the leftover budget to screen cholesterol in as many people as the remaining dollars permit.

Under most circumstances, one of two strategies seems to dominate: Mass Media (or some population-wide program) when resources permit and Targeted Screening when resources are limited.

Since many of the parameters about which we have uncertainty affect all of our programs similarly, it is useful to look at the possible

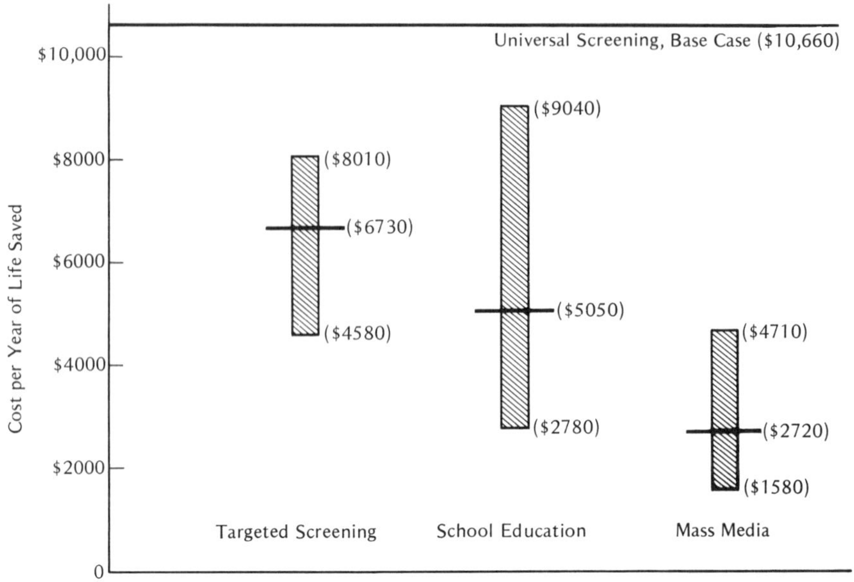

Figure 7-1. Confidence Intervals on Cost per Year of Life Saved Relative to Universal Screening, for Men. The intervals depicted are for the base case ± 1 SD. Calculations for the three indicated programs are done estimating error *only in* those parameters that do not simultaneously affect the cost-effectiveness of Universal Screening; thus the confidence intervals shown are for estimated cost per year of life saved *relative to* Universal Screening.

impact of *independent* uncertainties in changing the order of the programs. If we examine the uncertainty in cost-effectiveness of the three basic programs *relative to* Universal Screening, we see that it is unlikely that Universal Screening would ever emerge as more efficient than Targeted Screening or Mass Media (Figure 7-1).

RECOMMENDATIONS

Although the inherent uncertainties make us cautious, we are comfortable in making at least two recommendations. First, the Mass Media programs that we have analyzed appear so promising that the federal government should consider investing in further pilot or demonstration projects similar to the Stanford study in design and intent. These initial programs would prove more costly than our estimates suggest because they would and should include a substantial component of research directed principally at the following questions:

1. What forms of media intervention (television, newspaper, radio) are effective in changing behavior?
2. How large are the costs and effects of such programs over several years?
3. Which intervention designs—continuous campaigns, pulsed campaigns, or "one-shot" campaigns—are most effective and efficient?
4. Which subgroups of the population (defined by age or other risk factors) respond most readily to and benefit most from these campaigns?

Second, our results lead us to conclude that Targeted Screening is an especially promising type of screening program, especially if benefits can be achieved by such programs implemented among young adults instead of among school-aged children.* Because it is a program of limited scope, Targeted Screening is within the reach of local private or public agencies, such as a local heart association, that wish to address the problem of heart disease but lack the resources for a Population-wide Intervention program. We believe that early screening programs, like early Mass Media campaigns, should include efforts to resolve some of the remaining uncertainties about the efficacy of dietary changes in adulthood. We therefore recommend that the federal government encourage local agencies to undertake pilot Targeted Screening programs by offering to subsidize the research components of such projects. Among the key research questions for such pilot programs are these:

1. What forms of personal intervention (including dietary counseling) are effective?
2. What are the true costs and benefits over several years?
3. What levels of *long-term* compliance can be achieved?
4. How do health benefits decline with the age at which the dietary intervention begins?

With the information gleaned from the kinds of pilot program we have recommended, a second and more precise analytic look at Universal Screening and School Education programs should be possible. If, with new data, these programs then appear to be more promising than they do at first glance, they might be implemented also on a pilot basis.

*Many of the conclusions about Targeted Screening probably apply equally well to a Triggered Screening paradigm, but we have not analyzed the latter completely enough to make firm statements.

GENERAL CONCLUSIONS

Besides the specific recommendations just summarized, our work leads us to a few more global observations about preventive medical undertakings such as the reduction of cholesterol—observations suggested by our explorations, although not proven by them.

The high cost of prevention

It has become common to tout preventive medicine as a bargain when compared with "curative" medicine. Our figures on single factor intervention and screening suggest otherwise. Desirable though it may be on a moral or quality-of-life basis, the prevention of cardiovascular disease through cholesterol screening or dietary intervention on cholesterol is an expensive proposition. The expense may be lessened with a multifactorial approach, but it will still be true that health costs money, whether we seek to cure disease or to prevent it.

Economists use the label "opportunity costs" to denote what we give up when we choose to use our resources for one specific purpose and thereby forgo another. In the prevention of incurable disease, the meaning of this term may seem less obvious. Some argue that if cardiovascular disease cannot be cured but can be prevented, then it is meaningless to speak of what else we might do with the money spent on prevention. Dead people (so goes this argument) have no opportunities at all!

We do not subscribe to this chain of reasoning but believe instead that it is both meaningful and useful to consider alternative uses of resources that would be consumed in the prevention of disease—even of *fatal* disease. Decisions on prevention take place long before death, and rational people may well prefer to have public money spent for them on other enterprises than on disease prevention, even if their lives will thereby be shorter than they could be. In their private lives, people who are well informed of their risks continue to take chances—to drive, to ski, and even to smoke; the issue may not be one of rationality but rather one of preference.

The spending of money now to prolong life later directly and unavoidably raises issues of opportunities lost. Money is, to some extent, a determinant of quality of life in America, and it is far from absurd to ask how much money it is worth to each of us now in order to purchase some weeks or months or years of extra life in the distant future. Alexander the Great is said to have chosen a short and glorious life over a long and undistinguished one. Our individual preference may differ, but the possibility for choice remains.

The high cost of screening

Our investigation suggests that screening is an undertaking of limited value when treatment would be of positive benefit to the average member of the screened population. The mere existence of especially high-risk individuals does not automatically "prove" that screening is a useful strategy. Instead, its usefulness depends on the prevalence of the risk factor, on the exact relationship between risk and risk factor, and on the difference in benefit between treating a "positive" screenee and a random individual. It is simply not true that screening is efficient *whenever* a subgroup of a population is at high risk for a preventable condition.

When dealing with a continuously distributed risk variable like cholesterol, screening does have a peculiar form of insurance; namely its mistakes are not costly. In a search for a dichotomous disease whose natural history is bad or whose treatment is costly, a mistake in testing—a false-positive or a false-negative result—may be tragic; but for a continuous variable, such a tragedy is not likely. The screenee "mistakenly" placed just below or just above the cutoff for treatment suffers no irremediable loss. The person "mistakenly" treated thereby gains benefits not much different from those achieved by a "true positive." And the person who is "mistakenly" not treated is in a condition hardly distinguishable from a "true negative." If screening for such a risk variable is expensive, it is also rather immune to the consequences of error.

A corollary of this observation is that precision in measurement may be less critical in screening for continuous risk variables than for dichotomous disease states. This effect emerged in our analysis of Universal Rescreening in Chapter 4, a strategy that did, in fact, yield more precise cholesterol measurements than a single screen but resulted in a *decay,* not an improvement, in cost-effectiveness.

The critical role of discounting

We have stressed that the discount rate is the most powerful determinant of absolute cost-effectiveness and a frequent determinant of relative cost-effectiveness. It does not seem possible for rational policy to be made in the prevention of adult disease, especially through intervention in childhood, until discounting is both understood and agreed upon.

The importance of small effects

With a disease as prevalent as atherosclerosis and a risk factor as widespread as elevated cholesterol level, even tiny changes in risk are important. When we discussed Population-wide Intervention programs, we noted that reduction in average cholesterol level as small as 1 or 2 mg/dl would, under some quite plausible circumstances, be enough to make those programs cost-effective in comparison with screening. A small reduction in cardiovascular mortality rates (to 95 percent of their current level, for example) would avert more deaths yearly than are attributed to all motor vehicle accidents.

Figures like these pose a problem, namely that we *care* about effects that are too small to observe in experiments of reasonable size. We will have more to say about this in discussing public health research.

The contributions and limitations of research

Our journey through the volumes of information available on cholesterol and heart disease has made us aware of some thematic strengths and weaknesses in these accumulated data. Identifying some of those themes may help to direct future research efforts.

First, we notice that the *importance* of a research question to the evaluation and design of preventive strategies sometimes bears little relationship to the amount of research effort that has been devoted to answering that question. For example, we believe that the critical question, "How can physicians influence their clients to behave more healthfully?" has not received attention in the medical literature commensurate with its importance. Work on behavioral change that has been brought to the attention of physicians offers some attractive theoretical paradigms (e.g., the Health Belief Model), but few writers provide either specific instructions of direct applicability to clinical practice or specific intervention models that have been subjected to controlled scientific scrutiny. Recent experiments, especially the Stanford Heart Disease Prevention Program and the Multiple Risk Factor Intervention Trials, have woven into their designs rich collaborative efforts between behavioral scientists and medical researchers, but guidelines for generalizing their experience do not exist. We regard research into generalizable and cost-effective techniques for changing health-related behaviors, including both Mass Media and personal counseling, as an essential substrate for the design of rational preventive strategies.

Paradoxically, studies of compliance, intervention costs, and behavioral change, the results of which are observable over short time periods, are in theory easier to conduct than the massive longitudinal epidemiological trials that are well represented in our literature. The relative rarity of studies of behavioral change in medical journals probably implies that there has been little demand for them, not that they are difficult to carry out.

Suppose, for example, that we wish to compare two programs, Program A and Program B, both of which have the goal of reducing cardiovascular morbidity by reducing cholesterol levels. Suppose, further, that Program A is expected to achieve a compliance rate of 50 percent and an average cholesterol reduction of 4 percent, while Program B is expected to achieve 25 percent compliance and a cholesterol reduction of 2 percent. Finally, consistent with our model of benefits, suppose that the incidence of new ischemic heart disease under Program A over five years would be about 5 percent, and under Program B, about 5.1 percent.

We can calculate that in order to have an 80 percent chance of observing differences between these two programs which are statistically significant at the 5 percent level, we would need 47 people in each experimental program to test compliance, 540 people in each group to test change in cholesterol level, and 5890 people in each group to detect differences in heart disease incidence. Under these circumstances, an experiment on behavioral change would be both less costly and more quickly fruitful than one on cholesterol reduction or change in morbidity.

Second, in some areas we have noted a degree of redundancy that goes far beyond the bounds of reasonable and useful replication of research results. There seems little deterrent to generating studies whose marginal information content is small. On the other hand, in some instances, definitive work on important questions failed to emerge over decades even though the conceptual barriers to proper study design were minimal. Since the 1940s, for example, we find literally scores of reports of umbilical cord blood cholesterol levels in newborn infants in groups of 10 or 20 subjects; almost all of these studies could have been (and eventually were) supplanted by a single large series or two, which finally were reported in the early 1970s.

Meanwhile, through nearly three decades, not a single effective large study was mounted that tracked infant cholesterol levels into childhood. Even though the relationship between cholesterol and heart disease has been surmised for well over a generation, we do not, even today, have a single completed prospective study that simply follows children's lipid levels through adolescence and into middle adulthood. Only in the middle and late 1970s have we begun to accumulate meaningful information on the stability of cholesterol rank order even *within* childhood over as short a period as six years.

Third, we are impressed with the special value of two sorts of investigation—longitudinal epidemiological studies and exploration into biochemical mechanisms—in forming policy. Appropriately analyzed data from the former, of which the Framingham study is the archetype, seem to provide information with tighter confidence intervals and less vulnerability to criticism of methodology than do data from cross-sectional studies or observational comparisons of different populations. Biological research that provides a rational understanding of underlying physiological mechanisms, work such as that on dietary determinants of cholesterol or cellular control of lipoprotein levels, seems to hold the greatest ultimate promise of confidence in the efficacy of intervention.

Fourth, as noted above, we have become impressed with the smallness of the effects in which we are interested. As we try to change the public's health, alterations in average cholesterol level of a few milligrams per deciliter or changes in morbidity rates of a few percentage points may be all that we can realistically hope to achieve with available resources, at least in the short run. Such small effects are nonetheless important, and it is rational to try to maximize even these tiny changes.

A problem arises, however, when we seek to *measure* these small effects in population-based experiments. Sources of variance are so complex in social experimentation that investigations of enormous size and complexity would be required to detect with confidence the results about which we care. Under such circumstances, when we want to demonstrate small changes in the rates of rare events through interventions with delayed effects, null results or confounded results are to be expected and are, in fact, not very interesting. Such results tell us only that our experiment was insufficiently powerful; they offer little new information about the real world or about the fruits of our labors. In the preventive programs we have discussed, we must deal with the frustrating truth that *we both value and (if our assumptions about biology and behavior are not too errant) expect health outcomes that are often too small and too delayed to be measured reliably by experiments of reasonable size and cost.* Such frustration makes even more attractive the elucidation of biochemical or genetic mechanisms, which may give us more confidence that the small effects will occur, even if undetectable, and may identify intermediate outcome variables that correlate well with health outcomes but are easier to measure.

FINAL THOUGHTS: THE ROLE OF POLICY RESEARCH

The writing of this book has consumed many months of effort, and yet not a single new piece of empirical data is reported, not a single factual controversy is resolved. To what end, then, have we written? What is the contribution of our research?

Our contribution lies, we believe, in the *organization of information;* that is, we have sought to provide a useful way to organize a sometimes overwhelming body of scientific and quasi-scientific data to address a controversial and important question in health policy. In no sense does this kind of policy research *replace* scientific experimentation or clinical investigation. Indeed, in areas where results are clear-cut, the "right" policy may be obvious, and policy research may be a waste of time. In many health areas, however, such as in preventive cardiology, scientific results are far from clear-cut, and the medical research community may, in the midst of controversy, become so polarized that each new study serves not to clarify but to raise new uncertainties and to further fuel the flames of controversy. Sometimes such controversy over health management issues has no important impact on our national health policies, but when the costs are very high or the condition very common, policymakers do have a stake in resolving the uncertainty. How we decide to manage such costly treatments as dialysis for end-stage renal disease, bone marrow transplantation for leukemia, and coronary artery bypass surgery for ischemic heart disease will have important implications for our national health care costs and opportunities. Similar challenges in the proper management of uncertainty will be taking shape rapidly, we believe, in the field of disease prevention.

In such cases as these, policy research may play an important role. In the process of organizing and reviewing what is known, the reasons for uncertainty may be clarified, and the research and policy communities may become more fully informed about exactly what further studies are most needed.

When the potential areas for research are many, as is the case with cholesterol, policy research can help to shape research priorities *from the perspective of policy,* which may not coincide with the perspective of science. We have little reason to believe that those issues that seem most important to a biomedical scientist will necessarily be pivotal in formulating a sound national policy toward cholesterol. On the other hand, scientifically mundane issues that fail to excite the biomedical research community may have important consequences for policy. The exact incidence of monogenic hyperlipidemia, for example, is of far more importance to geneticists than it is in determining the cost-effectiveness of screening programs for cholesterol. On the other hand, how well people comply with dietary changes over several years is a critical policy question that has not yet been thoroughly explored.

The justifiable interest of our government in promoting those forms of scientific research that help us to understand our world has a long and successful tradition. Government stops short of its best opportunities, however, if it encourages the *creation* of information without providing for the systematic *organization* of that information. Public policy should promote research that will help to formulate long-term and short-term policies, even when that research does not seem to be of prime importance to scientists. As our world grows more technical and complex, and as government takes a more active role in shaping, regulating, and financing what we do, the need grows not just to expand our technical knowledge but also to organize it and place it at the service of human societal goals. Meeting that need is both the real objective and the ultimate test of policy research.

Appendix A. The benefits model

Our analysis employs three different measures of the benefit of lowering serum cholesterol levels: added years of life, added years of life *prior* to the first coronary heart disease, and added years of life *prior* to the first stroke. To predict the values of these three measures associated with a particular program, we employ variations of one basic model of the effects of lowering cholesterol level on cardiovascular morbidity and mortality.

The basic idea of all three models is the same. If we know (1) the sex- and age-specific cardiovascular mortality (or the sex- and age-specific incidence of first coronary heart disease (CHD) or first stroke) associated with a given cholesterol level, and (2) the sex- and age-specific mortality from noncardiovascular causes (which are assumed to be independent of cholesterol level), then we can use a life-table calculation to estimate for 30-year-old men and women the remaining life expectancy (or the expected time to the first coronary disease event or first stroke) as a function of cholesterol level. It is then an easy matter to estimate the change in life expectancy associated with a specific change in cholesterol level. In using this model, we assume that an individual's true cholesterol level stabilizes at age 30 and (owing to the infrequency of atherosclerotic cardiovascular events before that age) that all significant benefits accrue after age 30.

The primary source for the needed age- and cholesterol-specific risk data is the Framingham study, a longitudinal study of approximately 5000 adults (ages 30 to 62 at the initiation of the study) who have been followed closely, with biennial examinations, since 1948 (Kannel and Gordon, 1970a, 1970b). Ideally, such a study would directly supply the needed estimates of age-, sex-, and cholesterol-specific risks. Despite the size of the panel, however, the number of individuals in each age, sex, and cholesterol level group is too small to produce reliable estimates of the risks in that group. Instead, the Framingham analysts assumed that the general functional form relating risk and cholesterol level was of a special type called a "logistic function" (see Figure A-1), and the data were pooled over these broad age groups to estimate the parameters of this logistic function. The logistic function is a log-linear model that well represents many risk relationships.

The logistic equation is

$$\log\left(\frac{P}{1-P}\right) = (\alpha + \beta X)$$

where P is the probability of an event (death, myocardial infarction, or stroke), X is the standardized cholesterol score, and α and β are the logistic parameters. Solving for P, we get

$$P = \frac{\exp(\alpha + \beta X)}{1 + \exp(\alpha + \beta X)}$$

Figure A-1 shows the general form of the function. When P is very small, the relationship between P and X is approximately exponential. In this case,

$$\frac{P}{1-P} \simeq P$$

therefore,

$$\log\left(\frac{P}{1-P}\right) \simeq \log(P) \simeq (\alpha + \beta X)$$

$$P \simeq \exp(\alpha + \beta X)$$

The advantage of the logistic model over a simple exponential model is that the logistic model results in a natural upper bound on P of 1, while the exponential model has no such bound. When P is less than .05, however, the error introduced by using an exponential approximation to the logistic function is less than 5 percent.

After deciding to represent the risk of heart disease by a logistic model based on the Framingham data, we must choose a statistical method to estimate the parameters α and β. First, we consider the problem of estimating α.

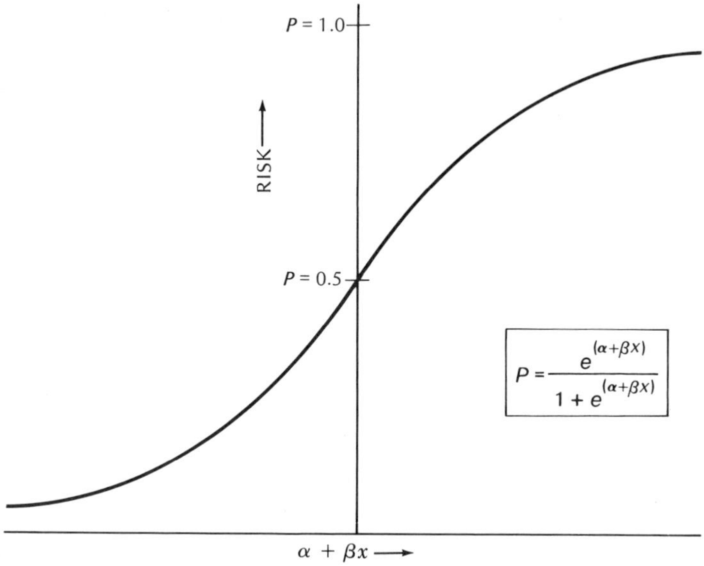

Figure A-1. General Form of the Logistic Function for Risk.

The Framingham data were collected in the years 1950 to 1970. During that time, the Framingham population was observed to be healthier than the U.S. population as a whole. There are several possible reasons for this: for example, individuals with preexisting heart disease were intentionally excluded from the study, and in addition, institutionalized or bedridden individuals were unable to appear for the intake examination. We make the assumption that while the Framingham population may not reflect the average mortality and morbidity experience of the population as a whole, it does accurately reflect the multiplicative effects of cholesterol level on mortality and morbidity. In other words, we apply the Framingham logistic model of risk of cardiovascular disease to the U.S. population as a whole, using the β parameters estimated from the Framingham data, but we reestimate the α parameters to conform to nationally observed mortality.

In order to reestimate the α parameters, we must first describe the relationship between the logistic parameters and the average mortality rates in a specific age and sex group. The expected or average mortality $\overline{M}_i$ is given by

$$\overline{M}_i = \int_{-\infty}^{+\infty} M_{i|X} F_i(X)\, dx \qquad \text{(A.1)}$$

where $\overline{M}_i$ is the average mortality in the ith age–sex group,
X is the standardized cholesterol score,

$M_{i|X}$ is the mortality in the ith age–sex group given a cholesterol level of X, and

$F_i(X)$ is the distribution of cholesterol in the ith age–sex group.

Assuming that $M_{i|X}$ is given by the logistic model

$$M_{i|X} = \frac{\exp(\alpha + \beta X)}{1 + \exp(\alpha + \beta X)}$$

and that $F_i(X)$ is normally distributed with mean of 0 and standard deviation of 1 (i.e., X is a standardized variable), then

$$F_i(X) = \frac{1}{\sqrt{2\pi}} \exp\left(\frac{-X^2}{2}\right)$$

and we can rewrite equation A.1 as

$$\overline{M}_i = \int_{-\infty}^{+\infty} \frac{\exp(\alpha + \beta X)}{1 + \exp(\alpha + \beta X)} \frac{1}{\sqrt{2\pi}} \exp\left(\frac{-X^2}{2}\right) dX$$

For the values of α and β observed in the Framingham data and for X in the range -3 to $+3$ SD, the logistic is well approximated by the exponential equation

$$\overline{M}_{i|X} \cong \exp(\alpha + \beta X)$$

Outside this range of X values (-3 to $+3$ SD) the approximation begins to degrade, but the value of the normal density function rapidly goes to zero, so that the average mortality may be approximated by

$$\overline{M}_i \cong \exp(\alpha) \int_{-\infty}^{+\infty} \frac{1}{\sqrt{2\pi}} \exp\left(-\frac{X^2}{2} + \beta X\right) dX$$

Completing the square, we have

$$\overline{M}_i \cong \exp(\alpha) \int_{-\infty}^{+\infty} \frac{1}{\sqrt{2\pi}} \exp\left(\frac{-(X^2 - 2\beta X + \beta^2 - \beta^2)}{2}\right) dX$$

$$\cong \exp(\alpha) \int_{-\infty}^{+\infty} \frac{1}{\sqrt{2\pi}} \exp\left(\frac{-(X^2 - \beta)^2}{2}\right) \exp\left(\frac{\beta^2}{2}\right) dX$$

$$\cong \exp\left(\alpha + \frac{\beta^2}{2}\right) \int_{-\infty}^{+\infty} \frac{1}{\sqrt{2\pi}} \exp\left(\frac{-(X - \beta)^2}{2}\right) dX$$

Since the expression to the right of the integral is just the normal density with a mean of β,

$$\int_{-\infty}^{+\infty} \frac{1}{\sqrt{2\pi}} \exp\left\{\frac{-(X - \beta)^2}{2}\right\} = 1$$

And

$$\overline{M}_i \cong \exp(\alpha + \beta^2/2)$$

This expression is just the exponential approximation to the logistic evaluation at $X = \beta/2$. Thus the average cardiovascular mortality is approximately equal to the cardiovascular mortality for an individual with a cholesterol level at $\beta/2$ standard deviations above the mean. Using this fact, we can then use the Framingham β parameters in conjunction with cardiovascular mortality reported in the Vital Statistics of the United States (1977) to estimate population-wide mortality as a function of cholesterol. In particular,

$$\exp(\alpha) \cong \frac{\overline{M}_i}{\exp(\beta^2/2)}$$

since

$$M_{i|X} = \exp(\alpha + \beta X) = \exp(\alpha) \cdot \exp(\beta X)$$

$$M_{i|X} = \frac{\overline{M}_i \exp(\beta X)}{\exp(\beta^2/2)}.$$

where $\overline{M}_i$ for one-year age intervals is derived from the five-year interval, age-specific coronary heart disease mortality reported in *Vital Statistics of the United States* (Table A-1). This derivation assumes that the proportion of coronary deaths for each one-year interval within a five-year group is the same as the proportion of all deaths for each year within the five-year group. Information on the number of deaths for each year is obtained from the National Center for Health Statistics complete life table (see Table A-2).

Estimating β presents a more complex problem, since there are several statistical methods that may be applied. We will describe four different approaches to estimation below and explain our choice among them.

The Framingham analysts used Berkson's "minimum logit Chi-squared" technique for all their reported results (Berkson, 1955). These estimates can be used for nonnormal or noncontinuous

Table A–1. Age-specific mortality rates from diseases of the heart (Rates reported per 100,000 population)

Age	*Males*	*Females*
30–34	19.6	9.1
35–39	54.6	19.9
40–44	130.5	39.0
45–49	265.4	72.2
50–54	449.3	130.3
55–59	766.7	243.1
60–64	1,169.4	429.2
65–69	1,709.3	722.6
70–74	2,581.1	1,349.5
75–79	3,897.0	2,423.6
80–84	5,544.4	3,928.5
85 +	9,308.6	7,916.8

Source. Vital Statistics of the United States, vol. II, Mortality, Part A, 1973. Rockville, Md.: U.S. Dept. of Health, Education and Welfare, Health Resources Administration, National Center for Health Statistics, 1977, adapted from Table 1–8.

explanatory variables, such as smoking status, and such yes-no variables as suspicious electrocardiogram (ECG) findings and glucose intolerance. These estimates perform better than maximum likelihood estimates (MLE) even for normally distributed explanatory variables, except when the probability of the events being analyzed is very small ($p = .02$) or very large ($p = .98$). Intuitively, what goes wrong with this method for very rare events is that its technique of adding 0.5 fictitious

Table A–2. Number of survivors at single years of age, out of 100,000 born alive, by sex: United States, 1973

Age	*Male*	*Female*
30	94,354	96,833
31	94,158	96,742
32	93,958	96,644
33	93,752	96,539
34	93,536	96,425
35	93,307	96,301
36	93,063	96,165
37	92,801	96,017
38	92,520	95,856
39	92,219	95,680
40	91,896	95,489
41	91,550	95,282
42	91,177	95,057
43	90,770	94,812

Table A–2 (Continued)

Age	*Male*	*Female*
44	90,323	94,544
45	89,830	94,251
46	89,285	93,929
47	88,687	93,578
48	88,037	93,199
49	87,338	92,794
50	86,592	92,363
51	85,798	91,906
52	84,949	91,419
53	84,032	90,896
54	83,032	90,329
55	81,936	89,711
56	80,739	89,038
57	79,441	88,310
58	78,041	87,526
59	76,540	86,689
60	74,940	85,800
61	73,238	84,854
62	71,435	83,846
63	69,533	82,775
64	67,537	81,640
65	65,450	80,439
66	63,276	79,169
67	61,018	77,821
68	58,672	76,378
69	56,233	74,816
70	53,700	73,118
71	51,082	71,282
72	48,389	69,306
73	45,627	67,174
74	42,803	64,870
75	39,929	62,383
76	37,020	59,717
77	34,097	56,885
78	31,186	53,908
79	28,315	50,811
80	25,513	47,621
81	22,811	44,365
82	20,241	41,069
83	17,836	37,758
84	15,631	34,458
85	13,662	31,192

Source. Vital Statistics of the United States, vol. II., Mortality, Section 5: Life Tables, 1973. Rockville, Md.: U.S. Department of Health, Education, and Welfare, Health Resources Administration, National Center for Health Statistics, 1977, adapted from Table 5–2.

events to any category with zero events can understate true effects. For example, in women aged 45 to 54, the method attributes a total of two fictitious events to individuals with cholesterol levels below 234 mg/dl, when in fact there were no events below this level and only six real events above this level.

Maximum likelihood estimation, which in this case is normal discriminant analysis, assumes that the explanatory variable (in this case, cholesterol) is normally distributed and that the only difference in the distributions that characterize people with and without an event is a shift in the means. The number of events even in the older men in the Framingham study is too small to test conclusively as to whether those with events have a normal distribution of cholesterol values with the same variance as those without, although casual inspection makes this plausible. However, Goldstein's study of 500 survivors of myocardial infarction shows that those survivors, at least, do satisfy the assumption (Goldstein et al., 1973a, 1973b). In our particular situation— regression of rare events (such as we observe for deaths, heart attack, and stroke) on cholesterol—MLE should perform best, and it is these estimates we will use in our analysis (Efron, 1975).

We perform the estimation using log cholesterol values, since we assume cholesterol is log-normally distributed (see Appendix D).

Conditional maximum likelihood estimation (CMLE) is a third technique and is based on assumptions similar to those of MLE except that the independent variables are taken as fixed values and are not assumed to come from any particular distribution.

The fourth method could be called the "median method." We observe that the median or mean log cholesterol level of those people who have fatal events is approximately equal to β. The mean log cholesterol for those dying of coronary disease in the ith age–sex group, for example, is

$$E_i\,(X|\text{death}) = \int_{-\infty}^{+\infty} X\,f_i\,(X|\text{death})\,dX$$

where $f_i\,(X|\text{death})$ is the conditional distribution of log cholesterol in those who died.

But by Bayes' rule,

$$f_i\,(X|\text{death}) = \frac{M_{i|X} f_i(X)}{\overline{M}_i}$$

where $M_{i|X}$ is the conditional mortality for an individual in the ith age–sex group given a log cholesterol level X (the logistic), $f(X)$ is the distribution of log cholesterol (assumed normal), and $\overline{M}_i$ is the average mortality in the ith group. Thus,

$$E(X|\text{death}) = \int_{-\infty}^{+\infty} \frac{X\left[\dfrac{\exp(\alpha + \beta X)}{1 + \exp(\alpha + \beta X)}\right]\left[\dfrac{1}{\sqrt{2\pi}}\exp\left(\dfrac{-X^2}{2}\right)\right]dX}{\overline{M}_i}$$

If we substitute equation A.1 for the logistic, then

$$\overline{M}_i \cong \exp(\alpha + \beta^2/2)$$

$$E_i\,(X|\text{death}) \cong \frac{1}{\sqrt{2\pi}}\int_{-\infty}^{+\infty} \frac{X\exp(+\alpha + \beta X)}{\exp(+\alpha + \beta^2/2)}\exp\left(\frac{-X^2}{2}\right) dX$$

$$= \frac{1}{\sqrt{2\pi}}\int_{-\infty}^{+\infty} X\exp(-\beta^2/2 + \beta X - X^2/2)\,dX$$

which is the equation for the expected value of a normal with mean β. Therefore,

$$E_i\,(X|\text{death}) \cong \beta$$

To the extent that the conditional distribution is, in fact, symmetric:

$$\text{Median}\,(X|\text{death}) \cong \beta$$

When the results of these four estimation methods were compared, we found that the resulting β values were very similar, except in the case of young women where the maximum likelihood and conditional maximum likelihood methods resulted in larger estimates than Berkson's "minimum logit Chi-squared" method. The MLE results imply that cholesterol has its largest relative effects on women aged 45 to 54, which agrees with the studies discussed in Chapter 5 that strongly link events in young adults to parental history of ischemic heart disease. These studies found that children whose parents died youngest had the highest cholesterol levels.

We chose to use the results of the MLE based on log-normally distributed cholesterol levels. We standardized the results assuming an age-adjusted standard deviation of cholesterol of 44-mg/dl. We assign a value of zero to negative values of β which are not significantly different from zero, and we assume that for men over 75, β is zero. We also assume that premenopausal women (i.e., those under 45) have a β equal to zero. In extending the results to men under 45 years of age, we make the conservative assumption that the β is the same in the under-45 age group as in the 45 to 54 group. It is comforting to realize that those β's based on the scantiest data have little effect on the analysis, since the reason the data are so scanty is that few people in that age group suffer from coronary events.

The Framingham cholesterol levels are based on a single observation. As we will discuss in Appendix B, when the results of a single measurement are used to estimate true values, an adjustment is needed to correct for test error and for short-term variation in cholesterol levels. In fact, the best estimate of true value X_T based on a single observation X_0 is $X_T = .8X_0$. This means simply that the expected *true* level is somewhat closer to the population's mean (which is assigned a standard score of zero) than is the *observed* level. (All levels here are expressed in age-adjusted standardized scores.)

Our screening model predicts a 10-year-old screenee's *true value* of cholesterol at age 30, based on his screened value at age 10. Therefore, our benefit calculations from age 30 must be based on true, not observed, cholesterol levels. We can easily adjust the Framingham observed values, β_o, to true values, β_T.

$$\log\left(\frac{P}{1 - P}\right) = (\alpha + \beta_o X_o) = \left(\alpha + \beta_o \frac{X_T}{.8}\right) = (\alpha + \beta_T X_T)$$

Therefore,

$$\beta_T = \frac{\beta_o}{.8}$$

Table A–3 summarizes our estimated β's for men and women. As that table shows, cholesterol level was highly correlated with heart disease death for women in the Framingham study. Although the coefficients for fatal heart disease and for all heart disease are all significantly greater than zero, the standard error, particularly for women aged 45 to 54 is large. (Indeed, it is based on only six deaths in the entire Framingham sample.) For this reason, we checked our results against other data sources. With the exception of Patterson and Slack (1972), wherein young female survivors had cholesterol levels only 12 mg/dl over controls, all other sources indicated extremely high values for young women. In Goldstein et al. (1973a), 60 percent of females 40 to 49 years old who survived heart attacks were hyperlipidemic. In the Tromsø heart study (Miller et al., 1977), a history of "mother with

Table A-3. Estimated betas for log cholesterol on event [Calculated for "True" Beta (β_T) and "True" Cholesterol level (X_T)]

		Heart disease death	*Any heart disease*	*Cerebrovascular accident*
Sex	*Age (years)*	β_T*	β_T*	β_T*
Males	30–44	.63†	.68†	.27†
	45–54	.63 ± .30‡	.68 ± .14	.27 ± .34
	55–64	.48 ± .25	.31 ± .11	.15 ± .25
	65–74	0	.06	0
	75+	0	0	0
Females	30–44	0	0	0
	45–54	1.35 ± .56	.47 ± .21	.61 ± .38
	55–64	1.07 ± .37	.45 ± .13	.13 ± .26
	65–74	.73 ± .36	.57 ± .18	0
	75+	.73†	.57†	0

*β_T = coefficient of regression of incidence of event on log of true cholesterol level, where

$$\log\left(\frac{P}{1-p}\right) = \alpha + \beta_T X_T$$

†Extrapolated value.

‡Represents 1 SD of the estimate.

myocardial infarction" was much more significant than a history of "father with myocardial infarction."

A variation of this model is used in estimating the age- and sex-specific incidence of first stroke and first coronary heart disease. From the Framingham data, we are able to estimate the following age- and sex-specific rates:

1. Incidence of first stroke and of first coronary heart disease
2. Incidence of any stroke and of any coronary heart disease
3. Logistic parameters for incidence of any stroke or any coronary heart disease
4. Overall mortality from stroke and from coronary heart disease

National data are available for overall mortality from stroke and from coronary disease. We assume the following:

1. The ratio of incidence of first stroke (or first heart disease) to mortality from any stroke (or first heart disease) is the same in the total population as in the Framingham population.
2. The logistic parameter β relating incidence of first stroke (or heart disease) to cholesterol level is approximated by the reported β relating all stroke (or heart disease) to cholesterol level.

Our adjusted estimates of β for incidence of stroke and coronary disease are also reported in Table A–3.

Later we will be concerned with the effect of the standard deviations recorded in Table A-3 on our estimates of cost per YLS. The statistical errors for each age–sex group are independent, but it is, in addition, important to know whether there is additional systematic error in the Framingham β value deriving from unique characteristics of that particular city or from problems in the study's design. A recent publication compares the Framingham results for middle-aged men with the results of five other large longitudinal studies. In four of the five studies, the agreement with the Framingham data is so close that it seems unlikely that systematic bias in the Framingham study is a problem (American Heart Association, 1978). The fifth study (from Tecumseh, Michigan) measured a much higher value for β than did the Framingham study, but the Tecumseh estimate is based on considerably fewer cases.

The ratio of incidence of first stroke and coronary disease to mortality from stroke and coronary disease is summarized in Table A-4. These figures were derived from the Framingham study and from the *Vital Statistics of the United States.*

We now use our age-, sex-, and cholesterol-specific ischemic heart disease mortality rates along with the mortality rates for all other

Table A-4. Ratio of incidence of new events to incidence of fatal events

	Coronary heart disease		*Cardiovascular accident*	
Age (years)	*Male*	*Female*	*Male*	*Female*
30	6.0	6.5	3.0	3.0
35	5.5	6.5	3.0	3.0
40	5.0	6.5	3.0	3.0
45	4.0	6.5	3.5	3.0
50	3.0	5.0	4.5	3.0
55	2.5	5.0	2.0	4.0
60	2.0	4.5	2.5	4.0
65	2.0	4.0	2.0	4.0
70	1.5	3.0	1.5	3.0
75	1.5	2.0	1.5	2.0
80	1.5	1.5	1.5	1.5
85+	1.5	1.5	1.5	1.5

Sources: Vital Statistics of the United States, vol. II, Mortality, Part A, 1973. Rockville, Md.: U.S. Department of Health, Education and Welfare, Health Resources Administration, National Center for Health Statistics, 1977, and the Framingham study.

causes of death in a life-table calculation to estimate the remaining life expectancy from age 30 for men and women as a function of cholesterol level. The overall mortality rate for a given age, sex, and cholesterol group is calculated assuming that the mortality from other causes and the coronary mortality associated with the specified cholesterol level are independent of each other. The net life-table mortality from all causes is taken from the life-table data in Table A-2. Death rates from coronary disease are converted to life-table mortality rates and adjusted for cholesterol level using the logistic model. The standard life-table calculation is then carried out (Chiang, 1968), resulting in the remaining life expectancy as a function of a given value of cholesterol level for men and women. Similarly, the expected time to the first stroke and the expected time to the first coronary heart disease event are also calculated.

Appendix B. Stability of cholesterol rank order

Screening children for cholesterol level is of no value if their levels in childhood bear no relation to their adult levels. In this section, we discuss how individual variation in cholesterol level over time compares with the variation among individuals that we hope to detect by screening.

There is considerable day-to-day and month-to-month variation in the cholesterol test results of individuals. This variation is the result of short-term changes in diet, physiology, situation, and test error. Keys (1969) notes that even under the most rigidly controlled conditions, the standard error of adult cholesterol measurements separated by a few weeks is about 13 mg/dl. For free-living, healthy individuals, the standard error is about 20 mg/dl. From this and other information, we can compute the contribution of various factors to total variation of observed cholesterol level in a population of 40-year-old adult males. This is shown in Table B-1.

The top three components of the table, which add up to 20 percent of the total variation, represent the short-term variation in individual cholesterol values. To estimate the long-term variation, we use the Framingham results. The Framingham study reports the correlation coefficients for individual serum cholesterol levels between each pair of biennial examinations (with a maximum elapsed time of 18 years).

The reported coefficients are separated according to sex, but they include all ages (30 to 62). Individual cholesterol values rise slightly from the thirties to the fifties and fall thereafter, so correlations for an

Table B-1. Components of variation in measured population cholesterol

Source of variation	*Proportion of variation*	*Standard deviation (mg/dl)*
Test error (Abell method)	.01	5
Changes in individual physiology	.06	11
Changes in individual life-style	.13	16
Differences among individuals	.80	39
Total	1.00	44

age cohort are somewhat higher than the overall correlations. Because the rise and fall due to age is less than a fifth of the total standard error, the effect is noticeable only for widely separated exams, and even for the 18-year interval, the overestimate for men is less than 3 percent. Thus, we will use the Framingham correlation for all ages combined as a proxy for the cohort correlation that we need. The secular trend in average cholesterol values which peaked in 1964 was fairly uniform across all age groups, so it does not affect rank order.

Because the reported correlations are based on cholesterol values and not on the logarithm of cholesterol values, we assume for this computation that the distribution of values is normal instead of log-normal. As shown in Table B-2, the two distributions are very similar, except for the upper tail, which is the region of greatest interest in screening programs. The six grossly hypercholesterolemic inhabitants were excluded from the Framingham study, so our estimates should not be distorted by the assumption here of a normal, instead of log-normal, distribution.

To analyze these correlations, we assume that the variation in an individual's cholesterol level has two components, a short-term fluctuation about the true value and a long-term change in true value (Gardner and Heady, 1973). We will call the short-term fluctuation the

Table B-2. Comparison of normal and log-normal cholesterol distributions* (mg/dl)

	−1 SD	*Median*	*+1 SD*	*+2 SD*
Normal	176	220	264	308
Log-normal	177	216	263	320

*Normal (220, 44) becomes log-normal (5.37, .198).

noise. Formally, let X_i be the observed cholesterol level in year i, scaled to have mean 0 and variance 1. We assume X_i is the sum of the true value t_i plue the noise e_i. The true value and the noise are also distributed normally with mean 0 and variance σ^2 and ϵ^2, respectively. They are independent. The noise is such that successive measurements separated by a reasonable period of time (say one month) are independent. The correlation of true values R_l measures the long-term variations. The correlation of observed values after one month, R_s, depends purely on noise. If $X = t + e$ and $X' = t + e'$ are separated by three months,

$$R_s = \frac{\text{cov}(t + e, t + e')}{\sqrt{\text{cov}(t + e, t + e)\,\text{cov}(t + e', t + e')}} = \sigma^2 \qquad \text{(B.1)}$$

Finally, we assume that the long-term variation is Markovian; this means that R_l between true values of an individual over a T-year interval are the Tth power of the one-year correlation.

Summarizing, we assume

$$X_i = t_i + e_i, \quad \text{cov}(t_i, e_i) = 0, \quad \text{cov}(e_i, e_j) = 0 \qquad \text{(B.2)}$$

$$t_i \sim N(0, \sigma^2), \quad e_i \sim N(0, \epsilon^2), \quad X_i \sim N(0, 1), \quad R(t_i, t_0) = R_l^i$$

One simple consequence is that $\epsilon^2 + \sigma^2 = 1$. In addition,

$$R(X_i, X_0) = \frac{\text{cov}(X_i, X_0)}{\sqrt{\text{cov}(X_i, X_i)\,\text{cov}(X_0, X_0)}} = \text{cov}(t_i, t_0)$$

But since $\text{cov}(t_i, t_0) = R(t_i, t_0)\,\sigma^2$, we can substitute equations B.1 and B.2 to obtain

$$R(X_i, X_0) = R_l^i R_s \qquad \text{(B.3)}$$

Taking the logarithms, we get

$$\log R(X_i, X_0) = \log R_s + i \log R_l$$

Thus, we can estimate R_s and R_l from simple regression of the log of reported Framingham correlations. Table B-3 gives the results. The fit is good, and the residuals seem randomly scattered. The standard error of the estimate of the slope is .002, so the difference between men and women is not significant. For simplicity, and to match Keys' results in Table B-1, we will assume that the correlations for men and for women are the same and that $R_s = .8$, $R_l = .98$.

Thus equation B.3 becomes

$$R(X_i, X_0) = .8(.98)^i$$

Table B-3. Regression of correlations of log cholesterol on time

	Number of observations	*Slope*	*Intercept*	R_s	R_l	R^2
Men	28	.0176	−.2397	.79	.98	.89
Women	28	.0208	−.2085	.81	.98	.89

This is a reasonable estimate of long-term correlation between adults; an analysis of 12 years' experience of a cohort of West Point cadets shows a similar pattern, but with slightly more short-term variation (Clark et al., 1967). However, we are interested in the correlation between levels of children and their levels 20 years later. Results for 8-year-olds in the Bogalusa study give a one-year correlation of .75, and results for teenagers are even lower. Our analysis of McGandy's study of teenagers gives a one-year correlation of .76 (McGandy et al., 1972). The Muscatine study of Iowa found a six-year correlation coefficient of .61. (Clarke et al., 1978). Short-term variation thus may be higher in children—and we will test the effects of this in our analysis—but it is unlikely that the 20-year correlation will fall much below .5.

Over an 18-year period, the Framingham correlation coefficients do not level out. That is, the correlation between readings 16 years apart is higher than that of readings 18 years apart. It is possible that the increasing effect of age-related differences in these long intervals is masking a leveling of age-cohort correlations. In any event, we are confident that correlations between childhood and adult levels will eventually level off for age cohorts of children, since the genetic identity of the child and the later adult should set a floor on correlation. Indeed, the Tecumseh studies of sibling correlation suggest that genetic effects become stronger after age 40 (i.e., that environmental variation becomes less) than at ages earlier in adulthood (Deutscher et al., 1966). The floor on correlation within individuals is twice the correlation between first-degree relatives, after taking out the shared variance due to environment. (Of course, the child and later adult may have a similar environment, depending on how much food consumption and life-style also track.) From the studies discussed in Chapter 5, this floor is between .4 and .6.

Multiple measurements separated by a few weeks are a useful way of reducing the noise of short-term variation. Our model of variation implies that the average is the best statistic to estimate the true value and that the correlation between averages of k measurements is

$$R_s(k) = \sigma^2/ (\sigma^2 + \epsilon^2/k)$$

This correlation is .89 with two measurements, when R_s (with one measurement) is .8. In this case, the 20-year correlation is $.89\,(.98)^{20} = .594$.

We should note for a standardized initial observed value of X (i.e., a cholesterol value X standard deviations above the mean), a 20-year correlation of R implies that the expected observed value is RX. Since the noise in the twentieth year is independent of X, the expected true value 20 years later is also RX. Thus, our 20-year endpoints represent true values.

We have to correct the Framingham mortality results (based on observed values) by dividing their regression coefficients by $1/\sigma^2$. Studies of the differential effects of diet must also be adjusted to provide the differential effects of diet on true cholesterol levels. This can be done by a calculation of regression or by separating regression from diet in the experimental design. A second baseline measurement taken after sorting into cholesterol classes, but before treatment, will include all the regression. The difference between this measurement and the final results gives true differential effects of diet (Ederer, 1972).

Appendix C. Diet-cholesterol relationships

Although dietary intervention studies uniformly demonstrate the responsiveness of individual cholesterol levels to dietary changes, studies in free-living populations generally fail to find statistically significant correlation between nutrient intake and cholesterol levels. In this appendix, we seek to reconcile such negative findings with a quantitative model provided by Keys (1969) for the impact of diet constituents on cholesterol level.

In his article "Serum Cholesterol and the Question of 'Normal'," Ancel Keys (1969) suggested that a variety of diet studies on institutionalized patients could be summarized by the following formula:

$$\Delta \text{ Cholesterol} = 1.3\,(2\,\Delta S - \Delta P + \Delta Z) \qquad \text{(C.1)}$$

where S = percentage of calories supplied by saturated fat;
P = percentage of calories supplied by polyunsaturated fat;
Z = square root of dietary cholesterol in milligrams per 1000 calories.

Because of the large number of repeated cholesterol measurements taken in these studies, the formula can be assumed to represent the effects of true dietary changes on true cholesterol levels.

If we assume that the current diet in the United States can be estimated by the average consumption of foodstuffs in this country and that a therapeutic cholesterol-lowering diet would seek to supply about 35 percent of calories as fat, then the changes in the significant variables in the Keys formula would be as shown in Table C-1.

The changes shown in Table C-1 would result in an average cholesterol drop of

$$\begin{aligned} \Delta \text{ Chol} &= 1.3\ [2(15.9 - 9.4) - (5.4 - 8.1) + (\sqrt{240} - \sqrt{180})] \\ &= 1.3\ (13 + 2.7 + 2.1) \\ &= 23.1 \text{ mg/dl} \end{aligned}$$

Similar calculations based on a new diet with 40 percent of calories from fat yield an estimated cholesterol drop of 21 mg/dl.

With the help of the Keys formula, it is also possible to estimate the differences in dietary intake and cholesterol levels that we might expect to see in the studies of free-living populations, which in general report "negative" findings. Such studies have usually measured cholesterol levels in a large number of people and have then used dietary histories and observations to determine if people with high cholesterol levels consumed diets of different composition than people with low cholesterol levels. The formula allows us to estimate the differences in diet that are implied by the observed differences in cholesterol levels in those studies.

We may then ask whether the results are closer to what would have been expected if the Keys formula applied or are closer to the null hypothesis that there is no effect of diet on the cholesterol levels of free-living populations. This test of competing hypotheses prevents us from accepting the null hypothesis simply because the sample size is too small rather than because diet really has no effect.

We will examine the two most frequently cited studies: The Framingham Diet Study (Kannel and Gordon, 1970b, Section 24), and the Tecumseh study (Nichols et al., 1976a). In the Framingham study, participants were asked to describe their "usual" diet, and the population was then divided into high and low groups for a variety of diet measures, among them the ratio of vegetable fat to animal fat. The investigators then compared the mean serum cholesterol levels of these groups.

Table C–1. Changes in dietary constituents from average United States consumption as a result of a cholesterol-lowering diet

	Current diet	*New diet*
P	5.4% of calories	8.1% of calories
S	15.9% of calories	9.4% of calories
Z^2	240 mg/1000 calories	180 mg/1000 calories

In the Tecumseh study, conducted ten years later, the participants were stratified into three groups based on their serum cholesterol levels, and the investigators looked for differences in reported diet during the 24 hours preceding blood testing. Restricting the dietary history to the immediately preceding 24 hours reduces recall error, but to the extent that diet varies over time and that cholesterol levels depend on more than the intake of the preceding 24 hours, this technique neglects some relevant dietary information. Both studies showed a positive, but not statistically significant, relationship between saturated fats in the diet and serum cholesterol levels.

METHODS

The most powerful test of the diet-cholesterol hypothesis as formulated by Keys would be a regression of serum cholesterol level on a "diet index" of $2S - P + Z$. However, we will instead follow the stratification methods of the papers, which should be adequate to demonstrate a relationship under most circumstances. Instead of testing the usual null hypothesis, that the groups do not differ from each other, we will test the hypothesis that the differences between groups are those that would have been predicted by the Keys formula relating diet to serum cholesterol levels.

To carry out our analysis, we first need to estimate the variances of S, P, and Z. In reanalyzing the Framingham data, where the population was stratified by diet, we will need to estimate the differences between the mean values of $(2S - P + Z)$ in the groups. Assuming that $(2S - P + Z)$ is normally distributed, these differences are easily estimated from the variance of $(2S - P + Z)$. In reanalyzing the Tecumseh data, where the population was stratified by serum cholesterol level, we will need to estimate the fraction of the variation in serum cholesterol level which is attributable to diet. Again, the variance of $(2S - P + Z)$ is required to make this calculation.

We base our estimates of the variances of S, P, and Z on data from each study. Table C-2 summarizes the pertinent information from both Tecumseh (Nichols et al., 1976a, Table 5) and Framingham (Kannel and Gordon, 1970b, Section 24, Table 3).

In Tecumseh, since the standard deviation of grams of polyunsaturated fat is about 0.6 times the standard deviation of grams of saturated fat, we assume that the standard deviation of P is also about 0.6 times that of S. Assuming that the total number of calories consumed as fat is independent from the proportions from animal and vegetable sources (as is implied by the lack of correlation between those proportions and

Table C–2. Standard deviations of daily nutrient intake in diet studies

	Tecumseh		*Framingham*	
Nutrient	*Men*	*Women*	*Men*	*Women*
Calories	1066	719	702	561
Saturated fat (g)	25	17	*	*
Animal fat (g)	45	30	31	24
Plant fat (g)	36	23	18	16
Polyunsaturated fat (g)	14	10	*	*
Cholesterol (mg)	353	234	221	170
P:S ratio	.19	.24	.13	.13
Calories from saturated fat, S (%)	3.8	4.2	*	*
Estimated $2S - P$ (%)	8	9	5.5	7.2

*Not given in report.

total calories, shown in Kannel and Gordon, 1970b, Table 5), it can be shown that S and P are slightly negatively correlated. It follows that $2S - P$ in Tecumseh had a standard deviation of about 8 in men and 9 in women. Assuming that dietary cholesterol is correlated about .5 with calories (as it was in Framingham), Z has a standard deviation of about 2. Thus, in men in these populations, fat intake should contribute $(8/2)^2 = 16$ times as much as dietary cholesterol to variation in blood cholesterol. In what follows, we will therefore concentrate on $2S - P$ and ignore Z.

The Framingham study reported much smaller standard deviations in grams of fat than did the Tecumseh study and a higher, but less variable, level of consumption of calories per day. (This reduction in variation is to be expected since the Framingham investigators were asking about average diet instead of only a 24-hour history.) Assuming conservatively that the standard deviation of $2S - P$ in Framingham is equal to that of Tecumseh multiplied by the ratio of the standard deviations of animal fat, this value is 5.5 for men and 7.2 for women. (Using the ratio of percentage of calories from fat as the multiplier leads to slightly lower estimates.)

RESULTS

Framingham results

The strongest test of Keys' formula is found in Table 15 of the Framingham (Kannel and Gordon, 1970b) report. There, subjects are split into two groups according to their plant/animal fat ratio. Since this ratio has a very high negative correlation with $2S - P$, we will assume conservatively that the division of subjects was on the basis of $2S - P$. The expected difference between the two groups, shown in Table C-3, is about 1.6 SD of $2S - P$.

Equation C.1 is based on true diet, but there are reporting errors when diet is estimated by recall. For calories, the reliability in such studies has varied from .55 (Ederer, 1972) to .84 (Burke, 1947). One would guess that the error in estimating diet components by recall methods would be greater than the error in estimating calories, since there is less opportunity for errors in estimating components to balance each other out. Suppose, then, that the reliability of $2S - P$ is P_d. Let the symbol Δ denote differences. As shown in Appendix B, E[true $\Delta(2S - \text{P})$|observed $\Delta(2S - \text{P})] = P_d \cdot$ obs. $\Delta(2S - \text{P})$. Also, the standard deviation of true $\Delta(2S - \text{P}) = \sqrt{P_d} \cdot$ SD[obs. $\Delta(2S - \text{P})$]. Finally, E(observed blood cholesterol|true cholesterol) = true cholesterol.

From these formulas, we can compute the value of P_d for which the predictions of Keys' formula exactly fit the observed results. We simply solve Δ(observed cholesterol) = 1.3 [P_d obs. $\Delta(2S - \text{P})$] for P_d. As shown in Table C-3 this value is .51 for men and .47 for women. Since these are approximately .5, even if P_d for the diet index were 1 (i.e., even if diet were perfectly and reliably measured), these data would support the Keys formula as much as the null hypothesis. Since P_d is probably about .75, the Keys formula is a better explanation of the experimental results than the hypothesis that there is no effect of diet on serum cholesterol.

Tecumseh results

In the Tecumseh study, the population was stratified by cholesterol. Diet differences in such a design seem small because diet explains such a small part of cholesterol variation within a group with reasonably a homogeneous diet. Let us denote the cholesterol level by X, its mean by $\overline{X}$, the contribution of diet by d, and the contribution of everything else by g. Age-adjusted cholesterol has a standard deviation of about 40 mg/dl, and from our earlier results the effect of diet on cholesterol has a standard deviation of about $1.3\sqrt{P_d} \cdot 8$. We expect day-to-day variation in diet to make P_d for 24-hour intervals of diet quite small. By comparing the standard deviation in Tecumseh with those in Framingham, we can estimate how much smaller the Tecumseh P_d is. This estimate assumes the true variation in average diet between individuals, σ_b^2, and the measurement error, σ_e^2, is the same in both studies, but the larger variances in Tecumseh are the result of variation within individuals over time, σ_w^2.

$$\text{Then, } P_d \text{ in Tecumseh} = \frac{\sigma_b^2}{\sigma_b^2+\sigma_e^2+\sigma_w^2}$$

$$= \frac{\sigma_b^2+\sigma_e^2}{\sigma_b^2+\sigma_e^2+\sigma_w^2} P_d \text{ in Framingham.}$$

But $\dfrac{(\sigma_b^2+\sigma_e^2)}{(\sigma_b^2+\sigma_e^2+\sigma_w^2)}$ is just the ratio of the observed population variances. By squaring the entries in the two sides of Table C-2 and dividing, we see that ratio is about $(2/3)^2$ for most components of diet. Thus the reliability of diet measures P_d in Tecumseh should be less than half the value in Framingham.

Assume that everything is normally distributed, for simplicity. Then (for men):

$$(X-\overline{X}) \sim N(0, 40^2)$$

$$d \sim N[0, P_d(10.4)^2]$$

and hence

$$g \sim N(0, 40^2 - P_d \cdot 10.4^2) \simeq N(0, 39^2)$$

In other words, little of the observed variation in cholesterol is due to diet. The regression of d on X is thus

$$d = \left(\frac{\sigma_d^2}{\sigma_x^2}\right) \cdot X = \frac{P_d\,(10.4)^2}{40^2} \cdot X$$

We can again solve for P_d, using the first and third tertiles of the blood cholesterol levels in Tecumseh. The Keys formula and the null hypothesis both predict that the average diet on the middle tertile will be the same as the overall average diet, so it is not useful for distinguishing the hypotheses. We can approximate (from detailed data kindly supplied by D. Lamphiear) the average values of $2S - P$ for the tertiles, using the assumption that S and P are given by the total grams of saturated and unsaturated fat divided by the total calories in each tertile.

The results are shown in Table C-3. Since the groups were stratified by observed cholesterol, we expect their true cholesterol differences to be 0.8 times the observed differences. The best-fitting P_d for the Tecumseh data is shown in Table C-3 to be about .16, so the break-

Table C–3. Correlation between diet and observed serum cholesterol level and implied reliability of the measure of diet

Study and group	*Number in group*	*Observed serum cholesterol level*	*Difference of estimated diet index from average* $\Delta(2S-P)$	*Implied reliability of diet measure,* P_d
Framingham				
Men, low diet	129	233	−6.4*	.51
high diet	302	239	+2.8*	
Women, low diet	186	239	−6.7*	.47
high diet	256	246	+4.8*	
Tecumseh				
Men, low cholesterol	320	170	−.24†	.15
high cholesterol	318	246	+.34†	
Women, low cholesterol	362	173	−.81†	.17
high cholesterol	359	245	−.16†	

*Estimated by assuming that the split on plant fat/animal fat is a split on levels of $2S–P$ and that $2S–P$ is normally distributed with standard deviation 5.5 in men, and 7.2 in women.

†Estimated by the approximation that $2S–P$ = [(18 × average grams of saturated fat) − (9 × average grams of polyunsaturated fat)]/average calories, and with data kindly supplied by D. Lamphiear.

even value for deciding between the Keys formula and the null hypothesis is twice that, or .32. Since we guess that the reliability in Framingham diet measures is about .75, the reliability for Tecumseh should be about $(2/3)^2$ .75 = .33, almost exactly the breakeven value. Thus, we would rate this study as equivocal, favoring neither the null hypothesis nor the Keys formula.

SUMMARY

Both studies show a connection between serum cholesterol level and diet, but the connection is less than would be observed if the diet surveys measured average diet perfectly and if Keys' formula applied. Because of the importance of nondietary factors in determining cholesterol levels, even these large sample sizes were not large enough to reject either the null hypothesis of no connection between diet and cholesterol or the Keys formula for the effect of diet. If forced to choose one hypothesis or the other, one would have to say that the Framingham data definitely support the Keys formula, but that the Tecumseh data are equivocal. Our analysis shows that the smallness of observed differences in diet in Tecumseh between high and low cholesterol groups derives mainly from the statistical design and from the variability of individual diet over time.

A similar critique of the cross-sectional diet-cholesterol studies was suggested by Jacobs et al. (1979). They tested the model by looking at cholesterol and diet index measurements of 91 MRFIT participants before and after they received three to six weeks of help in changing their eating habits. Although the correlation between diet and cholesterol was insignificant at both points in time, the correlation of changes in cholesterol levels with changes in diet index over time was .4. Looking at changes reduces the confounding caused by intrinsic population differences in cholesterol levels and allows the impact of diet to be observed.

Appendix D. The distribution of cholesterol in the population

In the United States and other Western countries, the average cholesterol level remains fairly constant from ages 4 to 17 and then rises over time until late in life. For example, the 20,000 people studied in the 1971–1974 Health and Nutrition Examination Survey (HANES) had the pattern shown in Figure D-1. The same pattern is seen in the Tecumseh, Busselton, Bogalusa and Framingham studies.

At the same time, the distribution of cholesterol levels in Americans of the same age and sex is a bell-shaped curve with a slight skew to the right as was shown in Figure 4-6. This pattern emerges for the overall population if cholesterol levels are adjusted to remove the effects of age and sex. For precise information on the upper tail of the distribution, which is most important to screening programs, very large sample surveys are required. In the Tecumseh study, age-adjusted cholesterol levels were used to permit calculations on the entire sample, and a log-normal approximation fit the resulting data best. (The log-normal distribution also appeared to be the best to fit the results from the 1960–1962 National Health Examination Survey and the Bogalusa and Muscatine studies of children.)

The log-normal has the familiar bell-shaped form if cholesterol values are plotted on a log scale, in which equal increments represent equal percentage increases in cholesterol rather than equal absolute amounts. The spread of the distribution is small—one standard deviation is .18 for males, which means that 68 percent of the values lie between 84 and 120 percent of the median. In such a case, the normal

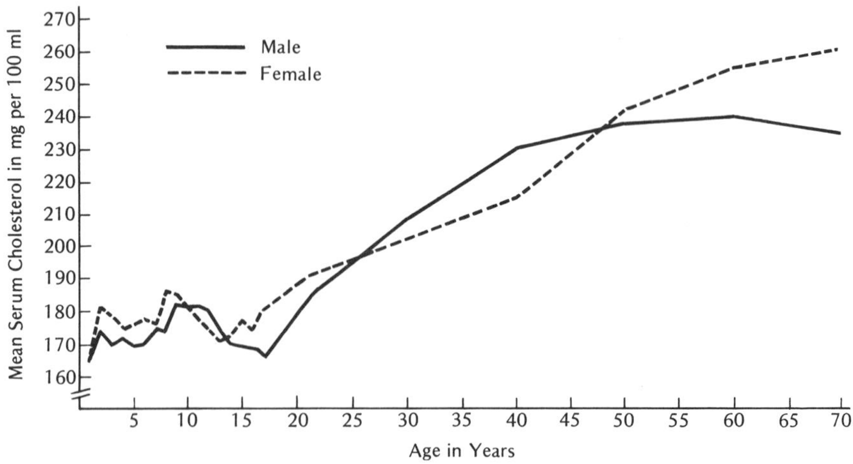

Figure D-1. Mean Serum Cholesterol Level by Age, U.S. Population. (Reproduced with permission from S. Abraham, Total serum cholesterol levels in children,4–17 years, United States, 1971–1974, Vital and Health Statistics, Series 11: Data from National Health Survey, No. 207. DHEW pub. no. (PHS)78-1655. Washington, D.C.: Government Printing Office, 1978.)

distribution is almost as good an approximation as the log-normal, and many early studies of cholesterol level used the assumption of normality without a conversion to logarithms. The results of studies that treat cholesterol level, itself, as a normally distributed variable can be roughly adapted to log cholesterol results by the following adjustment: $M = \exp(m + s^2/2)$, $S/M = \sqrt{\exp(s^2) - 1} \sim s$, where M and S are the mean and standard deviation of cholesterol, and m and s are the mean and standard deviation of the logarithm.

In addition to fitting the data well, the log-normal distribution has some other advantages for our analysis. All of the major studies show that as cholesterol levels rise over time, the spread of levels (measured by the standard deviation) rises proportionately. With the log-normal, this is easily modeled by a simple shift in the mean of log cholesterol. The most probable effect of diet on levels is a reduction in cholesterol that is proportional to the initial level. A proportional reduction is, again, easily represented as a simple shift in the mean of log cholesterol.

There may be a small bump in the distribution at very high levels caused by a relatively rare genetic condition. We discuss the evidence for this condition at length in Chapter 5, as it can strongly affect the results of the programs analyzed there. In the mass screening programs, such single-gene conditions can be ignored because we believe that less than 5 percent of hypercholesterolemics fall into this category, and little is known to distinguish their risks and benefits from people without the genetic condition but with equally high cholesterol levels.

Actual cholesterol values are quite sensitive to the laboratory method used for their determination. For example, results from the HANES study for children are about 6 percent higher than the Bogalusa values, and results from the Muscatine study are over 10 percent higher. When the latter two studies are standardized to the Abell-Kendall standards used in the Bogalusa study, the differences are greatly reduced. All our specific values will be based on the Abell-Kendall standard, which is generally acknowledged to be close to true cholesterol values.

Our recommendations for 10-year-olds will be based on a mean log cholesterol of 5.1 and a standard deviation of .18.* These figures, which represent a compromise of the Bogalusa, Tecumseh, and HANES, values, correspond to a mean level of 166 mg/dl and a standard deviation of 30. Where standardization is a problem, it will be better to ignore the specific recommended values and assume that any large group has a distribution similar to the national average and intervene on the recommended fraction.

A comparison of results from two National Health surveys shows about a 5 mg/dl decline in cholesterol levels in the 1960s for adults at all ages over 25. Figure D-2 shows these results. Unfortunately, children were not included in the 1960 survey, so we must guess what their results might have been. We will assume that the levels of children were about the same as now and that only the levels in adulthood changed. This assumption is based on the values from the Tecumseh study at the time of the earlier National Health survey, on the lack of difference in cholesterol values for children on vastly different diets around the world, and on the apparent convergence of the two curves for adults at age 18.

The decline in adult levels can also be seen in Framingham levels over that same decade and in comparisons of the original Framingham participants with their recently tested offspring (now adults). The decline may be explained in part by the drop in per capita consumption of eggs and beef and may help to explain why heart attack mortality has also fallen.

*All logarithms mentioned are in natural logarithmic units, that is, log to the base *e*.

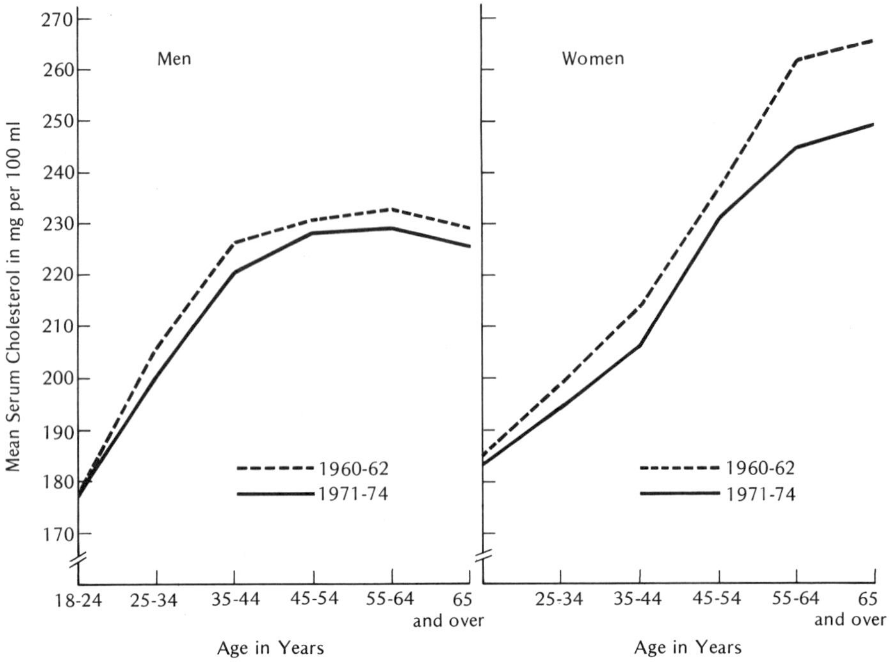

Figure D-2. Mean Serum Cholesterol Level of Adults 18–74 years by Age: United States, 1960–1962 and 1971–1974. (Reproduced with permission from S. Abraham et al., A comparison of levels of serum cholesterol of adults 18–74 years of age in the United States in 1960–62 and 1971–74. Advancedata no. 5, February 22, 1977. DHEW pub. no. (HRA)77-1250. Rockville, MD: National Center for Health Statistics, 1977.)

Appendix E. Estimating the food costs of cholesterol-lowering diets

Dietary changes to lower cholesterol levels can be as highly individualized as any dietary choices. Although cholesterol-reducing diets all strike common themes—reduction of saturated fat, substitution of polyunsaturated for saturated fats, and restriction of ingested cholesterol—they can differ widely in their specific features. A nutrition counselor seeking to help an individual reduce his or her cholesterol can and should exploit the variety of potential strategies to find those goals and changes most acceptable to the individual and therefore most likely to be followed.

From the perspectives of both cost and taste, the most important differences in low-cholesterol, low-fat diets lie in the methods used to reduce saturated fat intake. Two basic approaches are possible. The most obvious is to replace fatty red meats, a major source of saturated fat in the American diet, with lean red meats. Such a shift results in only a moderate dislocation in the taste and appearance of foods, but it is expensive. A second approach is to replace at least some meats with vegetable protein sources such as legumes and nuts. This results in a more dramatic alteration in the taste and appearance of the diet but is less expensive than "meat-for-meat" substitutions.

Since some cholesterol-lowering diets are more expensive than the "typical" American diet and some are cheaper, it is impossible to speak of *the* cost of a cholesterol-lowering diet. Instead, as we seek a range of such cost estimates, we will examine two diets that represent reasonable upper and lower bounds on cost. The first diet, the more expensive one, uses lean meats, poultry, and fish to replace fatty meats. The second, and cheaper, diet makes extensive use of legumes and nuts to replace fatty meats.

CHOLESTEROL-LOWERING DIET I: AN UPPER BOUND ON COST

The basic diet to reduce cholesterol recommended in Appendix C has several components. First, fats and oils in the diet are replaced by polyunsaturated oils, mainly corn oil and corn oil margarine. Second, the consumption of saturated meat fats is reduced by substituting veal, fish, poultry, and lean beef for current consumption of beef, lamb, and pork. Textured protein substitutes may also be used, especially for items such as bacon or breakfast sausages. Third, skim milk or low-fat milk is used instead of whole milk. Finally, the ingestion of cholesterol is reduced by restricting egg consumption or possibly by using low-cholesterol manufactured egg substitutes.

To estimate the costs of these dietary changes, we used U.S. Department of Agriculture sources (1, 2, 3)* to determine the average per capita consumption of fats and oils, meats, and eggs. The average consumptions of the recommended substitute products were also obtained from the *Commodity Yearbook* (4) and the USDA sources already cited. The costs per pound of substitutions were calculated from USDA (1, 2, 3) and Bureau of Labor Statistics (5) reports and, where necessary, from a survey of local grocery store prices. For fats and oils, this was relatively straightforward. In 1975, corn oil cost 68 cents a pound and salad oil with less polyunsaturated fat cost 56 cents a pound. The cost per pound of substitution was therefore 12 cents. For the meat products, further assumptions must be made as to the fractions of veal, poultry, fish, and lean beef that will be used to replace fatty meats. Assuming that 50 percent of the nonbeef meat consumption will be replaced by lean beef and the other half will be replaced by veal, poultry, and fish in proportion to their current consumption, we arrive at the lean meat mixture shown in Table E-1.

The net cost per pound of meat replacements is very sensitive to the mix of items used in the replacement. If more chicken and less lean beef were used, for example, the costs would be substantially lower. Clearly, the assistance of skilled nutritionists would be important in arriving at the most acceptable and efficient mix.

*See references at end of Appendix E.

Table E-1. Replacement meats in Cholesterol-lowering Diet I

Food item	*Projected replacement fraction*	*Cost per pound**
Lean beef	.500	$2.02
Veal	.023	1.77
Poultry	.385	0.64
Fish	.092	1.45

*Prices given as of 1975.

To find the annual cost of dietary change requires yet another assumption about the *degree* to which substitution occurs. For example, it may not be a realistic goal to replace *all* cooking and salad oil in the diet with corn oil. In particular, an individual would have some difficulty controlling the type of oil used in commercially prepared foods. Thus, it may perhaps be reasonable to assume that only 50 percent of the consumption of eggs, milk, and fats and oils will be altered. With meat products, on the other hand, given the nature of the substitution, it may be feasible to substitute for 100 percent of the consumption. Table E-2 summarizes the components of the food cost estimations.

The annual per capita cost of cholesterol-lowering diet I is approximately $20, which we take as an upper bound on the cost of a cholesterol-reducing diet.

CHOLESTEROL-LOWERING DIET II†: A LOWER BOUND ON COST

Another way to reduce the fat and cholesterol content of the "typical" American diet is to reduce the meat intake and increase the use of legumes and nuts as a source of protein. Table E-3 presents a low-fat, low-cholesterol diet that would involve a two-thirds decrease in the amount of meat consumed and a fourfold increase in the amount of beans and nuts consumed. Based on 1975 prices, this diet prepared at home would have cost a 20- to 54-year-old man $10.40 per week. The U.S. Department of Agriculture has prepared estimates of the costs of providing nutritious meals at four levels of expenditure: Thrifty, low cost, moderate cost, and liberal (Table E-4). For men in the 20- to 54-year age group, even the thrifty diet is more costly than the low-cholesterol diet proposed here (see Table E-4).

†We are deeply indebted to Dr. John W. Farquhar and Ms. Nancy Ellsworth who designed and analyzed the diet presented in this section.

Table E-2. Components of food costs in Cholesterol-lowering Diet I

Diet item	*Price per pound* (cents)*	*Recommended substitution*	*Price per pound of substitute (cents)*	*Per capita consumption of item (pounds), 1976*	*Per capita consumption of substitute (pounds), 1976*	*Net alterable consumption (pounds)*	*Fraction of alterable consumption assumed changed*	*Cost per pound of change (cents)*	*Annual cost of dietary substitutions (dollars)*
Fats and oils									
1. Cooking and salad oil	56	Corn oil	68	19.4	1.4	18.0	.50	+12	+1.08
2. Shortening	54	Corn oil and margarine	69	17.0	—	17.0	.50	+15	+1.28
3. Lard	30	Corn oil and margarine	69	3.2	—	3.2	.50	+39	+0.62
4. Margarine	52	Corn oil and margarine	69	9.1	0.9	8.2	All	+17	+1.32
5. Butter	110	Corn oil and margarine	69	4.6	—	4.6	All	−41	−0.94
Fatty meats									
6a. Pork (excluding lard, bacon, and breakfast sausage)	136	Lean meat mixture†	143†		—	47.3‡	.50	+8	+1.89

6b. Bacon and breakfast sausage	174	Textured protein substitute	99§	52.6	—	5.3‡	All	−75	−1.99
7. Beef	141	Lean beef and lean meat mixture†	202 143†	93.9	—	93.9	.20 .80	+61 +02	+11.46 1.50
8. Lamb	193	Lean meat mixture†	143†	1.7	—	1.7	All	−50	−0.43
9. Offal	134	Lean meat mixture†	143†	10.7	—	10.7	All	+9	+0.48
Lean meats and fish									
10. Poultry	64	None	—	50.3	—	—	—	—	
11. Fish	145	None	—	12.0	—	—	—	—	
12. Veal	177	None	—	3.0	—	—	—	—	
Milk and eggs									
13. Milk	20.5	Skim or low-fat milk	19.5	278.6	78.6	200.0	All	−1	−2.00
14. Eggs	6.2¢ each	Manufactured substitute	9.7¢ each	287 eggs	—	287 eggs	.50	+3.5 each	+5.02
Total annual cost of dietary substitutions									$19.29

†"Lean meat mixture" and its pricing are described in text.
§Price for amount of protein substitute that is equivalent to 1 pound of bacon.
‡Assumes 10% of pork is consumed as bacon and breakfast sausage.
*All prices are estimated as of 1975.

Table E-3. Components of a low-cholesterol and low-fat diet: Cholesterol-lowering Diet II

Foods	*Size of serving*	*Amount to be consumed per week*	*Cost Per week (cents), 1975*
Milk and milk products		14 servings	145
Low-fat or skim milk	8 oz		
Low-fat cottage cheese	1.5 cup		
Cheese (no more than 2 oz/wk)			
Animal protein			
Red meat: beef, pork, lamb, veal (All should be trimmed before cooking and degreased.) (Bacon, sausage, and organ meats should be omitted.)	3 oz	3 servings	138
Poultry: chicken, turkey	3 oz	3 servings	93
1. Organ meats should be omitted.			
Fish	3 oz	1 serving	50
Eggs	1 egg	≤ 3 eggs	19
Complementary protein foods			
Legumes and nuts		18 servings	112
Dried beans	.75 cup	11 servings	
Nuts	2 tbs	7 servings	
Whole grains		28 servings	107
Whole grain bread	1 slice	16 servings	
Rice, bulgar, cornmeal, etc.	.66 cup	14 servings	
(Legumes, nuts, grains, and dairy products should be combined and eaten in portion sizes that best form complete proteins.)			
Fruits and vegetables	.5 cup	28 servings	365
One vitamin C rich			
One dark green leafy			
One dark green or yellow			
One starchy			
Fats and/or oils	1 tbs	7 servings	12
Vegetable oil (except coconut or palm oil) based margarine, shortening, salad, and cooking oil			
No butter or lard			
Total cost per week			$10.41

Comments Regarding Cost Figures and General Remarks

1. Cost of fats and oils is averaged from the average prices of margarine and salad or cooking oil, assuming an equal consumption of each. The prices for each of these is that listed by the Bureau of Labor Statistics and is not specific for those margarines or oils made without coconut or palm oil.
2. Costs are based on 1975 retail prices compiled from Bureau of Labor Statistics data.
3. Milk cost is based on the prices of fresh grocery milk, not whole, low-fat, or nonfat milk specifically. Base cost could be decreased by the use of dried milk or increased by use of cottage cheese or store-bought yogurt. Because of the limited amounts of cheese allowed, only the most expensive varieties would affect the cost.

4. Red meat prices are based on an average of the average prices of choice grade beef, retail cuts of veal, pork, and choice grade lamb, with each of the four adjusted according to the amount consumed per capita in 1976.
5. Poultry prices are based on an average of the average prices of frying chicken in retail stores and turkeys in retail stores. This is an average price adjusted according to the amount consumed per capita of each in 1976. Costs would be increased considerably by buying specific cuts of chicken or turkey.
6. Fish prices are averaged from the average prices for frozen haddock fillets and canned tuna. Since these represented the consumption of many other types of fish, a straight average price of these was figured.
7. Serving weights of red meats, poultry, and fish were adjusted to retail weights before weekly cost figures were calculated.
8. Egg costs are based on a cost of $0.75 per dozen.
9. The cost of legumes and nuts is based on average prices for dried beans and peanut butter and for an 11-serving/7-serving ratio, respectively.
10. Whole grain prices are averaged from the average prices for whole wheat bread and long grain rice based on 14 servings of each per week.
11. Fruits and vegetable prices are based on commonly eaten representative produce. The cost per week is based on 7 servings of spinach, 3.5 servings each of fresh tomatoes, carrots, oranges, and grapefruits, and 7 servings of potatoes.
12. A cholesterol-lowering diet had been suggested here that would provide a balanced diet for a man 20 to 54 years of age. The foods on which the weekly cost has been based were chosen for their common usage and for their believed representativeness of costs for foods in that group. The total cost of this diet could be increased or decreased depending upon the particular food choices of an individual.

Table E–4. Cost of food for a week, all meals and snacks prepared at home* (U.S. average, July 1976)

Individual	*Thrifty plan*	*Low-cost plan*	*Moderate-cost plan*	*Liberal plan*
Women:				
20–54 years	$ 9.20	$12.00	$14.90	$17.90
55 years and over	8.30	10.70	13.30	15.80
Pregnant	11.50	14.80	18.30	21.80
Nursing	12.20	15.70	19.60	23.40
Men:				
20–54 years	11.30	14.80	18.80	22.70
55 years and over	10.00	13.00	16.20	19.50
Children:				
1–2 years	5.20	6.60	8.20	9.80
3–5 years	6.20	7.90	9.80	11.90
6–8 years	8.00	10.30	12.90	15.60
9–11 years	10.00	12.90	16.20	19.50
Girls 12–19 years	9.50	12.30	15.20	18.20
Boys 12–19 years	11.20	14.40	18.20	21.80

*These costs are for combinations of foods that will provide nutritious meals for a week at four levels of cost. Costs are for individuals eating in a family of four persons. Costs are estimated monthly by the Consumer and Food Economics Institute, Agriculture Research Service, U.S. Department of Agriculture, Hyattsville, Md. 20782. Current cost figures are available from above address on request.

Translated into terms of annual per capita consumption, diet II represents a *reduction* in annual per capita food costs of nearly $100 (Table E-5) and provides a lower bound on the dietary cost of cholesterol reduction.

It should be remembered that if *mass* changes in diet occurred, the demands for different foods would be altered and the prices of the products would reflect the changing demands. In evaluating screening programs that would only recommend dietary changes for about one individual in 20, neglecting the impact of shifting demand on price is acceptable. For mass interventions, however, it may not be. The economic consequences of mass shifts in diet are sure to be com-

Table E–5. Cost analysis of a low-cholesterol and low-fat diet: Cholesterol-lowering Diet II

	Price per pound (cents), 1975	*Per capita consumption of item (pounds), 1976*	*Recommended per capita consumption (pounds)*	*Annual cost of dietary change (dollars)*
Cooking and salad oil, vegetable oil, shortening vegetable oil, margarine	55*	50.2	11.5	−$21.29
Butter and lard	74	7.2	0	− 5.33
Red meat: beef, pork, lamb, veal, organ meats, bacon, sausage	141†	155	52	−145.23
Poultry	64	50.5	78.0	+ 17.60
Fish	145‡	12.9	12.9	—
Beans, peas, nuts, soy products	72§	17.0	70.0	+ 38.16
Milk	20.5	278.6	370.0	+ 18.74
Eggs	6.2 per egg	276 eggs	156 eggs	− 7.44
Cheese	173	15.9	6.4	− 16.44
Flour and cereal	52¶	142	187	+ 23.40
Total savings				$97.83

*Average of prices for margarine and salad or cooking oil.

†Average of prices for red meats based on consumption of various foods listed.

‡Average of prices for frozen haddock fillets and canned tuna.

§Average of prices for red kidney beans and peanut butter.

¶Average of prices based on an assumed consumption of 70% bread and 30% other grain and cereal products.

plex. A sudden increase in the demand for a product would result in an increase in price, but suppliers would respond by increasing production, and if there were substantial economies of scale, the equilibrium price might be below the initial price. Government intervention and price supports further complicate the picture in ways that we cannot now estimate.

REFERENCES FOR APPENDIX E

1. *Food Consumption, Prices, Expenditures,* Supplement for 1974 to Agricultural Economic Report No. 138. Washington, D.C.: U.S. Department of Agriculture, Economic Research Service, January 1976.
2. *Livestock and Meat Situation,* Washington, D.C.: U.S. Department of Agriculture, Economic Research Service, August 1976.
3. *Poultry and Egg Situation,* Washington, D.C.: U.S. Department of Agriculture, Economic Research Service, June 1976.
4. *Commodity Yearbook 1975,* New York: Commodity Research Bureau, Inc. 1975.
5. *Estimated Retail Food Prices by City,* Washington, D.C.: U.S. Department of Labor, Bureau of Labor Statistics, May 1976.
6. Economic Research Service, U.S. Department of Agriculture, *National Food Situation,* September 1977.
7. Economic Research Service, U.S. Department of Agriculture, *Fats and Oils Situation,* February, 1978.
8. King JC, Cohenour SH, Corruccini CG, Schneeman P. Evaluation and modification of the basic four food guide, Nutr Educ, vol. 10, no. 1, January–March 1978.
9. American Home Economics Association, *Handbook of Food Preparation,* 1964.
10. Farquhar JW. *The American Way of Life Need Not Be Hazardous To Your Health,* New York: W. W. Norton, 1978.
11. Taylor CB, et al. Nutrition and Weight Control Program Planning Guide for the Community Studies Education Program of Stanford Heart Disease Prevention Program, April 6, 1979.
12. Your money's worth in foods, *Home and Garden Bulletin,* No. 183, Washington, D.C.: U.S. Department of Agriculture, Agricultural Research Service, 1976.

Appendix F. Formal development of the screening model

We can now bring together the assumptions discussed earlier to compute the cost-effectiveness of screening programs under various assumptions. Suppose we have chosen the program we wish to evaluate, with values for all the necessary parameters as given in Table 4-4.

BENEFITS

From the Benefits Model, we obtain $\Lambda(x)$, the discounted life expectancy at age 30 of a person with true log cholesterol value of x. $\Lambda(x)$ is derived empirically and cannot be represented exactly as a simple closed-form function of x. However, it is approximately quadratic in the region of interest, and we approximate it by the quadratic function

$$\Lambda(x) = -Qx^2/2 - Lx + A \tag{F.1}$$

Without such an approximation, we would have to represent Λ by a list of values for each point and simulate various screening programs using a large representative set of children. Then, computed results would be somewhat more in accord with our beliefs, but the numbers are less easy to generate and much harder to interpret. Making sense of what is going on in such simulations is no easier than making sense of experiments in the real world.

With the quadratic approximation, we can generate results in closed form, and sensitivity analysis becomes a simple matter of algebraic manipulation. The equations, furthermore, show the logic of the program, which makes interpretation clear and simple. We will fit the quadratic form by weighted least squares on the values of Λ from $X = -1.5$ to $X = +2.5$. The weights are chosen to match the probability of age 30 cholesterol rank for a child who is at the 96th percentile at age 10 and complies with treatment. (The unweighted ordinary least-squares fit on the same X values is quite similar.) The fit between the quadratic approximation and the actual life-table predictions for the base case of life expectancy at age 30 discounted at 5 percent is shown in Table F-1. For the purposes of finding the optimal point to screen and computing cost-effectiveness, the limited fit in Table F-1 is adequate because lower values of cholesterol do not affect the screening decision and higher values are so rare that the error in the fit of risk changes results only slightly.

Let x_0 represent the log cholesterol level at the time of the screen. Let x and x_0 be rescaled so that observed values at each time have mean 0 and variance 1. From our assumptions on stability of level, the distribution of final values of x conditioned on an initial value of x_0 is normal with mean Rx_0 and variance $1 - R^2$. If the child complies with intervention, the mean is reduced to $Rx_0 - J$. The benefits of intervention are reduced by the fraction complying K, the fraction of benefit F, and the need to discount the gains back 20 years to the time of screening. In sum, if $b(x_0)$ is the expected benefit of intervention on a child with level x_0,

$$b(x_0) = FK/(1 + D)^{20} \cdot \int [\Lambda(x - J) - \Lambda(x)]\, dP(x|x_0)$$

Table F-1. Quadratic fit of discounted life expectancy at age 30

True age 30 cholesterol in SD	*Weight*	*Value (mg/dl) standardized to men at age 40*	*Males Life expectancy (years) Predicted‡*	*Males Life expectancy (years) Fitted**	*Females Life expectancy (years) Predicted‡*	*Females Life expectancy (years) Fitted†*
−1.5	0.1	160	17.60	17.56	18.42	18.30
−1.0	0.3	177	17.54	17.54	18.39	18.37
− .5	0.6	195	17.47	17.48	18.36	18.39
0	1.0	216	17.38	17.39	18.31	18.34
0.5	1.0	238	17.26	17.26	18.23	18.24
1	1.0	263	17.11	17.10	18.10	18.07
1.5	0.6	290	16.91	16.90	17.89	17.85
2	0.3	321	16.66	16.66	17.56	17.56
2.5	0.1	354	16.34	16.39	17.06	17.21
			$R^2 = 1.00$		$R^2 = .98$	

*Standardized values of male life expectancy = $17.39 - .218\,x - .073\,x^2$.

†Standardized values of female life expectancy = $18.34 - .151\,x - .119\,x^2$.

‡Predicted from life-table models.

For simplicity, let $k = FK/(1 + D)^{20}$. Combining with equation F.1, we get

$$b(x_0) = k(QJRx_0 - QJ^2/2 + LJ)$$

Since $b(x_0)$ is linear in x_0, the benefit of intervening on the child with median cholesterol $b(0)$ is also the benefit of intervening on a randomly selected child. In addition,

$$b(x_0) = \mathrm{b}(0) + kQJRx_0 \qquad \text{(F.2)}$$

Let $B(d)$ be the average benefit of selecting a person from the initial screen at random and intervening if his log cholesterol level is greater than d standard deviations above the mean. Since x_0 is log-normally distributed, we can compute B from the equation

$$B(d) = \int_d^\infty b(x_0)\, \phi\, (x_0)\, dx_0 \qquad \text{(F.3)}$$

where ϕ is the standard normal density function $\phi(d) = 1/\sqrt{2\pi}$ exp $(-d^2/2)$. Let $\Phi(d)$ denote the cumulative normal distribution $\Phi(d) = \int_{-\infty}^{d} \phi\, (t)\, dt$. Then substituting equation F.2 into F.3, we obtain

$$B(d) = b(0)\, [1 - \Phi(d)] + kQJR\phi(d) \qquad \text{(F.4)}$$

COSTS

The cost of screening C_S is one of the parameters given in Table 4-4. The costs of intervention C_I are computed from the assumptions of level of program and compliance. Intervention costs must be discounted back to the time of screening. The average cost of selecting a person from the initial screen at random and intervening if his standardized log cholesterol level is above d is $C_S + C_I\, [1 - \Phi(d)]$.

SELECTION OF THE OPTIMAL CUTOFF FOR INTERVENTION

We know that at the optimal cutoff level for intervention, the marginal cost-effectiveness of intervening on the highest remaining child must equal the marginal cost-effectiveness of screening one more child and intervening if the level is above d. The former is $C_I/b(d)$ and the latter is $\{C_S + C_I[1 - \Phi(d)]\}/B(d)$. Equating these expressions and dividing by C_I, we get

$$B(d) = b(d)\, C_S/C_I + [1 - \Phi(d)]$$

After substitution of equation F.2 and F.4, this becomes

$$kQJR\{\phi(d) - d[1 - \Phi(d)]\} = C_S/C_I\, [b(0) + kJQR\, d] \qquad \text{(F.5)}$$

Table F-2. Elasticities: Sensitivity of cutoff and cost-effectiveness to assumptions

Parameter			
Symbol	*Meaning*	*Derivative of* d *with respect to proportional change in parameter*	*Elasticity of* C *with respect to change in parameter*
d	Cutoff point	—	0
F	Fraction of benefit	0	-1
K	Compliance (if noncompliers pay C_I)	0	-1
K	If noncompliers pay no charge	$(b + d)S$	$-S$
C_S	Cost of screening	$-(b + d)S$	S
C_I	Cost of intervention	$(b + d)S$	$1 - S$
$\frac{1}{1+D} = r$	Rate of Discount	$rS\left[\frac{C_I'(b + d)}{C_I} - b'\right]$	$r\left[\frac{C_I'}{C_I} - \frac{b'}{b + d}\right]$ $(1 - S) - \frac{rQ'}{Q} - 20$
J	Dietary reduction	$+JS/2R$	$-1 + \frac{J(1 - S)}{2R(b + d)}$
R	20-year correlation	bS	$-1 + b(1 - S)/(b + d)$
Q	Curviness of risk	LS/QR	$-1 + \frac{L(1 - S)}{(b + d)QR}$
L	Linear slope of risk	$-LS/QR$	$-L(1 - S)/(b + d)QR$

To simplify further computations, let $b = b(0)/kQJR$. Then equation F.5 can be written as

$$\phi(d) - d[1 - \Phi(d)] = C_S/C_I\,(b + d) \qquad \text{(F.6)}$$

As d increases, the left-hand side decreases and the right-hand side increases, so equation F.6 has a unique solution for all values of the parameters. Since the overall cost-effectiveness C is the same as the cost-effectiveness of intervening on a child at d, C is easily computed by substituting the optimal d into $C_I/b(d)$.

SENSITIVITY ANALYSIS

We can apply differential calculus to equation F.6 to compute what happens to the cutoff d and the cost-effectiveness C as we vary the assumed values of the parameters. In such analyses, economists generally present "elasticities," which measure the proportional change in results that follow from a proportional change in the parameter. For example, Table F-2 shows that the elasticity of C with respect to F is

-1. This means that a 10 percent increase in the fraction of benefit to dieters leads to a 10 percent decrease in the cost per year of life saved. The advantage of elasticities over derivatives is that they are unit-free, which makes it easy to switch from consideration of individuals to whole programs. In symbols, the elasticity of C with respect to x is $(x/C)\, dC/dx$.

Our computations are summarized in Table F-2. The proportion of program costs that goes to screening is $C_S/\{C_S + C_I[1 - \Phi(d)]\}$. This ratio appears in almost every expression in the table, so it will be convenient to denote it by S. The numerical values in Table 4-10 are computed by substituting the base values for all parameters and multiplying the derivative of d by $d(\log[1 - \Phi(d)])/dd = -\phi(d)/(1 - \Phi(d))$.

Appendix G. The model for repeated tests

For this analysis, we assume that every child has cholesterol levels measured twice, at an interval of about one month. Then we may assume we have two independent measurements. Let R_s be the correlation of measurements a month apart, and let R_l be the correlation of true values in a cohort over a 20-year interval. From Appendix B, we know that the average of the two measurements is the best predictor and $R'_s = \sigma^2/(\sigma^2 + \epsilon^2/2) = 2R_s/(1 + R_s)$, where R'_s is the correlation between two averages of two measurements. The development of Appendix F remains the same with $R'_s R_l = R'$ substituted for R until we get to equation F.3. Since the distribution of the average of two measurements has variance $\sigma^2 + \epsilon^2/2 = (\sigma^2 + \epsilon^2)(1 + R_s)/2$. Equation F.3 becomes

$$B(d) = \int_d^\infty b(x_o)\,\phi\,[x_0/\sqrt{(1 + R_s)/2}]\,dx_0 \qquad \text{(G.1)}$$

If we set $d' = d/\sqrt{(1 + R_s)/2}$, we can integrate equation G.1 to obtain,

$$B(d) = b(o)[1 - \Phi(d')] + kQJR'\sqrt{(1 + R_s)/2)}\,\phi(d')$$

Continuing as in Appendix F, the optimal cutoff occurs when

$$\sqrt{(1 + R_s)/2}\cdot\phi(d') - d[1 - \Phi(\mathrm{d}')] = C_s/C_I(b + d)$$

Appendix H. The formal model of an optimal rescreening strategy

The model of rescreening is an extension of the model presented in Appendix F, and our discussion here will utilize the same assumptions and notations. In addition, we will require a few new calculations on the characteristics of repeated cholesterol measurements.

Recall that observed log cholesterol values are standardized in our model to a mean of 0 and a variance of 1. Given any two measurements (X_1 and X_2) on the same individual, the expected true value is

$$E(t|X_1, X_2) = (X_1 + X_2)/2 \cdot \sigma^2/(\sigma^2 + \epsilon^2/2)$$

Even if X_2 is a measurement from rescreening a selected initial screenee, the average of X_1 and X_2 still provides the best measure of true cholesterol.

We define R_s as the short-term correlation coefficient of cholesterol

$$R_s = \sigma^2/(\sigma^2 + \epsilon^2)$$

The distribution of a second measurement, X_2, given an initial measurement of X_1, is normal, with mean $R_s X_1$ and a variance of $1 - R_s^2$. The correlation, σ, between the average of two measurements now and true cholesterol level 20 years from now is given by

$$\sigma = R_l \cdot \sigma^2/(\sigma^2 + \epsilon^2/2)$$

We represent the cutoff level for intervention by d. In a selective rescreening program, we wish to define a new cutoff level d_R above which children are retested. In an optimal program, three cost-effectiveness ratios are equal to each other:

The cost-effectiveness of intervening on a child at d

The cost-effectiveness of rescreening a child whose level in the initial screen is d_R

The cost-effectiveness of the program as a whole

Setting these three ratios equal permits us to solve for d and d_R and gives us the overall cost-effectiveness.

The average cost per screenee for the whole program depends on the sum of the cost of the initial screening, the cost of rescreening if the child is above d_R, and the cost of intervention if the average of the two measurements is above d.

For notational ease, let

$$A(X_1) \equiv \phi(X_2 - R_s X_1)/\sqrt{(1 - R_s^2)}$$

Then,

$$\text{Cost} = C_S + C_S[1 - \Phi(d_R)] + C_I \int_{d_R}^{\infty} \int_{2d - x_1}^{\infty} A(x_1)\, dx_2\, \phi(x_1)\, dx_1 \qquad \text{(H.1)}$$

Similarly,

$$\text{Benefits} = \int_{d_R}^{\infty} \int_{2d - x_1}^{\infty} \left[b(\text{o}) + kJQR' \frac{x_1 + x_2}{2} \right] A(x_1)\, dx_2\, \phi(x_1)\, dx_1 \qquad \text{(H.2)}$$

The other required formulas are simpler. The average cost of retesting a child whose initial measurement is d_R is given by

$$C_S + C_I \int_{2d-d_R}^{\infty} A(d_R)\, dx_2 \qquad \text{(H.3)}$$

while the benefits are

$$\int_{2d-d_R}^{\infty} \left[b(\text{o}) + kJQR' \frac{(d_R + x_2)}{2} \right] A(d_R)\, dx_2 \qquad \text{(H.4)}$$

Finally the cost-effectiveness of treating at d is $b(d)/C_I$.

Equating H.3/H.4 with $b(d)/C_I$, we can solve for d_R as a function of d. Each pair (d, d_R) is substituted into equations H.1/H.2. We can thus search for a value of d to make the three cost-effectiveness ratios equal.

If the cost of screening includes some fixed costs in each screening site, then the only changes needed in the computational procedure are to let C_S be the variable cost per screenee and to add a sum to equation H.1 equal to the fixed costs per site divided by the number of screenees per site.

Appendix I. The formal model of case-finding

The model that we use to describe and evaluate the efficiency of an optimal Case-finding program to supplement Universal Screening makes several tacit assumptions. First, it assumes that siblings of a positive screenee are close in age to the propositus and, in particular, that their ages are similar enough that no adjustment needs to be made for either fraction of benefit or effect of discounting over slightly different time periods. Second, we assume that the screening costs for siblings, once found, are small. Finally, our evaluation of Case-finding applies rigorously only to the first year of the program and thereby makes the implicit assumption that siblings of positive screenees have not themselves been screened in school as primary screenees.

We extend the linear additive model described in Appendixes A through F by dividing the variance of cholesterol level into two components: one resulting from shared attributes of siblings and one resulting from all other effects. Correlations that bear on the first component of the variance are derived from the literature on age- and sex-adjusted cholesterol levels. In the analysis that follows, we assume that the cholesterol level is measured only once, so that the Case-finding model can be compared directly to the model in Appendix F, in which a similar assumption was made.

Our Case-finding model thus assumes that an individual's standardized age- and sex-adjusted log cholesterol value is the sum of three independent, random, normally distributed variables: (1) the genetic and environmental effects shared by siblings (which have a variance that we denote by s); (2) other real effects; and (3) random fluctuation, or noise.

Further analysis requires two estimates. First, we must know the expected distribution of cholesterol levels in the siblings of screenees. Given a screenee's cholesterol level of X, then his or her sibling has an expected level with a mean of sX and a variance of $1 - s^2$. Second, we must estimate the *true* cholesterol level of a sibling of screenee, which will be some weighted combination of the sibling's measured level and the screenee's measured level. In particular, if a screenee has a measured cholesterol level of b and a sibling of that screenee has a measured level of a, then the best estimate of the sibling's *true* level is not a but rather

$$\text{“True cholesterol”} = \frac{(R_s - s^2)a}{1 - s^2} + \frac{s(1 - R_s)b}{1 - s^2}$$

Even if monogenic forms of hypercholesterolemia did not exist, we might expect from the discussion so far that Case-finding would make a valuable contribution to cost-effectiveness for at least two reasons: (1) the average observed cholesterol levels of siblings of positive screenees will be higher than that of the general population, and (2) the expected *true* values of siblings, given their observed values, will also be higher than would be the case for the general population.

For a Case-finding program, we would seek to set the optimal levels for three cutoff levels:

The level at which to intervene on positive screenees (d)

The level at which to intervene on siblings of positive screenees (t)

The level at which to initiate a search among the siblings of an initial screenee (d_1)

At the optimum cutoff levels, the following four cost-effectiveness ratios would be equal to each other:

The cost-effectiveness of treatment of initial screenees at d

The cost-effectiveness of treatment of siblings at t

The cost-effectiveness of initiating a search among siblings of initial screenees at d_1

The cost-effectiveness of the screening and Case-finding program as a whole

If one of these ratios were higher than the others, then the relevant cutoff level should be changed so that resources are shifted toward the more efficient enterprises. At the optimum, the ratios must be equal.

The existence of monogenic forms of hypercholesterolemia (MHC) creates a problem for the analysis of Case-finding. We know very little about the distribution of cholesterol levels among people with MHC, but we assume that their mean cholesterol levels are 65 percent above normal, with a standard deviation of 10 percent. Moreover, we will simplify our work by assuming that each child with MHC would receive the same benefit from intervention and that the unaffected members of an affected family are not hypercholesterolemic. In the equations below, we represent the benefits from intervention to a child with MHC as the product of a factor k multiplied by the benefit from intervention to a child without MHC whose cholesterol level is 65 percent above normal.

The optimizing equations for Case-finding are considerably more complicated than for other programs, and to ease the computational chores, we make a few further assumptions. Although a sibling's true cholesterol level does depend on the value of the initial screenee's level (as can be seen in Table I-1), we assume that the same correction to the sibling's measured level applies in all cases. In particular, we will adjust the sibling's observed level by an expression that uses the factor $d_1 + 0.5$ to represent the initial screenee level instead of using the initial screenee's actual measured level. Table I-1 shows how a sibling's measured cholesterol level can be adjusted to a better estimate of his "true" level by using a weighted sum of his own cholesterol score and his sibling's (the initial screenee's) score.

Because we assume that intervention costs are the same for initial screenees and for treated siblings, the relative cost-effectiveness ratios of treatment depend only on the true cholesterol levels of each. Thus, an optimum Case-finding program would employ cutoff levels for treatment of initial screenees (d) and of siblings (t) that satisfy the following equations for the equality of the true levels assuming $R_{\text{SIB}} = .35$ and $R_s = .8$:

$$.8\,d = .77t + .08(d_1 + .5)$$

The ideal proportion of cases to treat depends partly on the probability that an initial screenee at cholesterol level d_1 has MHC. Using an assumption that children with MHC have normally distributed log cholesterol levels, with a mean of 2.5 and a standard deviation of .5, this probability is

Table I-1. Weights for estimating the true cholesterol level from an individual's measured level and his or her sibling's measured level (assuming $R_s = .8$)

Correlation coefficient between siblings (R_{SIB})	*Weight on the individual's measured level*	*Weight on the sibling's measured level*
.25	.79	.05
.35	.77	.08
.45	.75	.11

Note. For example, if an individual has a true level X_T and a measured level X_i and a sibling with a measured level X_s, and if $R_{SIB} = .35$ and $r = .8$, then $X_T = .77X_i + .08X_s$ provides the best estimate of X_T.

$$p(d_1) = 2f\ [\exp(-2.5 - d_1)^2/.5] \div \exp(-d_1^2/2)$$

where f is the proportion of the whole population who have MHC.

The cost of Case-finding in a sibling at d_1 and intervening at cholesterol levels above t is thus

$$C_F + C_I\ \{(1 - p)\ [1 - \Phi\ (t')] + p/2\}$$

where

$$t' = (t - sd_1)/\sqrt{1 - s^2}$$

If we assume that the benefits for treated siblings who do not have MHC have the same distribution as the benefits for initial screenees and that the benefits for children with MHC are k times the corresponding benefits to a nonheterozygote at the same cholesterol level, then the benefits of Case-finding at d_1 are given by

$$[1 - p(d_1)][1 - \Phi(t')][b + \phi(d)/1 - \Phi(d)] + (b + 2.5)\cdot k\cdot p(d_1)/2 \qquad \text{(I.2)}$$

We can solve for d_1 by equating I.1/I.2 with $C_I/b(d)$.

Finally, let A be the expected number of siblings investigated for each positive initial screenee, let s_1 denote the treated siblings in each search who do not have MHC, and let s_2 denote the treated siblings in each search who do have MHC.

$$s_1 = \int_{d_1}^{\infty} [1 - p(x_1)]\{1 - \phi\ [(t - sx_1)/\sqrt{1 - s^2}]\}\ \phi\ (x_1)\ dx_1$$

$$s_2 = \tfrac{1}{2} \int_{d_1}^{\infty} p(x_1) \cdot \phi(x_1) dx_1$$

The expected costs of screening one child and proceeding with the Case-finding program are

$$C_s + C_I\ [1 - \Phi(d)] + C_F A\ [1 - \Phi(d_1)] + C_I A(s_1 + s_2) \qquad \text{(I.3)}$$

The expected benefits of such action are

$$[b + \phi(d)/1 - \Phi(d)][1 - \Phi(d) + As_1] + (b + 2{\cdot}5)kAs_2 \qquad \text{(I.4)}$$

Equating equations I.3/I.4 with $C_I/b(d)$, we can find the optimal values of d, t, and d_1.

Appendix J. Derivation of estimates for use in evaluating targeted screening programs

Evaluation of targeted screening programs that attempt to capitalize on the high risk associated with positive family histories or premature coronary disease requires the estimation of several new parameters, including the yield of family history questionnaires of several sorts and the risk and cholesterol levels that can be expected to characterize those children who respond positively to the questionnaire. This appendix discusses the derivation of three of those estimates, which are summarized briefly in the text of Chapter 5.

YIELD OF QUESTIONS ON FAMILY HISTORY OF MYOCARDIAL INFARCTION

The potential yield of family history questionnaires can be estimated from data on the incidence of first heart attack by age and sex combined with data on the age distribution of parents and grandparents of 10-year-old children.

From the Framingham study, we have some estimates for the risk of first myocardial infarction for people who are alive at a given age. Using the stationary population generated by 1976 death rates (*Monthly Vital Statistics Report,* March 1978), we can estimate how many people out of 100 born would be alive and free of infarction at each age if current death rates were to continue to apply in the future. We can then use the Framingham risks to estimate the probability that a random person will have a heart attack before each specified age. The results are shown in Table J-1.

Table J-1. Risk and cumulative incidence of first myocardial infarction (MI) at various ages

Sex	*Age range*	*Risk of first MI in period* (%)*	*Cumulative incidence of first MI per 100 thirty-year-olds (at end of period)†*
Men	30–34	0.5	0.5
	35–39	0.7	1.1
	40–44	1.3	2.4
	45–49	2.0	4.2
	50–54	2.8	6.7
	55–59	4.8	10.6
	60–64	6.5	15.3
	65–69	6.0	19.1
Women	40–44	0.2	0.2
	45–49	0.4	0.6
	50–54	0.5	1.1
	55–59	0.8	1.8
	60–64	1.3	2.9
	65–69	1.8	4.4

Source. Monthly Vital Statistics Report, March 1978.
* Framingham data
†Assuming 100 born each year.

The next computation, that of the age of parents and grandparents of 10-year-old children, must be done in steps. First, from the 1968 vital statistics on birth, we can determine the age distribution of mothers of 10-year-olds. The distribution of fathers' ages is then estimated, assuming that fathers are, on the average, two years older than mothers (with a standard deviation of three years). Their grandparents ages are then estimated assuming that the 1968 distribution of parents' ages at birth applied to the earlier years when the parents themselves were born. The results are shown in Table J-2. Since a questionnaire would yield information on both dead and living relatives, the numbers in Table J-2 include parents and grandparents who would have, in fact, died.

Finally, to estimate the yield of a questionnaire, we combine the information in Tables J-1 and J-2. In order to reduce the complexity of later benefits calculations, we categorize children by the most significant part of their history. Thus, among children with a positive history of heart attack in a parent, we make no further distinctions according

Table J-2. Age distribution of parents and grandparents of 10-year-olds, including those who have died

Age (years)	*Father*	*Mother*	*Age (years)*	*Grandfather*	*Grandmother*
<30	.11	.17	<50	.02	.03
30–34	.36	.37	50–54	.08	.10
35–39	.29	.26	55–59	.19	.21
40–44	.14	.12	60–64	.24	.23
45+	.10	.08	65–69	.20	.19
			70–74	.15	.14
			75+	.12	.10
Total	1.00	1.00		1.00	1.00

to grandparent history. If several grandparents have had heart attacks, we take into account only the history of the youngest of these. We assume that the probabilities of heart attacks of spouses are independent of each other, but we do make adjustments for the expected correlation between coronary disease events in parents and grandparents. The results are shown in Table 5-8 of Chapter 5.

RELATIVE RISK OF CORONARY HEART DISEASE OF OFFSPRING OF VICTIMS OF MYOCARDIAL INFARCTION

Our estimates of the relative risks of coronary disease in persons with a positive parental history are derived from studies of risk among first-degree relatives of people with myocardial infarction. We first estimate the risks relative to a negative family history and then use data on the incidence of heart attack to adjust these to risks relative to the population average. Finally, we estimate the relative risks given a positive history in grandparents by extrapolation from the results for parents. Because of this extrapolation, the estimates of risk, given a positive history in grandparents, must be regarded as especially speculative.

There are several studies of coronary risk among first-degree relatives of people with myocardial infarction. The best of these for our purposes is that of Slack and Evans (1966), whose data are aggregated and displayed in Table J-3.

The relative risks in Table J-3 are quite high. For example, the risk of death compared to the average in the youngest relatives of the youngest index patients is 7/.5 or 14. However, the 95 percent confidence interval for this risk is large, ranging approximately from 6.7 to

Table J-3. Ischemic heart disease deaths in relatives of index patients*

Age of relatives' CHD death	*Age of CHD in index patient*					
	Males < 45 Females < 55		*Males 45–54 Females 55–64*		*Males 55–64 Females 64–69*	
	Observed	*Expected*	*Observed*	*Expected*	*Observed*	*Expected*
Males < 45 Females < 55	7	.5	2	.6	0	.5
Males 45–54 Females 55–64	9	1.4	15	2.9	3	1
Males 55–64 Females 65–69	9	3.7	12	6.2	2	2.2

*Calculated from data in Slack and Evans, 1966.

30. The results calculated from the work of Slack and Evans are corroborated by three large population studies. Deutscher et al. (1970) showed that the risk of fatal coronary disease in men aged 40 to 59 in the Tecumseh study was about eight times higher for those with a parent who died of coronary disease before 65 than for those whose parents died of other causes. Sholtz et al. (1975) showed a relative risk of 2.02 for symptomatic myocardial infarction before the age of 50 years for those with a positive parental history of ischemic heart disease compared with those whose family histories were negative.

Finally, Førde and Thelle (1977) showed a relative risk of 5.5 for heart attack under the age of 50 for people with a positive history in a male family member and a risk of 13 for people with a positive history in a female. The lower value in the Sholtz study is probably the result of its less restrictive definition of a positive history. The other studies reported results based on "hard," early events. Combining these results, we obtain our estimates for the relative risk of coronary death at various ages as a function of age of onset of disease in parents (Table J-4).

As a last step in our risk calculations, the risks relative to negative family history are converted to risks relative to the population average using data on the incidence of infarction before each age to determine how people would be apportioned among history categories. For this estimate, we must assume that the children we screened are old enough so that their parents have had a chance to run through all the age categories, since this *was* the case in the studies from which the relative risks that we use are derived. By adjusting for the distribution of the population among parental history categories for 50-year-olds,

Table J-4. Risk of death from heart disease in people with a positive parental history relative to people with a negative parental history

	Age of parents' first MI			
Age of child's CHD death	*Males < 45 Females < 55*	*45–54 55–64*	*55–64 65–69*	*Other*
Males < 45 Females < 55	10	6	2	1
Males 45–54 Females 55–64	6	6	2	1
Males 55–64 Females 65–69	2	2	2	1

Table J-4 can be reexpressed as risks relative to the population average, with the results shown in Table 5-9.

In the absence of detailed empirical data on the effect of a positive history of myocardial infarction in grandparents on future coronary heart disease mortality in grandchildren, we have been forced to estimate this risk from the observed risks from a positive parental history. The results gleaned therefrom seem plausible but are based on several unsupported assumptions, and are the least empirically founded of any parameters used in the analysis.

Basically our model assumes that the effects of a positive history in paternal grandparents are completely communicated through the elevated risk of the father. In other words, we use the matrix of relative risks of positive parents' history twice—first to compute the impact of a positive history in a grandparent on the chances that the father will have an early heart attack, and then to estimate the effects of that putative paternal history on the relative coronary risk of the child. We assume that the impact of a positive history in a maternal grandparent is the same as in a paternal grandparent, even though the excess risk would not be expressed phenotypically as often in the mother as in the father.

For simplicity, we also assume that the risk to the child depends on the single riskiest part of his or her history. Thus, in the unlikely event that a parent had already had a heart attack, the grandparents' experience is ignored. If one grandparent had a premature myocardial infarction and another had a later infarction, only the impact of the former is considered. This simplification renders computation much easier, and our results are, on the whole, so tentative that it would not be productive to grapple with the complication that would be introduced by trying to adjust for the fairly rare occurrence of multiple positive family histories. However, we should in fairness note that Deutscher, for example, showed that the risk of coronary disease at young ages in the Tecumseh study was three times as high for men with *both* parents dead from heart disease than for men with only *one* parent dead from heart disease. Some of that difference can be reconciled with our simplifying assumption by the fact that the younger of two dead parents will have died several years younger, on the average, than a single parent victim of coronary disease. Our calculations yield the results shown in Table 5-10.

CHOLESTEROL LEVELS IN OFFSPRING OF VICTIMS

The children of victims of early heart attack can be expected to have higher cholesterol values than the population at large, because the victims themselves have higher values than normal and because correlations in lipid levels among family members are generally positive.

In Appendix A we showed that the approximate cholesterol level of victims of heart disease is β standard deviations over the mean, where β is the regression coefficient of cholesterol in the mathematical expression for risk as a function of cholesterol. From this we can infer that the children of victims of early heart attack should have levels of $.3\beta$ and the grandchildren should have levels of $.15\beta$, using Sing's linear model G (Sing and Orr, 1978) and his empirical results from the Tecumseh study.

These predictions can be verified by comparison with the many studies of cholesterol levels in survivors of myocardial infarction and their children. Table J-5 shows the Framingham betas, which are in good agreement with the measured cholesterol levels of heart attack survivors, except for those with the earliest infarctions. Apparently cholesterol level becomes an extremely important risk factor at very young ages, but these events are so rare that they could not be estimated in the Framingham study.

The cholesterol levels for first-degree relatives of victims of myocardial infarction are shown in Table J-6. Except for the study by Tamir et al. (1972), the agreement is good between the empirical data and the predictions of our mathematical model. Large retrospective population studies (such as the one by Sholtz et al. [1975]) yield lower values than do studies from specialized centers (such as the reports by Jensen et al. [1967] and Stone et al. [1974]). This might follow from

Table J-5. Cholesterol levels of victims of myocardial infarction

Study	*Number of events*	*Age (years)*	*Results (standard deviations from the mean)*		*Central value (mg/dl)*
			Men	*Women*	
Framingham*		45–54	0.54	0.76	
		55–64	0.33	0.57	
		65–74	0.27	0.54	
Goldstein et al†	401 M	30–39	0.95	—	
(1973a, 1973b)	99 W	40–49	0.7	1.0	
		50–59	0.45	0.6	
		60–69	0.3	0.6	
		70–79	0.3	0.4	
Patterson & Slack	108 M	30–39	1.1	—	
(1972)	85 W	40–49	0.8‡	0.2	
		50–59	0.7	0.5	
		60–69	0.7	0.7	
Nikkilä & Arö (1973)	101	<50	0.7		301
Tamir et al. (1972)	64 M	<41	1.1		263
Blumenthal et al. (1975)	28	<50	0.6§		251
Glueck et al. (1974)	70	<50	1.4§		284 (median)

*Maximum likelihood estimate for regression coefficient of log cholesterol on event.

†Estimated from percentage hyperlipidemic assuming log-normality of cholesterol and no interaction between age and proportion of hyperlipidemics that were hypercholesterolemic.

‡Assuming cholesterol values for 40-year-olds are no greater than those for 50-year-olds.

§Controlled by U.S. males aged 35 to 44 at time of study.

Table J-6. Levels of cholesterol in children of victims of myocardial infarction

Study	*Number of subjects*	*Parent's event*	*Measured central cholesterol level (standard deviations from the mean*	*Predicted cholesterol level from the model (standard deviations from the mean)*
Nikkilä and Arô (1973)	412	MI < 50	0.4	0.3
Tamir et al. (1972)	140	MI < 41	1.4	0.4
Hennekens et al. (1976)	90	MI < 50	0.5	0.3
Glueck et al. (1974)	223	MI < 50	0.3	0.3
Sholtz et al. (1975)	578	CHD	0.19	0.15
Førde and Thelle (1977)	749	MI < 60	0.14	0.19
		MI ⩾ 60	0.05	0.11

two likely sources of error; namely poor recall in reported family history in population studies, which would dilute the observed effects of family history, and bias in the selection of patients for the specialized centers, which would inflate the effects that these centers observe.

Appendix K. The population-wide intervention model

In the previously analyzed screening programs, cholesterol-lowering diets were recommended to individuals whose serum cholesterol levels were above a specified cutoff point. The programs saved life-years because those with relatively high cholesterol levels were able to lower their levels. In the screening models, no benefits derived from individuals with lower cholesterol levels, since they remained untreated and their levels were assumed to remain unchanged. In both the School Education and the Mass Media programs, in contrast, we assume that all individuals will be advised to adopt a "prudent" (or cholesterol-lowering) diet without regard to their initial cholesterol levels. Benefits from these population-wide programs will accrue because the entire distribution of cholesterol shifts downward or, from a different perspective, because some fraction of the population, P, chosen *independent* of cholesterol level, achieve lower lipid levels, while the remainder $(1 - P)$ remain unchanged.

In our previous analyses, we approximated an individual's life expectancy as a function of cholesterol level using a quadratic function of log cholesterol (see Appendix A):

$$\Lambda(X) = A - LX - QX^2/2 \tag{K.1}$$

where X is the normalized log cholesterol level; A, L, and Q are constants to be fitted; and $\Lambda(X)$ is the life expectancy (or expected years to first coronary event) for an individual at X.

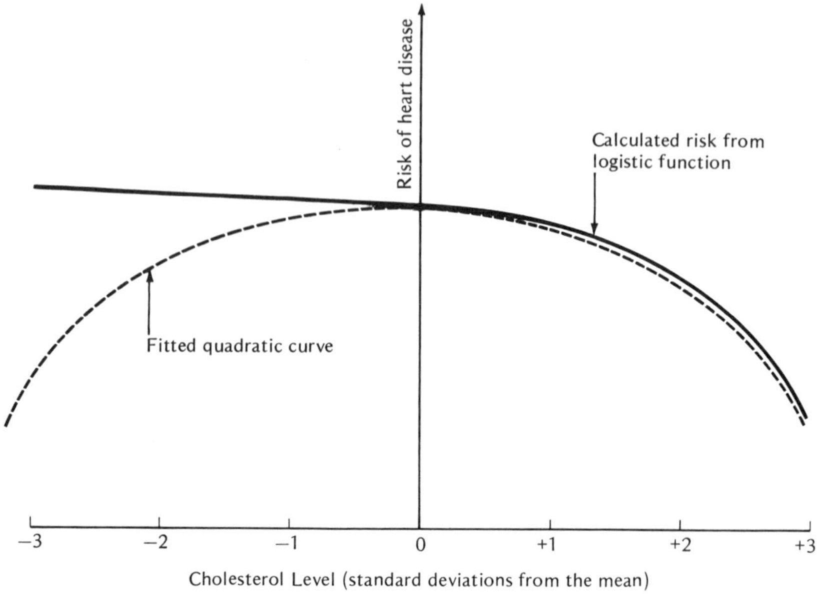

Figure K-1. The Accuracy of the Quadratic Approximation for Calculated Risk at Various Cholesterol Levels.

While this model resulted in a good fit to our computed risk curve for individuals with levels above the mean, the fit deteriorated for individuals with levels below the mean. The *computed* life expectancy curve is a monotonic function of X that increases as X becomes more negative; however, for sufficiently large negative values of X, the quadratic *approximation* of life expectancy $\Lambda(X)$ begins to decrease (see Figure K-1).

As long as our programs recommended interventions only on individuals well above the mean, this deterioration of fit made little difference to our estimates of overall benefits. Mass Media and School Education programs, however, will be intervening on individuals both above and below the mean. To achieve a better fit to the computed risks, we have replaced our quadratic model of risk with a cubic model:

$$\Lambda(X) = A + LX + QX^2 + CX^3 \qquad \text{(K.2)}$$

where X is the normalized log cholesterol level; A, L, Q, and C are constants to be fitted; and $\Lambda(X)$ is the life expectancy (or expected years to the first coronary event) for an individual at X. The cubic model, although somewhat more complex to work with, results in a better fit to the computed life expectancy curves for all values of X within 4 SD of the mean.

As before, we assume that cholesterol is log-normally distributed and that our intervention results in a constant proportional change in cholesterol level, which is the same thing as a constant shift in log cholesterol units of Δ standard deviations.

The change in life expectancy for an individual going from log cholesterol level X to level $(X - \Delta)$ is given by

$$\Lambda(X - \Delta) - \Lambda(X) = -L\,\Delta + Q\,\Delta^2 - C\,\Delta^3 - 2Q\,\Delta X + 3C\,\Delta^2 X - 3C\,\Delta X^2 \quad \text{(K.3)}$$

If log cholesterol is normally distributed with a mean of zero and a variance of one, the average benefit to the community of a community-wide shift of Δ is given by

$$\text{Benefit} = \int_{-\infty}^{+\infty} [\Lambda(X - \Delta) - \Lambda(X)]\, \mathrm{N}(0, 1)\, dX \quad \text{(K.4)}$$

where $N(0, 1)$ is the unit normal density function. This simplifies to

$$\text{Benefit} = -\,(L + 3C)\,\Delta + Q\,\Delta^2 - C\,\Delta^3 \quad \text{(K.5)}$$

Using the previously computed values for life expectancy and years free from heart disease, the constants for the cubic model were estimated using a least-squares regression, with the results shown in Table K-1. Benefits in terms of added years of life and added disease-free years were calculated using equation K.5 for several different levels of Δ. These benefits are tabulated in Table K-2.

To permit direct comparison with the program for 10-year-olds evaluated in Chapters 4 and 5, the benefits in Table K-2 have been adjusted by discounting from birth back to age 10. They are greater than benefits to newborns by a factor of $(1 + D)^{10}$.

The calculated benefits are for the case where 100 percent of the population undergoes a shift of Δ. Because the linear component dominates the benefit equation for small shifts, the benefits will be approximately the same when a fraction P of the population undergoes a shift of Δ/P and a fraction $1 - P$ of the population remains unchanged. In other words, the benefits reported in Table K-2 are a good approximation to the *average* benefits that might be expected to accompany a community-wide *average* shift of Δ.

Table K-1. Fitted constants for cubic model

		*Constants in cubic risk equation**		
Discount rate	*Sex*	*L*	*Q*	*C*
Life expectancy				
0%	F	−0.947	−0.499	−0.1342
	M	−1.033	−0.269	−0.0389
5%	F	−0.126	−0.0760	−0.0226
	M	−0.208	−0.0578	−0.0091
10%	F	−0.0216	−0.0151	−0.0049
	M	−0.0565	−0.0169	−0.0029
Heart-disease-free years				
0%	F	−1.677	−0.283	−0.0117
	M	−1.928	−0.327	−0.0147
5%	F	−0.253	−0.0460	−0.0031
	M	−0.330	−0.0621	−0.0049
10%	F	−0.0500	−0.0098	−0.00091
	M	−0.0824	−0.0172	−0.0019
Stroke-free years				
0%	F	−0.143	−0.032	−0.0060
	M	−0.117	−0.014	−0.0011
5%	F	−0.0264	−0.0067	−0.0012
	M	−0.0262	−0.0033	−0.00028
10%	F	−0.0063	−0.0017	−0.00033
	M	−0.0080	−0.0011	−0.00010

*$R(X) = A + LX + QX^2 + CX^3$

Table K-2. Health benefits from a population-wide shift in cholesterol (discounted to age 10)

Shift in cholesterol		*Men*			*Women*		
Δ *(standard deviations)*	J_M *(or* J_E*) percent*	*Days of life added*	*Heart-disease-free days added*	*Stroke-free days added*	*Days of life added*	*Heart-disease-free days added*	*Stroke-free days added*
Discount rate = 0%							
.01	0.2	4.0	7.3	0.4	4.7	6.2	0.6
.05	1.0	20.8	35.8	2.2	24.1	31.0	2.9
.10	2.0	40.9	70.8	4.3	47.5	61.5	5.8
.15	3.0	60.6	105.1	6.5	70.1	91.4	8.6
.20	4.0	79.9	139.1	8.6	91.6	120.9	11.3
.30	6.0	117.2	205.1	12.7	132.9	178.3	16.6
Discount rate = 5%							
.01	0.2	0.3	0.5	*	0.3	0.4	*
.05	1.0	1.6	2.2	0.2	1.3	1.8	0.2
.10	2.0	3.3	4.8	0.4	2.6	3.5	0.4
.15	3.0	4.8	6.9	0.6	3.8	5.3	0.6
.20	4.0	6.2	9.1	0.8	5.1	7.0	0.8
.30	6.0	9.1	13.5	1.2	7.3	10.3	1.2
Discount rate = 10%							
.01	0.2	*	0.1	*	*	*	*
.05	1.0	0.2	0.3	*	0.1	0.1	*
.10	2.0	0.3	0.5	*	0.2	0.3	*
.15	3.0	0.5	0.7	0.1	0.3	0.4	0.1
.20	4.0	0.7	0.9	0.1	0.4	0.6	0.1
.30	6.0	1.0	1.4	0.1	0.5	0.8	0.1

*Less than 0.1 days added.

Bibliography

Abraham S: Total serum cholesterol levels in children, 4–17 years, United States, 1971–1974, Vital and Health Statistics, Series 11: Data from National Health Survey, No. 207. DHEW pub. no. (PHS) 78-1655. Washington, D.C.: Government Printing Office, 1978.

Abraham S., Johnson CL, Carroll MD: A comparison of levels of serum cholesterol of adults 18-74 years of age in the United States in 1960–62 and 1971–74. Advancedata no. 5, February 22, 1977. DHEW pub. no. (HRA) 77-1250. Rockville, Md: National Center for Health Statistics, 1977.

Acton JP: Measuring the Social Impact of Heart and Circulatory Disease Programs. R-1697-NHLI. Santa Monica, Calif.: Rand Corporation, 1975.

Altschul AM: The potential for vegetable proteins in prudent diet foods. Prev Med 2:378-386, 1973.

American Academy of Pediatrics, Committee on Nutrition: Childhood diet and coronary heart disease. Pediatrics 49:305-307, 1972.

American Heart Association, Committee on Nutrition. Diet and Coronary Heart Disease. New York: American Heart Association, 1973(a).

American Heart Association: Coronary Risk Handbook: Estimating Risk of Coronary Heart Disease in Daily Practice. New York: American Heart Association, 1973(b).

American Heart Association, Pooling Project Research Group: Relationship of blood pressure serum cholesterol, smoking habit, relative weight and ECG abnormalities to incidence of major coronary events: Final report of the Pooling Project. American Heart Association Monograph Number 60. Dallas: American Heart Association, 1978.

Anitschkow N: Ueber die veranderungen der kaninchenaorta bei experimenteller cholesterinsteatose. Beitr Pathol Anat Allg Pathol 56: 379–404, 1913.

Antonis A, Bersohn I: Serum triglyceride levels in South African Europeans and Bantu and in ischaemic heart-disease. Lancet 1:998-1002, 1960.

Armstrong BK, Mann JI, Adelstein AM, Eskin F: Commodity consumption and ischemic heart disease mortality, with special reference to dietary practices. J Chronic Dis 28:455-469, 1975.

Armstrong ML, Megan MB, Warner ED: Intimal thickening in normocholesterolemic rhesus monkeys fed low supplements of dietary cholesterol. Circ Res 34:447–454, 1974.

Armstrong ML, Warner ED, Conner WE: Regression of coronary atheromatosis in rhesus monkeys. Circ Res 27:59–67, 1970.

Arö A: Serum lipids and lipoproteins in first degree relatives of young survivors of myocardial infarction. Acta Med Scand Suppl 553, 1973.

Aronow WS, Allen WH, De Cristofaro D, Ungermann S: Follow-up of mass screening for coronary risk factors in 1817 adults. Circulation 51:1038–1045, 1975.

Ashley FW, Kannel WB: Relation of weight change to changes in atherogenic traits: The Framingham study. J Chronic Dis 27:103–114, 1974.

Atlas P, Clejan S, Eshchar Y, Neufeld HN: Primary familial hyperlipoproteinemia in young adults with myocardial infarction and their relatives. Harefuah 89:145–147, 1975.

Axnick NW, Shavell SM, Witte JJ: Benefits due to immunization against measles. Public Health Rep 84:673–680, 1969.

Bailar JC III: Mammography: A contrary view. Ann Intern Med 84:77–84, 1976.

Baker H, Frank O, Feingold S, Christakis G, Ziffer H: Vitamins, total cholesterol, and triglycerides in 642 New York City school children. Am J Clin Nutr 20:850–857, 1967.

Ball KP, Hanington E, McAllen PM, Pilkington TRE, Richards JM, Sharland DE, Sowry SC, Wilkinson P, Clarke JAC, Murland C, Wood J: Low-fat diet in myocardial infarction. A controlled trial. Lancet 2:501–504, 1965.

Barboriak JJ, Rimm AA, Anderson AJ, Tristani FE, Walker JA, Flemma RJ: Coronary artery occlusion and blood lipids. Am Heart J 87:716–721, 1974.

Bauer RA: The obstinate audience: The influence process from the point of view of social communication. Am Psychol 19:319–328, 1964.

Baumol WJ: On the social rate of discount. Am Econ Rev 58: 788–802, 1968.

Baumol WJ: On the discount rate for public projects, in The Analysis and Evaluation of Public Expenditures: The PPB System, vol 1. U.S. Congress, Joint Economic Committee. Washington, DC: Government Printing Office, 1969.

Berenson GS, Foster TA, Frank GC, Frerichs RR, Srinivasan SR, Voors AW, Webber LS: Cardiovascular disease risk factor variables at the preschool age: The Bogalusa Heart Study. Circulation 57:603–612, 1978.

Berenson GS, Srinivasan SR, Dalfers ER, Puyau FA, O'Meallie LP, Hall RJ, Pargaonkar PS : Serum lipoproteins and coronary heart disease. Am J Cardiol 34:558–593, 1974.

Bergsma D: Ethical, Social and Legal Dimensions of Screening for Human Genetic Disease. New York: Stratton Intercontinental Medical Book Corporation, 1974.

Berkson J: Maximum likelihood and minimum χ^2 estimates of the logistic function. J Am Stat Assoc 50:130–162, 1955.

Bersohn I, Wayburne S: Serum cholesterol concentration in newborn African and European infants and their mothers. Am J Clin Nutr 4: 117–123, 1956.

Berwick DM, Keeler E, Cretin S: Screening for cholesterol: Costs and benefits, in Lubs HA, de la Cruz F (eds): Genetic Counseling. New York: Raven Press, 1977.

Bessman SP, Swazey JP: Phenylketonuria: A study of biomedical legislation, in Mendelsohn E, Swazey JP, Taviss I (eds): Human Aspects of Biomedical Innovation. Cambridge: Harvard University Press, 1971.

Bevans M, Davidson JD, Kendall FE: Regression of lesions in canine arteriosclerosis. Arch Pathol 51:288–292, 1951.

Bierenbaum ML, Fleischman AI, Raichelson RI, Hayton T, Watson PB: Ten-year experience of modified-fat diets on younger men with coronary heart-disease. Lancet 1:1404–1407, 1973.

Bierenbaum ML., Green DP, Florin A, Fleischman AI, Caldwell AB: Modified-fat dietary management of the young male with coronary disease. JAMA 202:1119–1123, 1967.

Bierenbaum ML, Green DP, Gherman C, Florin A, Caldwell AB: The effects of two low fat dietary patterns on the blood cholesterol level of young male coronary patients. J Chronic Dis 16:1073–1083, 1963.

Bierman EL, Shank RE: Homogenized milk and coronary artery disease. Theory not fact. JAMA 234:630–631, 1975.

Blackburn H: Multifactor prevention trials in coronary heart disease, in Steward GT (ed): Trends in Epidemiology: Application to Health Service Research and Training. Springfield, Ill: Charles C Thomas, 1972.

Blackburn H: Progress in the epidemiology and prevention of coronary heart disease. Prog Cardiol 3:1–6, 1974.

Blackburn H: Contrasting professional views on atherosclerosis and coronary disease. N Engl J Med 292:105–107, 1975.

Blumenthal S, Jesse MJ, Hennekens CH, Klein BE, Ferrer PL, Gourley JE: Risk factors for coronary artery disease in children of affected families. J Pediatr 87:1187–1192, 1975.

Bortz WM: Reversibility of atherosclerosis in cholesterol-fed rabbits. Circ Res 22:135–139, 1968.

Bortz WM: The pathogenesis of hypercholesterolemia. Ann Intern Med 80:738–746, 1974.

Böttiger LE, Carlson LA: The Stockholm Prospective Study 2: New events of coronary heart disease in men in relation to findings at initial examination, 9-year followup, Waldenstrom J, Larsson T, Ljunstedt N (eds): Early Phases of Coronary Heart Disease: The Possibility of Prediction. Seventh Skania International Symposia. Stockholm: Nordiska Bokhandelns Forlag, 1973.

Bowen RE, Reid EF, Moshy RJ: Designing formulated foods for the cardiac-concerned. Prev Med 2:366–377, 1973.

Braun P, Weinstein MC, Farber M: An inventory for health care research. Working paper. Center for the Analysis of Health Practices, Harvard School of Public Health, 1976.

Breslow JL: Pediatric aspects of hyperlipidemia. Pediatrics 62: 510–520, 1978.

Bronte-Stewart B, Roberts B, Wells VM: Serum cholesterol in vitamin C deficiency in man. Br J Nutr 17:61–68, 1963.

Brook CG, Ball KP: Prevention of coronary heart disease starts in childhood. Arch Dis Child 52:904–906, 1977.

Brown DF, Daudiss K: Hyperlipoproteinemia. Prevalence in a free-living population in Albany, New York. Circulation 47:558–566, 1973.

Brown HB, Lewis LA, Page IH: Effects of clofibrate and a fat-modified diet on serum lipids. Clin Pharmacol Ther 17:171–178, 1975.

Brown MS, Goldstein JL: Expression of the familial hypercholesterolemia gene in heterozygotes: Mechanism for a dominant disorder in man. Science 61–63, 1974.

Brown MS, Goldstein JL: Familial hypercholesterolemia: A genetic defect in the low-density lipoprotein receptor. N Engl J Med 294:1386–1390, 1976(a).

Brown MS, Goldstein JL: Receptor-mediated control of cholesterol metabolism. Science 191:150–154, 1976(b).

Brunner D, Altman S, Posner L, Bearman J, Loebl K, Levin S: Heredity, environment, serum lipoprotein and serum uric acid: A study in a community without familial eating patterns. J Chronic Dis 23:763–773, 1971.

Bureau of Labor Statistics, U.S. Department of Labor: Estimated Retail Food Prices by City. Washington, D.C.: Bureau of Labor Statistics, May 1976.

Burke, B.S. The dietary history as a tool in research. J Am Diet Assoc 23:1041–1046, 1947.

Burkitt DP, Walker ARP, Painter NS: Dietary fiber and disease. JAMA 229:1068–1074, 1974.

Bush JW, Chen MM, Patrick DL: Health status index in cost-effectiveness: Analysis of PKU program, in Berg RL (ed): Health Status Indexes. Chicago: Hospital Research and Education Trust, 1973.

Bush JW, Fanshel S, Chen MM: Analysis of a tuberculin testing program using a health status index. Socio-Env Plan Sci 6:49–68, 1972.

Carlson J: Valuation of Life Saving. Ph.D. Dissertation. Harvard University, 1963.

Carlson LA, Böttiger LE: Ischaemic heart disease in relation to fasting values of plasma triglycerides and cholesterol. Lancet 1: 865–868, 1972.

Carlson LA, Lindstedt S: The Stockholm prospective study: 1. The initial values for plasma lipids. Acta Med Scand Suppl 493:1–135, 1968.

Carryer HM, Randall RV, Mankin HT, Carter ET: Executive health examinations: Analysis of 2,812 examinations on 569 subjects at Mayo Clinic. Mayo Clin Proc 46:742–746, 1971.

Cassel JC: Review of 1960 through 1962 cardiovascular disease prevalence study. Arch Intern Med 128:890–895, 1971 (a).

Cassel JC: Summary of major findings of the Evans County cardiovascular studies. Arch Intern Med 128:887–889, 1971 (b).

Cassel J, Heyden S, Bartel AG, Kaplan BH, Tyroler HA, Cornoni JC, Hames CG: Incidence of coronary heart disease by ethnic group, social class, and sex. Arch Intern Med 128:901–906, 1971 (a).

Cassel J, Heyden S, Bartel AG, Kaplan BH, Tyroler HA, Cornoni JC, Hames CG: Occupation and physical activity and coronary heart disease. Arch Intern Med 128:920–928, 1971 (b).

Chakravarti RN, Dumar BS, Nair CR, Kumar M: Reversibility of cholesterol-adrenaline-induced atherosclerosis in rhesus monkeys; evaluation of safflower oil and low-fat low-calorie diet. Atherosclerosis 28:405–416, 1977.

Chapman JM, Coulson AH, Clarke VA, Borun ER: The differential effect of serum cholesterol, blood pressure and weight on the incidence of myocardial infarction and angina pectoris. J Chronic Dis 23:631–645, 1971.

Chapman JM, Reeder LG, Massey FJ, Jr., Borun ER, Picken B, Browning GG, Coulson AH, Zimmerman DH: Relationships of stress, tranquilizers, and serum cholesterol levels in a sample population under study for coronary heart disease. Am J Epidemiol 83:537–547, 1966.

Chase HP, O'Quin RJ, O'Brian D: Screening for hyperlipidemia in childhood. JAMA 230:1535–1537, 1974.

Chiang CL: Introduction to Stochastic Processes and Their Applications. New York: Krieger, 1968.

Chong YH, Soh CC, Ho, GS, Rajaratnam R, Nonis P. Serum low density lipoproteins, triglycerides and cholesterol levels in Malaysia. Clin Chem Acta 34:85–92, 1971.

Christakis G, Rinzler SH, Archer M, Winslow G, Jampel S, Stephenson J, Friedman G, Fein H, Kraus H, James G: The anticoronary club. A dietary approach to the prevention of coronary heart disease—a seven year report. Am Public Health 56:229–314, 1966.

Clarenberg R, Kim Chung IS, Wakefield LM: Reducing the egg cholesterol by including emulsified sitosterol in standard chicken diets. J Nutr 101:289–298, 1971.

Clark DA, Allen MF, Wilson FH: Longitudinal study of serum lipids. Am J Clin Nutr 20:743–752, 1967.

Clarke RP, Merrow SB, Morse EH, Keyser DE: Interrelationships between plasma lipids, physical measurements, and body fatness of adolescents in Burlington, Vermont. Am J Clin Nutr 23:754–763, 1970.

Clarke WR, Schrott HG, Leaverton PE, Conner WE, Lauer RM: Tracking of blood lipids and blood pressures in school-age children: The Muscatine study. Circulation 58:626–634, 1978.

Cohen SI: The psychiatric effects of mass screening. Public Health 86:125–128, 1972.

Committee of Principal Investigators: A cooperative trial in the primary prevention of ischemic heart disease using clofibrate. Br Heart J 40:1069–1118, 1978.

Committee on Diet and Heart Disease of the National Heart Foundation of Australia: Dietary fat and coronary heart disease: A review. 1. Diet in the prevention of coronary heart diseae and some pathogenetic aspects. Med J Aust 1:575–579, 1974.

Committee on Nutrition: Childhood diet and coronary heart disease. Pediatrics 49:305–307, 1972.

Commodity Research Bureau, Inc.: Commodity Yearbook 1975. New York: Commodity Research Bureau, Inc., 1975.

Conner WE, Conner SL: The key role of nutritional factors in the prevention of coronary heart disease. Prev Med 1:49–83, 1972.

Cooper R, Stamler J, Dyer A, Garside D: The decline in mortality from coronary heart disease, U.S.A., 1968–1975. J Chronic Dis 31:709–720, 1978.

Cornfield J: Joint dependence of risk of coronary heart disease on serum cholesterol and systolic blood pressure: A discriminant function analysis. Fed Proc 21(suppl 11):58–61, 1962.

Cornfield J, Mitchell S: Selected risk factors in coronary disease. Arch Environ Health 19:382–394, 1969.

Court JM, Dunlop M: Neonatal plasma lipids. Med J Aust 2: 1387, 1972.

Court JM, Dunlop M: Plasma lipid values and lipoprotein patterns during adolescence in boys. J Pediatr 86:453–458, 1975.

Cretin S: Analysis of sequential screening strategies. Institute of Management Science Bulletin (Operations Research Society of America) No. 4, 1977 (a).

Cretin S: Cost/benefit analysis of treatment and prevention of myocardial infarction. Health Serv Res 12:174–189, 1977 (b).

Dalderup LM, Doornbos R, den Hartog C, Van Haard WB, de Vries JE, Keller GHM: A practical method for decreasing the serum cholesterol level in man. Am Clin Nutr 22:1521–1530, 1969.

Darmady JM, Fosbrooke AS, Lloyd JK: Prospective study of serum cholesterol levels during first year of life. Br Med J 2:685–688, 1972.

Davies JDG, Newson J: Ascorbic acid and cholesterol levels in pastoral peoples in Kenya. Am J Clin Nutr 27:1039–1042, 1974.

Dayton S, Pearce ML, Goldman H, Harnish A, Plotkin D, Shickman M, Winfield M, Zager A, Dixon W: Controlled trial of a diet high in unsaturated fat for prevention of atherosclerotic complications. Lancet 2:1060–1062, 1968.

Dayton S, Pearce ML, Hashimoto S, Dixon WJ, Tomiyasu U: A controlled clinical trial of a diet high in unsaturated fat in preventing complications of atherosclerosis. Circulation 40 (suppl 2):1–63, 1969.

Deutscher S, Epstein FH, Kjelsberg MO: Familial aggregation of factors associated with coronary heart disease. Circulation 33:911–924, 1966.

Deutscher S, Ostrander LD, Epstein FH: Familial factors in premature coronary heart disease—a preliminary report from the Tecumseh community health study. Am J Epidemiol 91:233–237, 1970.

Dewailly P: Hypercholesterolemia and cardiovascular disease incidence. Lille Med 20:374–376, 1975.

Dick TBS, Stone MC: Prevalence of three major risk factors in random sample of men and women, and in patients with ischaemic heart disease. Br Heart J 40:617–626, 1978.

Dolder MA, Oliver MF: Myocardial infarction in young men. Study of risk factors in nine countries. Br Heart J 37:493–503, 1975.

Doyle JT: Risk factors in coronary heart disesase. NY State J Med 63:1317–1320, 1963.

Drash A: Atherosclerosis, cholesterol, and the pediatrician. J Pediatr 80:693–696, 1972.

Drash A, Hengstenberg F: The identification of risk factors in normal children in the development of arteriosclerosis. Ann Clin Lab Sci 2:348–359, 1972.

du Plessis JP, Vivier FS, de Lange DJ: The biochemical evaluation of the nutrition status of urban school children aged 7-15 years: Serum cholesterol and phospholipid levels and serum and urinary amylase activities. S Afr Med J 41:1216–1222, 1967.

Dyer AR: An analysis of the relationship of systolic blood pressure, serum cholesterol, and smoking to 14-year mortality in the Chicago Peoples Gas Company Study—II. Coronary and cardiovascular-renal mortality in two competing risk models. J Chronic Dis 28:571–578, 1975.

Dyer AR, Stamler J, Paul O, Berkson DM, Lepper MH, McKean H, Shekelle RB, Lindberg HA, Garside D: Alcohol consumption, cardiovascular risk factors, and mortality in two Chicago epidemiologic studies. Circulation 56:1067–1074, 1977.

Economic Research Service, United States Department of Agriculture: Food Consumption, Prices, Expenditures. Supplement for 1974 to Agricultural Economic Report No. 138. Washington, D.C.: Economic Research Service, anuary 1976 (a).

Economic Research Service, United States Department of Agriculture: Livestock and Meat Situation. Washington, D.C.: Economic Research Service, August 1976 (b).

Economic Research Service, United States Department of Agriculture: Poultry and Egg Situation. Washington, D.C.: Economic Research Service, June 1976 (c).

Eddy DM: Screening for Cancer: Theory, Analysis, and Design (draft, March 1978).

Ederer F: Serum cholesterol changes: Effects of diet and regression toward the mean. J Chronic Dis 25:277–289, 1972.

Ederer F, Leren P, Turpeinen O, Frantz ID Jr: Cancer among men on cholesterol-lowering diets. Experience from five clinical trials. Lancet 2:203–206, 1971.

Editorial: Screening for hyperlipidaemia in childhood. Br Med J 4:367–368, 1974.

Efron B: The efficiency of logistic regression compared to normal discriminant analysis. J Am Stat Assoc 70:892–898, 1975.

Egdahl RH, Gertman PM (eds): Technology and the Quality of Health Care. Germantown, MD: Aspen Systems Corporation, 1978.

Ellefson RD, Elveback LR, Hodgson PA, Weidman WH: Cholesterol and triglycerides in serum lipoproteins of young persons in Rochester, Minnesota. Mayo Clin Proc 53:307–320, 1978.

Elston RC, Namboodiri KK, Glueck CJ, Fallat R, Tsang R, Leuba V: Study of the genetic transmission of hypercholesterolemia and hypertriglyceridemia in a 195 member kindred. Ann Hum Genet 39:67–87, 1975.

Engel HJ, Page HL, Campbell WB: Coronary artery disease in young women. JAMA 230:1531–1534, 1974.

Enos WF, Holmes RH, Beyer J: Coronary disease among United States soldiers killed in action in Korea. JAMA 152:1090–1093, 1953.

Enthoven AC: Shattuck lecture—cutting cost without cutting the quality of care. N Engl J Med 298:1229–1238, 1978.

Epstein FH: The epidemiology of coronary heart dissease. J Chronic Dis 18:735–774, 1965.

Epstein FH: Multiple risk factors and the prediction of coronary heart disease. Bull NY Acad Med 44:916–935, 1968.

Epstein FH: Epidemiologic aspects of atherosclerosis. Atherosclerosis 14:1–11, 1971.

Epstein FH: Genetics of ischaemic heart disease. Postgrad Med J 52:477–480, 1976.

Epstein FH, Ostrander LD Jr, Johnson BC, Payne MW, Hayner NS, Keller JB, Francis T Jr: Epidemiological studies of cardiovascular disease in a total community—Tecumseh, Michigan. Ann Intern Med 62:1170–1187, 1965.

Evans DW, Turner SM, Gnosh P : Feasibility of long-term plasma-cholesterol reduction by diet. Lancet 1:172–174, 1972.

Evans RI, Rozelle RM, Lasater TM, Allen BP: Fear arousal, persuasion and actual versus implied behavioral change: New perspective utilizing a real-life dental hygiene program. J Pers Soc Psychol 16:220–227, 1970.

Fallat RW, Tsang RC, Glueck CJ: Hypercholesterolemia and hypertriglyceridemia in children. Prev Med 3:390–405, 1974.

Farquhar JW, Maccoby N, Wood PD, Alexander JK, Breitrose H, Brown BW, Jr, Haskell WL, McAlister AL, Meyer AJ, Nash JD, Stern MP: Community eduction for cardiovascular health. Lancet 1:1192–1195, 1977.

Farquhar J, Maccoby N, Wood P, Brown B Jr: Results of a two-year health education campaign on cardiovascular risk: Stanford Three Community Study. Circulation 51 and 52 (suppl 2):117, 1975.

Feldstein MS: The social time preference discount rate in cost-benefit analysis. Econ J 74:360–379, 1964.

Fleischman AI, Hayton T, Bierenbaum ML: Serum lipids and certain dietary factors in young men with coronary heart disease. J Am Diet Assoc 50:112–115, 1967.

Florey C Du V, McDonald H, Miall WE, Milner RDG: Serum lipids and their relation to blood glucose and cardiovascular measurements in a rural population of Jamaican adults. J Chronic Dis 26:85–100, 1973.

Fomon SJ: A pediatrician looks at early nutrition. Bull NY Acad Med 47:569–578, 1971.

Fomon SJ: What are infants fed in the United States? Pediatrics 56:530–354, 1975.

Fomon SJ, Bartels DJ: Concentrations of cholesterol in serum of infants in relation to diet. Am J Dis Child 99:27–30, 1960.

Food and Nutrition Board, Division of Biology and Agriculture, National Academy of Sciences, National Research Council, and the Council on Foods and Nutrition, American Medical Association: A joint statement: Diet and coronary heart disease. Prev Med 1:559–561, 1972.

Ford CH, McGandy RB, Stare FJ: An institutional approach to the dietary regulation of blood cholesterol in adolescent males. Prev Med 1:426–445, 1972.

Førde OH, Thelle DS: The Tromsø heart study: Risk factors for coronary heart disease related to the occurrence of myocardial infarction in first degree relatives. Am J Epidemiol 105:192–199, 1977.

Fox SM III, Haskell WL: Physical activity and the prevention of coronary heart disease. Bull NY Acad Med 44:950–967, 1968.

Frank CW: The course of coronary heart disease: Factors relating to prognosis. Bull NY Acad Med 44:900–915, 1968.

Fredrickson DS, Goldstein JL, Brown MS: The familial hyperlipoproteinemias, in Stanbury JB, Wyngaarden JB, Fredrickson DS (eds): The Metabolic Basis of Inherited Disease. New York: McGraw-Hill Book Company, 1978, pp. 604–655.

Fredrickson DS: The field trial: Some thoughts on the indispensable ordeal. Bull NY Acad Med 44:985–993, 1968.

Fredrickson DS: Factors in childhood that influence the development of atherosclerosis and hypertension. Introduction. Am J Clin Nutr 25: 221–223, 1972.

Fredrickson DS, Breslow JL: Primary hyperlipoproteinemia in infants. Annu Rev Med 24:315–324, 1973.

Fredrickson DS, Levy RI, Lees RS: Fat transport in lipoproteins—an integrated approach to mechanisms and disorders. N Engl J Med 276:34–42, passim, 1967.

Frerichs RR, Srinivasan SR, Webber LS, Berenson GS: Serum cholesterol and triglyceride levels in 3,446 children from a biracial community: The Bogalusa Heart Study. Circulation 54:302–309, 1976.

Friedman G, Goldberg SJ: Normal serum cholesterol values. Percentile ranking in a middle-class pediatric population. JAMA 225:610–612, 1973.

Friedman G, Goldberg SJ: Concurrent and subsequent serum cholesterols of breast and formula-fed infants. Am J Clin Nutr 28:42–45, 1975.

Friss-Hansen B, Clausen J: Studies on serum lipoprotein in the neonatal period. Z Ernahrungswiss 10:253–263, 1971.

Fuchs VR: Who Shall Live? Health, Economics, and Social Change. New York: Basic Books, 1974.

Garcia-Palmieri MR: Precursors of coronary artery disease in Puerto Rico. Am Clin Nutr 26:1133–1137, 1973.

Garcia-Palmieri MR, Costas R, Schiffman J, Colon AA, Torres R, Nazario E: Interrelationship of serum lipids with relative weight, blood glucose, and physical activity. Circulation 45:829–836, 1972.

Gardner MJ, Heady JA: Some effects of within-person variability in epidemiological studies. J Chronic Dis 26:781–795, 1973.

Garrison R, Castelli WP, Feinlieb M, Kannel WB, Hovlik R, Padgett S, McNamara P: The association of total cholesterol, triglycerides, and plasma lipoprotein cholesterol levels in first degree relatives and spouse pairs. Am J Epidemiol, in press.

Gibson RM: National health care expenditures, 1978. Health Care Financing Review 1:1–36, 1979.

Gibson RM, Fisher CR: National health expenditures, fiscal year 1977. Soc Secur Bull 41:3–20, 1978.

Ginter E, Kajaba I, Nizner O: The effect of ascorbic acid on cholesterolemia in healthy subjects with seasonal deficit of vitamin C. Nutr Metab 12:76–86, 1970.

Glasunov IS, Dowd JE, Jaksic Z, Kesic B, Ray D, Steinberger C, Stromberg J, Vuletic S: Repetitive health examinations as an intervention measure. Bull WHO 49:423–432, 1973.

Glueck CJ: Neonatal familial type II hyperlipoproteinemia: Cord blood cholesterol in 1660 births. Circulation 40 and 41(suppl 3): 11, 1970.

Glueck CJ, Conner WE: Diet-coronary heart disease relationships reconnoitered. Am J Clin Nutr 31:727–737, 1978.

Glueck CJ, Fallat R, Buncher CR, Tsang R, Steiner P: Familial combined hyperlipoproteinemia: Studies in 91 adults and 95 children from 33 kindreds. Metabolism 22:1403–1428, 1973 (a).

Glueck CJ, Fallat R, Tsang R: Pediatric familial type II hyperlipoproteinemia: Therapy with diet and cholestyramine resin. Pediatrics 52:669–677, 1973 (b).

Glueck CJ, Fallat RW, Tsang R, Buncher CR: Hyperlipidemia in progeny of parents with myocardial infarction before age 50. Am J Dis Child 127:70–75, 1974.

Glueck CJ, Kelly K, Mellies MJ, Gartside PS, Steiner PM: Hypercholesterolemia and hyper-alpha-lipoproteinemia in schoolchildren. Pediatrics 62:478–487, 1978 (a).

Glueck CJ, McGill NC, Jr, Shank RE, Lauer RM: The value and safety of diet modification to control hyperlipidemia in childhood and adolescence: A statement for physicians. Circulation 58:381A–387A, 1978 (b).

Glueck CJ, Steiner PM, Tsang RC: A pediatric approach to prevention of atherosclerosis. Circulation 43 and 44 (suppl 2):3, 1971.

Goalwin A, Pomeranze J: Serum cholesterol studies in infants. Arch Pediatr 79:58–62, 1962.

Godfrey RC, Stenhouse NS, Cullen KJ, Blackman V: Cholesterol and the child: Studies of the cholesterol levels of Busselton school children and their parents. Aust Paediatr J 8:72–78, 1972.

Goldbourt U, Medalie JH, Neufeld HN: Clinical myocardial infarction over a five-year period—III. A multivariate analysis of incidence, the Israel ischemic heart disease study. J Chronic Dis 28:217–237, 1975.

Goldstein JL, Albers JJ, Schrott HG, Hazzard WR, Bierman EL, Motulsky AG: Plasma lipid levels and coronary heart disease in adult relatives of newborns with normal and elevated cord blood lipids. Am J Hum Genet 26:727–735, 1974(a).

Goldstein JL, Brown MS: Familial hypercholesterolemia: Identification of a defect in the regulation of 3-hydroxy-3-methylglutaryl coenzyme a reductase activity associated with overproduction of cholesterol. Proc Natl Acad Sci USA 70:2804–2808, 1973.

Goldstein JL, Brown MS: Familial hypercholesterolemia: A genetic regulatory defect in cholesterol metabolism. Am J Med 58:147–150, 1975(a).

Goldstein JL, Brown MS: Hyperlipidemia in coronary heart disease: A biochemical genetic approach. J Lab Clin Med 85:15–25, 1975 (b).

Goldstein JL, Harrod MJ, Brown MS: Homozygous familial hypercholesterolemia: Specificity of the biochemical defect in cultured cells and feasibility of prenatal detection. Am J Hum Genet 26:199–206, 1974 (b.)

Goldstein JL, Hazzard WR, Schrott HG, Bierman EL, Motulsky AG: Genetics of hyperlipidemia in coronary heart disease. Trans Assoc Am Physicians 85:120–150, 1972.

Goldstein JL, Hazzard WR, Schrott HG, Bierman EL, Motulsky AG: Hyperlipidemia in coronary heart disease. I. Lipid levels in 500 survivors of myocardial infarction. J Clin Invest 52:1533–1543, 1973 (a).

Goldstein JL, Schrott HG, Hazzard WR, Bierman EL, Motulsky AG: Hyperlipidemia in coronary heart disease. II. Genetic analysis of lipid levels in

176 families and delineation of a new inherited disorder, combined hyperlipidemia. J Clin Invest 52-1544–1568, 1973 (b).

Golubjatnikov R, Paskey T, Inhorn SL: Serum cholesterol levels of Mexican and Wisconsin school children: Am J Epidemiol 96:36–39, 1972.

Gordon T: Hazards in the use of the logistic function with special reference to data from prospective cardiovascular studies. J Chronic Dis 27:97–102, 1974.

Gordon T, Garcia-Palmieri MR, Kagan A, Kannel WB, Schiffman J: Differences in coronary heart disease in Framingham, Honolulu and Puerto Rico. J Chronic Dis 27:329–344, 1974.

Gordon T, Kannel WB: Multiple contributors to coronary risk: Implications for screening and prevention. J Chronic Dis 25:561–565, 1972 (a).

Gordon T, Kannel WB: The prospective study of cardiovascular disase, in Steward GT (ed): Trends in Epidemiology: Application to Health Service Research and Training. Springfield, Ill: Charles C Thomas, 1972 (b).

Gordon T, Thom T: The recent decrease in CHD mortality. Prev Med 4:115–125, 1975.

Gori GB, Richter BJ: Macroeconomics of disease prevention in the United States. Science 200:1124–1130, 1978.

Gotto AM, De Bakey ME, Foreyt JP, Scott LW, Thornby JI: Dietary treatment of type IV hyperlipoproteinemia. JAMA 237:1212–1215, 1977.

Greek Vital Statistics, 1941–1947. Athens, Greece.

Green HP, Capron AM: Issues of law and public policy in genetic screening, Bergsma D (ed): Ethical, Social and Legal Dimensions of Screening for Human Genetic Disease. New York: Stratton Intercontinental Medical Book Corp., 1974.

Groen JJ: Effect of bread in the diet on serum cholesterol. Am J Clin Nutr 20:191–197, 1967.

Gross LP: Can we influence behavior to promote good nutrition? Bull NY Acad Med 47:613–623, 1971.

Gustafson A, Elmfeldt D, Wilhelmsen L, Tibblin G: Serum lipids and lipoproteins in men after myocardial infarction compared with representative population sample. Circulation 46:709–716, 1972.

Guthrie R: Blood screening for phenylketonuria. JAMA 178:863, 1961.

Haefner DP, Kirscht JP: Motivational and behavioral effects of modifying health beliefs. Public Health Rep 85:478–484, 1970.

Hall Y, Stamler J, Cohen DB, Mojonnier L, Epstein MB, Berkson DM, Whipple IT, Catchings S: Effectiveness of a low saturated fat, low cholesterol, weight-reducing diet for the control of hypertriglyceridemia. Atherosclerosis 16:389–403, 1972.

Hames CG, Greenberg BG: A comparative study of serum cholesterol levels in school children and their possible relation to atherogenesis. Am J Public Health 51:374–385, 1961.

Hampton ML, Anderson J, Lavizzo BS, Bergman AB: Sickle-cell "nondisease." A potentially serious public health problem. Am J Dis Child 128:58–61, 1974.

Hansen PF, Geill T, Lund E: Dietary fats and thrombosis. Lancet 2:1193–1194, 1962.

Hapgood F: Risk-benefit analysis. Atlantic, January 1979, pp 33–38.

Harberger A: Economic analysis at public investment decisions: Interest rate policy and discounting analysis. Remarks before subcommittee on Economy in Government, Joint Economic Committee, 90th Congress, 2nd Session, 1968.

Hartroft WS, Thomas WA: Pathogenesis of atherosclerosis and myocardial infarction. Fed Proc 18:36–46, 1959.

Hatch FT, Abell LL, Kendall FE: Effects of restriction of dietary fat and cholesterol upon serum lipids and lipoproteins in patients with hypertension. Am J Med 19:48–60, 1955.

Hatch FT, Reissell PK, Poon-King TMW, Canellos GP, Lees RS, Hagopian LM: A study of coronary heart disease in young men. Characteristics and metabolic studies of the patients and comparison with age-matched healthy men. Circulation 33:679–703, 1966.

Haveman RH: The opportunity cost of displaced private spending and the social discount rate. Water Resources Research 5:947–956, 1969.

Haynes RB, Sackett DL, Taylor DW, Gibson ES, Johnson AC: Increased absenteeism from work after detection and labeling of hypertensive patients. N Engl J Med 299:741–744, 1978.

Hazemann JJ, Rossinol Cl, Vesin Cl, Farnier MA: Our experience with early lipid measurements. Ann Pediatr 22:565–573, 1975.

Hazzard WR, Goldstein JL, Schrott HG, Motulsky AG, Bierman EL: Hyperlipidemia in coronary heart disease. III. Evaluation of lipoprotein phenotypes of 156 genetically defined survivors of myocardial infarction. J Clin Inpest 52:1569–1577, 1973.

Heiberg A: The heritability of serum lipoprotein and lipid concentrations. A twin study. Clin Genet 6:307–316, 1974.

Hennekens CH, Jesse MJ, Klein BE, Gourley JE, Blumenthal S: Cholesterol among children of men with myocardial infarction. Pediatrics 58:211–217, 1976.

Heydon S, Walker L, Hames CG, Tyroler HA: Decrease of serum cholesterol level and blood pressure in the community. Seven to nine years of observation in the Evans County study. Arch Intern Med 128:982–986, 1971.

Heywood PF: The public health significance of fat-modified ruminant foods. Am J Clin Nutr 30:1726–1733, 1977.

Hitchcock NE, Gracey M: Diet and serum cholesterol. Arch Dis Child 52:790–793, 1977.

Hodges RE, Krehl WA: Nutritional status of teenagers in Iowa. Am J Clin Nutr 17:200–210, 1965.

Hodges RE, Krehl WA, Stone DB, Lopez A: Dietary carbohydrates and low cholesterol diets: Effects on serum lipids of man. Am J Clin Nutr 20:198–208, 1967.

Hodgson PA, Ellefson RD, Elveback LR, Harris LE, Nelson RA, Weidman WH: Comparison of serum cholesterol in children fed high, moderate, or low cholesterol milk diets during neonatal period. Metabolism 25:739–746, 1976.

Holtzman NA: Screening for phenylketonuria and its problems, in Motulsky AG, Lentz W (eds): Birth Defects: Proceedings of the Fourth International Conference, Vienna, Austria, 2-8 September 1973. New York: Elsevier, 1974.

Hood B, Sanne H, Orndahl G, Ahlstrom M, Welin G: Long-term prognosis in essential hypercholesterolemia. The effect of strict diet. Acta Med Scand 178:161–173, 1965.

Hoover SR: Proceedings: Research into foods from animal sources. I. Controlling level and type of fat. II. Recent developments in beef and dairy products. Prev Med 2:346–360, 361–365, 1973.

Hopper PF: Food industry view of the regulatory climate for prudent diet foods. Prev Med 2:397–402, 1973.

Horlic L, Katz LN: Retrogression of atherosclerotic lesions on cessation of cholesterol feeding in the chick. J Lab Clin Med 34:1427–1442, 1949.

Hulley SB, Cohen R, Widdowson G: Plasma high-density lipoprotein cholesterol level: Influence of risk factor intervention. JAMA 238:2269–2271, 1977.

Hunter JD: Diet, body build, blood pressure, and serum cholesterol levels in coconut-eating Polynesians. Fed Proc 21(suppl 11):36–43, 1962.

Hurter R, Swale J, Peyman MS, Barnett CWH: Some immediate and long-term effects of exercise on the plasma-lipids. Lancet 2:671–674, 1972.

Illich I: Medical Nemesis: The Expropriation of Health. New York: Random House, 1976.

Inter-Society Commission for Heart Disease Resources: Report of Inter-Society Commission for Heart Disease Resources: Primary prevention of the atherosclerotic diseases. Circulation 42:A55–A59, 1970.

Inter-Society Commission for Heart Disease Resources: Primary prevention of the atherosclerotic diseases. Circulation 42:1–44, 1972.

Jacobs DR, Anderson JT, Blackburn H: Diet and serum cholesterol: Do zero correlations negate the relationship? Am J Epid 110:77–87, 1979.

Jahnke KS, Breitbach A: Statistical connection between nutrition and arteriosclerosis, in Arteriosclerosis and Nutrition. (Will, Veroffentl. Deut. Ges. Erhahrung.) Darmstadt: Deitrich Steinkopk, 1959.

Jenkins CD: Psychologic and social precursors of coronary disease (II). N Engl J Med 284:307–317, 1971.

Jensen J, Blankenhorn DH: The inheritance of familial hypercholesterolemia. Am J Med 52:499–516, 1972.

Jensen J, Blankenhorn DH, Kornerup V: Coronary disease in hypercholesterolemia. Circulation 36:77–82, 1967.

Johansson BW, Persson B: Coronary heart disease in Malmo, in Waldenstrom J, Larsson T, Ljundstedt N (eds): Early Phases of Coronary Heart Disease: The Possiblity of Prediction. Seventh Skania International Symposia. Stockholm: Nordiska Bokhandelns Forlag, 1973.

Johnson BC, Epstein FH, Kjelsberg MO: Distributions and familial studies of blood pressure and serum cholesterol levels in a total community—Tecumseh, Michigan. J Chronic Dis 18:147–160, 1965.

Johnson OC: Present and proposed regulations affecting the marketing of prudent diet foods. Prev Med 2:403–406, 1973.

Jolliffe N, Archer M: Statistical associations between international coronary heart disease death rates and certain environmental factors. J Chronic Dis 9:636–652, 1959.

Kahn HA: Change in serum cholesterol associated with changes in the United States civilian diet, 1909, 1965. Am Clin Nutr 23:879–882, 1970.

Kahn HA, Dawber TR: The development of coronary heart disease in relation to sequential biennial measures of cholesterol in the Framingham study. J Chronic Dis 19:611–620, 1966.

Kannel WB: The role of cholesterol in coronary atherogenesis. Med Clin North Am 58:363–379, 1974.

Kannel WB, Castelli WP: The Framingham study of coronary disease in women. Med Times 100:173–175 passim, 1972.

Kannel WB, Castelli WP, Gordon T: Cholesterol in the prediction of atherosclerotic disease. New perspectives on the Framingham study. Ann Intern Med 90:85–91, 1979.

Kannel WB, Castelli WP, Gordon T, McNamara PM: Serum cholesterol, lipoproteins and risk of coronary heart disease. The Framingham study. Ann Intern Med 74:1–12, 1971(a).

Kannel WB, Dawber TR: Atherosclerosis as a pediatric problem. J. Pediatr 80:544–554, 1972.

Kannel WB, Garcia MJ, McNamara PM, Pearson G: Serum lipid precursors of coronary heart disease. Hum Pathol 2:129–151, 1971(b).

Kannel WB, Gordon T (eds): The Framingham Study: An Epidemiological Investigation of Cardiovascular Disease. Sections 1–32. Washington, D.C.: Government Printing Office, 1970–1977(a).

Kannel WB, Gordon T (eds): The Framingham Study: An Epidemiologic Investigation of Cardiovascular Disease. Section 24. The Framingham Diet Study: Diet and the regulation of serum cholesterol. Washington, D.C.: Government Printing Office.

Karvonen MJ: Epidemiology of ischaemic heart disease in Finland, in de Haas JH, Hemker HC, Snellen HA (eds): Ischaemic Heart Disease. Baltimore: Williams & Wilkins, 1970.

Karvonen MJ: Primary prevention of coronary heart disease. Acta Cardiol (Brux) Suppl 20:159–173, 1974.

Katz LN, Stamler J: Experimental Atherosclerosis. Springfield, Ill: Charles C Thomas, 1953.

Keys A: Prevention of coronary heart disease. Official recommendations from Scandinavia. Circulation 38:227–228, 1968.

Keys A: Serum cholesterol and the question of "normal." In Benson ES, Straudjord PE (eds): Multiple Laboratory Screening. New York: Academic Press, 1969.

Keys A (ed): Coronary heart disease in seven countries. Circulation 41(suppl 1):1–211, 1970.

Keys A: Coronary heart disease—the global picture. Atherosclerosis 22:149–192, 1975.

Keys A, Anderson JT, Grande F: Serum cholesterol response to changes in the diet. I. Iodine value of dietary fat versus 2S-P. Metabolism 14:747–758, 1965 (a).

Keys A, Anderson JT, Grande F: Serum cholesterol response to changes in diet. II. The effect of cholesterol in the diet. Metabolism 14:758–765, 1965 (b).

Keys A, Anderson JT, Grande F: Serum cholesterol response to changes in diet. III. Differences among individuals. Metabolism 14: 766–775, 1965 (c).

Keys A, Anderson JT, Grande F: Serum cholesterol response to changes in the diet. IV. Particular saturated fatty acids in the diet. Metabolism 14:776–787, 1965 (d).

Keys A, Aravanis C, Blackburn W, van Buchem FSP, Buzina R, Djordjevic BS, Dontas SA, Fidanza F, Karvonen MJ, Kimura N, Lekos D, Monti M, Puddu V, Taylor HL: Epidemiological studies related to coronary heart disease: Characteristics of men aged 40–59 in seven countries. Acta Med Scan Suppl 460:1–392, 1966.

Keys A, Aravanis C, Blackburn H, van Buchem FSP, Buzina R, Djordjevic BS, Fidanza F, Karvonen MJ, Menotti A, Puddu V, Taylor HL: Probability of middle-aged men developing coronary heart disease in five years. Circulation 45:815–828, 1972.

Keys A, Kimura N, Kusukawa A, Bronte-Stewart B, Larsen N, Keys MH: Lessons from serum cholesterol studies in Japan, Hawaii and Los Angeles. Ann Intern Med 83–94, 1958.

Keys A, Mickelsen O, Miller EVO, Hayes ER, Todd RL: The concentration of cholesterol in the blood serum of normal man and its relation to age. Clin Invest 29:1347–1353, 1950.

Keys A, Taylor HL, Blackburn H, Brozek J, Anderson JT, Simonson E: Mortality and coronary heart disease among men studied for 23 years. Arch Intern Med 128:201–204, 1971.

Kimura N, Keys A: Coronary heart disease in seven countries. X. Rural southern Japan. Circulation 41(suppl 1):101–112, 1970.

Kisch A, Keeler E: Breast cancer mortality. Algorithms for Health Planners: vol 3. Rand R-2215/3 HEW. Santa Monica: Rand Corporation, 1977.

Knox EG: Foods and diseases. Br J Prev Soc Med 31:71–80, 1977.

Krasilnikoff PA, Vesterdahl J: Serum lipids in premature infants on vegetable fat diet. Acta Paediatr Scand 55:505–509, 1966.

Kromhout D, van der Harr F, Hautvast JG: Coronary heart disease risk factors in Dutch schoolchildren—results of a pilot-study. Prev Med 6:500–513, 1977.

Krueger DE, Moriyama IM: Mortality of the foreign born. Am J Public Health 57:496–503, 1967.

Kwiterovich PO Jr: Neonatal screening for hyperlipidemia. Pedatrics 53:455–457, 1974.

Kwiterovich PO Jr, Levy RI, Fredrickson DS: Early detection and treatment of familial type II hyperlipoproteinemia. Circulation 40 and 41(suppl 3):11, 1970.

Kwiterovich PO Jr, Levy RI, Fredrickson DS: Neonatal diagnosis of familial type II hyperlipoproteinaemia. Lancet 1:118–122, 1973.

Laird WP: Childhood and diet as related to atherosclerosis. Clin Pediatr 14:485–494, 1975.

Lau R, Kane R, Berry S, Ware J, Roy R: Channeling Health: A Review of the Evaluation of Televised Health Campaigns. Rand/P-6262. Santa Monica: Rand Corporation, 1978.

Lauer RM, Connor WE, Leaverton PE, Reiter MA, Clarke WR: Coronary heart disease risk factors in school children: The Muscatine study. J Pediatr 86:697–706, 1975.

Lee VA: Individual trends in the total serum cholesterol of children and adolescents over a ten-year period. Am J Clin Nutr 20:5–12, 1967.

Leelarthaepin B, Woodhill JM, Palmer AJ, Blacket RB: Obesity, diet, and type-II hyperlipidaemia. Lancet 2:1217–1221, 1974.

Leren P: The effect of plasma cholesterol lowering diet in male survivors of myocardial infarction. A controlled clinical trial. Acta Med Scand Suppl 466:1–92, 1966.

Leren P: The effect of plasma-cholesterol-lowering diet in male survivors of myocardial infarction. A controlled clinical trial. Bull NY Acad Med 44:1012–1020, 1968.,

Leren P, Haabrekke O: Blood lipids in patients with coronary heart disease. Acta Med Scand 189:505–509, 1971.

Leventhal H: Changing attitudes and habits to reduce risk factors in chronic disease. Am J Cardiol 31:571–580, 1973.

Levy HL: Newborn screening for metabolic disorders. N Engl J Med 1299–1300, 1973.

Levy RI, Rifkind BM: Diagnosis and management of hyperlipoproteinemia in infants and children. Am J Cardiol 31:547–556, 1973.

Lewis B, Chait A, Oakley CM, Wooton IDP, Krikler DM, Onitiri A, Sigurdsson G, February A: Serum lipoprotein abnormalities in patients with ischaemic heart disease: Comparisons with a control population. Br Med J 3:489–493, 1974 (a).

Lewis B, Chait A, Wootton ID, Oakley DM, Krikler DM, Sigurdsson G, February A, Maurer B, Birkhead J: Frequency of risk factors for ischaemic heart-disease in a healthy British population. With particular reference to serum-lipoprotein levels. Lancet 1: 141–146, 1974 (b).

Lewis LA, Olmstead F, Page IH, Lawry EY, Mann GV, Stare FJ, Hanig M, Lauffer MA, Gordon T, Moore FE: Serum lipid levels in normal persons. Findings of a cooperative study of lipoproteins and atherosclerosis. Circulation 16:227–245, 1957.

Lindquist B, Malmcrona R: Dietary fat in relation to serum lipids in the normal infant. Am J Dis Child 99:39–49, 1960.

Lisovskii VA, Mikushkin MS: The effect of oxygen on the development of experimental atherosclerosis in rabbits. Pathol Physiol Exp Ther 6:33–36, 1962.

Little JA, Shanoff HM, Roe RD, Csima A, Yano R: Studies of male survivors of myocardial infarction. IV. Serum lipids and five-year survival. Circulation 31:854–862, 1965.

Lloyd JK: Hyperlipidaemia in children. Br Heart J 37:105–114, 1975.

Lloyd JK, Fosbrooke AS, West R, Wolff OH: Screening for hyperlipidaemia in childhood. Br Med J 1:35, 1975.

Lloyd JK, Wolff OH: A paediatric approach to the prevention of atherosclerosis. J Atheroscler Res 10:135–138, 1969.

LNA Multi-Media Report Service: Class/Brand YTDS, vol 4, no 3. New York: Leading National Advertisers, Inc., January–December 1977.

Looney G: Television as a major factor in the ecology of childhood. Clin Pediatr 10:445–446, 1971.

Lowe CU: Research in infant nutrition: The untapped well. Am J Clin Nutr 25:245–254, 1972.

Lowenstein FW: Epidemiologic investigations in relation to diet in groups who show little atherosclerosis and are almost free of coronary ischaemic heart disease. Am J Clin Nutr 15:175–186, 1964.

Lyon TP, Yankley A, Gofman JW, Strisower B: Lipoproteins and diet in coronary heart disease; 5-year study. Calif Med 84:325–328, 1956.

Maccoby N, Farquhar JW: Communication for health: Unselling heart disease. J Commun 25:114–126, 1975.

Malmros H: The relation of nutrition to health; a statistical study of the effect of wartime on atherosclerosis, cardiosclerosis, tuberculosis, and diabetes. Acta Med Scand Suppl 246:137–153, 1950.

Malmros H: Dietary prevention of atherosclerosis. Lancet 2:479–484, 1969.

Mann GV: Diet-heart: End of an era. N Engl J Med 297:644–650, 1977.

Mann GV, Andrus SB: Xanthomatosis and atherosclerosis produced by diet in an adult rhesus monkey. J Lab Med 48:533–550, 1956.

Mann GV, Roels OA, Price DL, Merrill JM: Cardiovascular disease in African pygmies. A survey of the health status, serum lipids, and diet of pygmies in the Congo. J Chronic Dis 15:341–371, 1962.

Mann GV, Spoerry A, Gray M, Jarashow D: Atherosclerosis in the Masai. Am J Epidemiol 95:26–37, 1972.

Mann JI, Thorogood M: Serum lipids in young female survivors of myocardial infarction. Br Heart J 37:790–794, 1975.

Manoff RK: Potential uses of mass media in nutrition programs. J Nutr Educ 5:125–129, 1973.

Marglin SA: The social rate of discount and the optimal rate of investment. Q J Econ 77:95–112, 1963.

Margolis JR, Gillum RF, Feinleib M, Brasch R, Fabsitz R: Community surveillance for coronary heart disease: The Framingham Cardiovascular Disease Survey. Am J Cardiol 37:61–67, 1976.

Marktl W, Rudas B: Screening for risks of cardiovascular disease in children. A preliminary report. Br J Nutr 35:223–227, 1976.

Marmot MG, Syme SL, Kagan A, Kato H, Cohen JB, Belsky J: Epidemiologic studies of coronary heart disease and stroke in Japanese men living in Japan, Hawaii and California: Prevalence of coronary and hypertensive heart disease and associated risk factors. Am J Epidemiol 102:514–525, 1975.

Martin AO, Kurczynski TW, Steinberg AG: Familial studies of medical and anthropometric variables in a human isolate. Am J Hum Genet 25:581–593, 1975.

Masironi R: Dietary factors and coronary heart disease. Bull WHO 42:;103–114, 1970.

Mason JK: Asymptomatic disease of coronary arteries in young men. Br Med J 2:1234–1237, 1963.

Matanoski GM, Henderson MM, Stine O, Courpas C, Hepner R, Walker S: Evaluation of a screening program for heart disease. Am J Public Health 67:609–611, 1977.

Mathew NT, Davis D, Meyer JS, Chandar K: Hyperlipoproteinemia in occlusive cerebrovascular disease. JAMA 232:262–266, 1975.

McAlister A, Meyer A, Maccoby N: Results of a two-year health education campaign on smoking behavior: Stanford Three Community Study. Circulation 51 and 52 (suppl 2):117, 1975.

McGandy RB: Adolescence and the onset of atherosclerosis. Bull NY Acad Med 47:590–600, 1971.

McGandy RB, Hegsted DM, Stare FJ: Dietary fats, carbohydrates and atherosclerotic vascular disease. N Engl J Med 277:186–192, 242–247, 1967.

McGandy RB, Hall BH, Ford C, Stare FJ: Dietary regulation of blood cholesterol in adolescent males: A pilot study. Am J Clin Nutr 25:61–66, 1972.

McGill HC, Arias-Stella J, Carbonell LM et al: General findings of the International Atherosclerosis Project. Lab Invest 18:498–502, 1968.

McKeown T: Validation of screening procedures, in McKeown T, Butterfield WJ, Cochrane AL et al (eds): Screening in Medical Care: Reviewing the Evidence, a Collection of Essays. London: Oxford University Press, 1968.

McMillan GC: Development of arteriosclerosis. Am J Cardiol 31:542–546, 1973.

McNamara JJ, Molot MA, Stremple JF, Cutting RT: Coronary artery disease in combat casualties in Vietnam. JAMA 216:1185–1187, 1971.

McNeil BJ, Weichselbaum R, Pauker SG: Fallacy of the five-year survival in lung cancer. N Engl J Med 299:1397–1401, 1978.

Medalie JH, Kahn HA, Neufeld HN, Riss E, Goldbourt U: Five-year myocardial infarction incidence. II Association of single variables to age and birthplace. J Chronic Dis 26:329–349, 1973 (a).

Medalie JH, Kahn N, Neufeld HN, Riss E, Goldbourt U, Perlstein T, Oron D: Myocardial infarction over a five-year period. I. Prevalence, incidence and mortality experience. J Chronic Dis 26:63–84, 1973 (b).

Medalie JH, Levene C, Papier C, Goldbourt U, Dreyfuss F, Oron D, Neufeld H, Riss E: Blood groups, myocardial infarction and angina pectoris among 10,000 adult males. N Engl J Med 285:1348–1353, 1971.

Meyer AJ, Henderson JB: Multiple risk factor reduction in the prevention of cardiovascular disease. Prev Med 3:225–236, 1974.

Meyer WH: Economic and other considerations bearing on marked and rapid changes in the fat composition of the diet. Prev Med 2:337–345, 1973.

Miettinen M, Turpeinen O, Karvonen MJ, Elosuo R, Paavilainen E: Effect of cholesterol-lowering diet on mortality from coronary heart-disease and other causes. Lancet 2:835–838, 1972.

Miller GJ, Miller NE: Plasma-high-density-lipoprotein concentration and development of ischaemic heart-disase. Lancet 1:16–19, 1975.

Miller NE, Førde OH, Thelle DS, Mjos OD: The Tromso heart study: High-density lipoprotein and coronary heart disease: A prospective case-control study. Lancet 1:965–967, 1977.

Milligan CA, Wilcox EB, Galloway LS: Serum cholesterol and physical characteristics of pre-adolescents and adolescents. J Am Diet Assoc 49:309–315, 1966.

Mishan EJ: Evaluation of life and limb: A theoretical approach. Journal of Political Economy 79:687–705, 1971.

Mitchell SC: Symposium on prevention of atherosclerosis at the pediatric level, including identification of potential risks and prophylaxis. Introduction. Am J Cardiol 31:539–541, 1973.

Mitchell SC, Jesse MJ: Risk factors of coronary heart disease—their genesis and pediatric implications. Am J Cardiol 31:588–590, 1973.

Morris JN: Physical inactivity and coronary heart disease. Acta Cardiol (Brux) Suppl 20:95–103, 1974.

Morris JN, Ball KP, Antonis A et al: Controlled trial of soya-bean oil in myocardial infarction. Lancet 2:693–699, 1968.

Morris JN, Kagan A, Pattison DC, Gardner MJ, Raffle PA: Incidence and prediction of ischaemic heart-disease in London businessmen. Lancet 2:553–559, 1966.

Morris JN, Marr JW, Clayton DG: Diet and heart: A postscript. Br Med J 2:1307–1314, 1977.

Morrison JA, Kelly KA, Mellies MJ, deGroot I, Glueck CJ: Parent-child associations at upper and lower ranges of plasma cholesterol and triglyceride levels. Pediatrics 62:468–477, 1978.

Morrison LM: Reduction of mortality rate in coronary atherosclerosis by a low cholesterol-low fat diet. Am Heart J 42:538–545, 1951.

Morrison LM: Diet in coronary atherosclerosis. JAMA 173:104–108, 1960.

Motulsky AG: Current concepts in genetics. The genetic hyperlipidemias. N Engl J Med 294:823–827, 1976.

Motulsky AG, Boman H: Screening for the hyperlipidemias, in Milunsky A (ed): The Prevention of Genetic Disease and Mental Retardation. Philadelphia: W. B. Saunders, 1975.

National Center for Health Statistics: Limitations of activity due to chronic conditions. United States, 1969 and 1970. Vital and Health Statistics, series 10, no. 80, table 19. DHEW pub. no. (HSM) 73-1506. Washington, D.C.: Government Printing Office, 1973(a).

National Center for Health Statistics: Serum cholesterol levels of adults. United States, 1960–1962. Vital and Health Statistics, series 11, no. 22. Washington, D.C.: Government Printing Office, 1973 (b).

National Center for Health Statistics: Vital Statistics of the United States, 1970. Vol II: Mortality, Part A. DHEW pub. no. (HRA) 75-1101. Washington, D.C.: Government Printing Office, 1974.

National Center for Health Statistics: Utilization of short-stay hospitals, by diagnosis: United sStates, 1973. Monthly Vital Statistics Report 24 (3) supp 2. DHEW pub. no. (HRA) 75–1120. Washington, D.C.: Government Printing Office, 1975 (a).

National Center for Health Statistics: Vital Statistics of the United States, 1971. Vol II: Mortality, Part A DHEW pub. no. (HRA) 75-1114. Washington, D.C.: Government Printing Office, 1975 (b).

National Center for Health Statistics: Health United States 1976–77. DHEW pub. no. (HRA) 77-1232. Washington, D.C.: Government Printing Office, 1977 (a).

National Center for Health Statistics: Vital Statistics of the United States, 1973. Vol II: Mortality, Part A. DHEW pub. no. (HRA) 77-1101. Washington, D.C.: Government Printing Office, 1977 (b).

National Center for Health Statistics: Advance report: Final mortality statistics, 1976. Monthly Vital Statistics Report 26 (12) suppl 2. DHEW pub. no. (PHS) 78-1120. Washington, D.C.: Government Printing Office, 1978.

National Diet-Heart Study Research Group: National Diet-Heart Study final report. Circulation 37(suppl 1):1–419, 1968.

National Heart and Lung Institute, Task Force on Arteriosclerosis: Arteriosclerosis: A report. Vol 2. DHEW pub. no. (NIH) 72-219. Washington, D.C.: Government Printing Office, 1972.

Nelson AM: Treatment of atherosclerosis by diet. I. Results in patients followed from 36 to 72 months. Northwest Med 55:643–649, 1956.

Neufeld HN: Eighth Edgar Mannheimer Lecture. Studies of the coronary arteries in children and their relevance to coronary heart disease. Eur J Cardiol 1:479–489, 1974.

Neufeld HN, Medalie JH, Riss E, Goldbourt U: Selected findings of the Israeli ischemic heart disease study. Geriatrics 28:134–136, 1973.

Newhouse JP: Medical care expenditure: A cross-national survey. Rand Paper Series No. P-5608. Santa Monica: Rand Corporation, 1976.

Nichaman MZ, Hamilton HB, Kagan A, Grier T, Sacks ST, Syme SL: Epidemiologic studies of coronary heart disease and stroke in Japanese men living in Japan, Hawaii and California: Distribution of biochemical risk factors. Am J Epidemiol 102:491–501, 1975.

Nichols AB, Ravenscroft DE, Lamphier DE, Ostrander LD, Jr: Daily nutritional intake and serum lipid levels. The Tecumseh study. Am J Clin Nutr 29:1384–1392, 1976(a).

Nichols AB, Ravenscroft C, Lamphier DE, Ostrander LD Jr: Independence of serum lipid levels and dietary habits: The Tecumseh study. JAMA 236:1948–1953, 1976(b).

Nikkilä EA, Arö A: Family study of serum lipids and lipoproteins in coronary heart-disease. Lancet 1:954–959, 1973.

Nitowsky HM: Prescriptive screening for inborn errors of metabolism: A critique. Am J Ment Defic 77:538–550, 1973.

North AF: Should pediatricians be concerned about children's cholesterol levels? The disadvantages outweigh the advantages except for children from high-risk families. Clin Pediatr 14:439–444, 1975.

O'Keefe MT: The anti-smoking commercials: A study of television's impact on behavior. Public Opinion Quarterly 35:242–248, 1971.

Oliver MF: The primary prevention of ischemic heart disease by means of Atromid–S (clofibrate). Bull NY Acad Med 44:1021–1027, 1968.

Oliver MF: Ischaemic heart disease in young women. Br Med J 4:253–259, 1974.

Oliver M: Dietary cholesterol, plasma cholesterol and coronary heart disease. Br Heart J 38:214–218, 1976.

Oliver MF, Nimmo IA, Cooke M, Carlson LA, Olsson AG: Ischaemic heart disease and associated risk factors in 40 year old men in Edinburgh and Stockholm. Eur J Clin Invest 5:507–514, 1975.

Orr JD, Sing CF, Block WD: Analysis of genetic and environmental sources of variation in serum cholesterol in Tecumseh, Michigan: II. The role of education, occupation, and income. Soc Biol 22:34–43, 1975.

Paffenbarger RS Jr, Hale WE, Brand RJ, Hyde RT: Work-energy level, personal characteristics, and fatal heart attack: A birth-cohort effect. Am J Epidemiol 105:200–213, 1977.

Paffenbarger RS Jr, Notkin J, Krueger DE, Wolf PA, Thorne MC, LeBauer EJ, Williams JL: Chronic disease in former college students. II. Methods of study and observations on mortality from coronary heart disease. Am J Public Health 56:962–971, 1966.

Page LB, Damon A, Moellering RC Jr: Antecedents of cardiovascular disease in six Solomon Island societies. Circulation 49:1132–1146, 1974.

Pagnan A, Donadon W, Ferrari S, Bruni EG, Tonolli E, Palu CD: Study on the risk factors of coronary heart disease in family aggregates of Verona. G Ital Cardiol 4:249–260, 1974.

Patterson D, Slack J: Lipid abnormalities in male and female survivors of myocardial infarction and their first-degree relatives. Lancet 1:393–399, 1972.

Paul O, Lepper MH, Phelan WH, Dupertuis GW, MacMillan A, McKean H, Park H: A longitudinal study of coronary heart disease. Circulation 28:20–31, 1963.

Pazzanese D, Portugal OP, Ramos OL, Finatti AAC, Lanfranchi W, Barreto HPCB, Sustovich DR: Serum-lipid levels in a Brazilian Indian population. Lancet 2:615–617, 1964.

Pearce ML, Dayton S: Incidence of cancer in men on a diet high in polyunsaturated fat. Lancet 1:464–467, 1971.

Pelkonen R, Nikkila EA, Kiskinen S, Penttinen K, Sarna S: Association of serum lipids and obesity with cardiovascular mortality. Br Med J 2:1185–1187, 1977.

Phelps CE: Illness prevention and medical insurance. J Hum Res 13 (suppl):183–207, 1978.

Pinckney ER: The potential toxicity of excessive polyunsaturates. Do not let the patient harm himself. J Am Heart J 85:723–726, 1973.

Podell RN: The politics of health behavior: Diet and heart disease. Am Fam Physician 10:67–69, 1974.

Podell RN: Physician's Guide to Compliance in Hypertension. Summit, N.J.: Merck and Co., 1975.

Pomeranze J: Serum cholesterol studies in infants. A comparison of infants fed breast milk, evaporated milk and prepared milk formulas. Am J Clin Nutr 9:570–572, 1961.

Pomeranze J, Goalwin A, Slobody LB: The effect of a corn oil-evaporated milk mixture on serum cholesterol levels in infancy. Am J Dis Child 95:622–625, 1958.

Pomerleau O, Bass F, Crown V: Role of behavior modification in preventive medicine. N Engl J Med 292:1277–1282, 1975.

Porter RR: The contribution of the biological and medical sciences to human welfare. Presidential addresses delivered at the Swansea meeting, 1971, British Association for the Advancement of Science, London, 1971.

Powles J: On the limitations of modern medicine. Sci Med Man 1:–30, 1973.

Puska P: North Karelia Project, A Programme for Community Control of Cardiovascular Diseases. Kuopio, Finland: University of Kuopio, 1974.

Puska P, Tuomilehto J, Nissinen A, et al: Changing the cardiovascular risk in an entire community: The North Karelia Project. Paper presented to the Chicago Heart Association, October 1978.

Puska P, Tuomilehto J, Salonen J, et al: Changes in coronary risk factors during comprehensive five-year community programme to control cardiovascular diseases (North Karelia Project). Br Med J 2:1173–1178, 1979.

Reiser R: Control of adult serum cholesterol by the nutrition of the suckling: A progress report. Circulation (suppl 2):44:3, 1971.

Rhoads GG, Gulbrandsen CL, Kagan A: Serum lipoproteins and coronary heart disease in a population study of Hawaii Japanese men. N Engl J Med 294:293–298, 1976.

Rifkind BM, Levy RI: Does hypolipidemic therapy prevent coronary heart disease?, in Melmon KL (ed): Cardiovascular Drug Therapy. Philadelphia: F.A. Davis, 1974.

Rigal RD, Lovell FW, Townsend FM: Pathologic findings in the cardiovascular systems of military flying personnel. Am J Cardiol 6:19–25, 1960.

Rinzler SH: Primary prevention of coronary heart disease by diet. Bull NY Acad Med 44:936–949, 1968.

Robertson CJ: The food service industry's requirement for prudent diet foods. Prev Med 2:387–396, 1973.

Robertson TL, Kato H, Rhoads GG, et al: Epidemiologic studies of coronary heart disease and stroke in Japanese men living in Japan, Hawaii, and California. Incidence of myocardial infarction and death from coronary heart disease. Am J Cardiol 39:239–243, 1977.

Rose G: Methodology of epidemiological surveys, in de Haas JH, Hemker HC, Snellen HA (eds): Ischaemic Heart Disease. Leiden, The Netherlands: Leiden University Press, 1970.

Rose GA, Thomson WB, Williams RT: Corn oil in treatment of ischaemic heart disease. Br Med J 1:1531–1533, 1965.

Rosenman RH, Friedman M, Jenkins CD, Straus R, Wurm M, Kositchek R: Recurring and fatal myocardial infarction in the Western Collaborative Group Study. Am J Cardiol 19:771–775, 1967.

Rosenman RH, Friedman M, Straus R, Jenkins CD, Zyzanski SJ, Wurm M: Coronary heart disease in the Western Collaborative Group Study. A follow-up experience of 4½ years. J Chronic Dis 23:173–190, 1970.

Rosenstock IM: Patients' compliance with health regimens. JAMA 234:402–403, 1975.

Sackett DL: Cardiovascular diseases. Lancet 2:1189–1191, 1974.

Sackett DL, Haynes RB: Compliance with Therapeutic Regimens. Baltimore: Johns Hopkins University Press, 1976.

Sackett DL, Haynes RB, Gibson ES, Hackett RC, Taylor DW, Roberts RS, Johnson AL: Randomized clinical trial of strategies for improving medication compliance in primary hypertension. Lancet 1:1205–1207, 1975.

Sackett DL, Holland WW: Controversy in the detection of disease. Lancet 2:357–359, 1975.

Sackett DL, Winkelstein W Jr: The epidemiology of aortic and peripheral atherosclerosis. A selective review. J Chronic Dis 18:775–795, 1965.

Sacks FM, Castelli WP, Donner A, Kass EG: Plasma lipids and lipoproteins in vegetarians and controls. N Engl J Med 292:1148–1151, 1975.

St Clair RW, Clarkson TB, Lofland HB: Effects of regression of atherosclerotic lesions on the content and esterification of cholesterol by cell-free preparations of pigeon aorta. Circ Res 31:664–671, 1972.

Salel AF, Fong A, Zelis R, Miller RR, Borhani NO, Mason DT: Accuracy of numerical coronary profile. Correlation of risk factors with arteriographically documented severity of atherosclerosis. N Engl J Med 296:1447–1450, 1977.

Salonen J, Puska P, Mustaniemi H: Changes in morbidity and mortality during comprehensive community programme to control cardiovascular diseases during 1972-7 in North Karelia. Br Med J 2:1178–1183, 1979.

Savage PJ, Hamman RF, Bartha G, Dippe SE, Miller M, Bennett PH: Serum cholesterol levels in American (Pima) Indian children and adolescents. Pediatrics 58:274–282, 1976.

Schaefer LE, Adlersberg D, Steinberg AG: Heredity, environment, and serum cholesterol. A study of 201 healthy families. Circulation 17:537–542, 1958.

Schaefer LE, Drachman SR, Steinberg AG, Adlersberg D: Genetic studies on hypercholesteremia: Frequency in a hospital population and in families of hypercholesteremic index patients. Am Heart J 46:99–116, 1953.

Schilling FJ, Christakis GJ, Bennett NJ, Coyle JF: Studies of serum cholesterol in 4,244 men and women: An epidemiological and pathogenetic interpretation. Am J Public Health 54:461–476, 1964.

Schornagel HE: The connection between nutrition and mortalty from coronary sclerosis during and after World War II. Docum Med Geogr Trop 5:173–183, 1953.

Schrott HG, Goldstein JL, Hazzard WR, McGoodwin MM, Motulsky AG: Familial hypercholesterolemia in a large kindred. Evidence for a monogenic mechanism. Ann Intern Med 76:711–720, 1972.

Schubert WK: Fat nutrition and diet in childhood. Am J Cardiol 31:581–587, 1973.

Schwartz MK, Hill P: Problems in the interpretation of serum cholesterol values. Prev Med 1:167–177, 1972.

Scott RF, Florentin RA, Daoud AS, Morrison ES, Jones RM, Hutt MSR: Coronary arteries of children and young adults. A comparison of lipids and anatomic features in New Yorkers and East Africans. Exp Mol Pathol 5:12–42, 1966.

Scrimshaw NS, Balsam A, Arroyave G: Serum cholesterol levels in school children from three socio-economic groups. Am J Clin Nutr 5:629–633, 1957.

Scrimshaw NS, Guzman MS: Diet and atherosclerosis. Lab Invest 18:623–628, 1968.

Segall MM, Fosbrooke AS, Lloyd JK, Wolff OH: Treatment of familial hypercholesterolaemia in children. Lancet 1:641–644, 1970.

Sepe SJ, Levy HL, Mount FW: Follow-up screening for phenylketonuria. N Engl J Med 300:606–609, 1979.

Shanoff HM, Little JA, Csima A: Studies of male survivors of myocardial infarction. XII. Relation of serum lipids and lipoproteins to survival over a 10-year period. Can Med Assoc J 103:927–933, 1970.

Shaper AG, Jones KW: Serum cholesterol in camel-herding nomads. Lancet 2:1305–1307, 1962.

Shaper AG, Jones KW, Jones M, Kyobe J: Serum lipids in three nomadic tribes in Northern Kenya. Am J Clin Nutr 13:135–146, 1963.

Shaper AG, Marr JW: Dietary recommendations for the community towards the postponement of coronary heart disease. Br Med J 1:867–871, 1977.

Shapiro S, Strax P, Venet L, Venet W: Changes in 5-year breast cancer mortality in a breast cancer screening program, in Proceedings, American Cancer Society 7th National Cancer Conference. Philadelphia: J. B. Lippincott, 1973.

Shear CL, Frerichs RR, Weinberg R, Berenson GS: Childhood sibling aggregation of coronary artery disease risk factor variables in a biracial community. Am J Epidemiol 107:522–528, 1978.

Sholtz RI, Rosenman RH, Brand RJ: The relationship of reported parental history to the incidence of coronary heart disease in the Wester Collaborative Group Study. Am J Epidemiol 102:350–356, 1975.

Shorey RL, Sewell B, O'Brien M: Efficacy of diet and exercise in the reduction of serum cholesterol and triglyceride in free-living adult males. Am J Clin Nutr 29:512–521, 1976.

Sing CF, Chamberlain MA, Block WD, Feiler S: Analysis of genetic and environmental sources of variation in serum cholesterol in Tecumseh, Michigan. I. Analysis of the frequency distribution for evidence of a genetic polymorphism. Am J Hum Genet 27:333–347, 1975.

Sing CF, Orr JD: Analysis of genetic and environmental sources of variation in serum cholesterol in Tecumseh, Michigan. IV. Separation of polygene from common environmental effects. Am J Hum Genet 30:491–504, 1978.

Sirtori CR, Agradi E, Conti F, Mantero O, Gatti E: Soybean-protein diet in the treatment of type-II hyperlipoproteinaemia. Lancet 1:275–277, 1977.

Slack J: Risks of ischaemic heart-disease in familial hyperlipoproteinaemic states. Lancet 2:1380–1382, 1969.

Slack J. Inheritance of familial hypercholesterolemia, in Paoletti R, Gotto AM Jr (eds): Atherosclerosis Reviews, Vol 5. New York: Raven Press, 1979.

Slack J, Evans KA: The increased risk of death from ischaemic heart disease in first degree relatives of 121 men and 96 women with ischaemic heart disease. J Med Genet 3:239–257, 1966.

Slack J, Noble N, Meade TW, North WRS: Lipid and lipoprotein concentrations in 1604 men and women in working populations in north-west London. Br Med J 2:353–356, 1977.

Stamler J: Prevention of atherosclerotic coronary heart disease by change of diet and mode of life, in de Haas JH, Hemker HC, Snellen HA (eds): Ischaemic Heart Disease. Baltimore: Williams and Wilkins, 1970.

Stamler J: Acute myocardial infarction—progress in primary prevention. Br Heart J 33 (suppl):145–164, 1971.

Stamler J: Lifestyle, major risk factors, proof and public policy. Circulation 58:3–19, 1978.

Stamler J, Berkson DM: Prospects with multifactorial approaches emphasizing improvement in life style, in Holmes WL, Paoletti R, Kritchevsky D (eds): Pharmacological Control of Lipid Metabolism. New York: Plenum Press, 1972.

Stamler J, Berkson DM, Lindber HA: Risk factors: Their role in the etiology and pathogenesis of the atherosclerotic diseases, in Wissler RW, Geer JC (eds): The Pathogenesis of Atherosclerosis. Baltimore: Williams and Wilkins, 1972.

Stamler J, Stamler R, Snekelle RB: Regional differences in prevalence, incidence and mortality from atherosclerotic coronary heart disease, in de Haas JH, Hemker HC, Sneken HA (eds): Ischaemic Heart Disease. Baltimore: Williams & Wilkins, 1970.

Stange PB, Sumner AT: Predicting treatment costs and life expectancy for end-stage renal disease. N Engl J Med 298:372–378, 1978.

Stare FJ: Summary of symposium and recommendations for food industry action. Prev Med 2:407–411, 1973.

Starr P: Hypercholesterolemia in school children: A preliminary report. Am J Clin Pathol 56:512–522, 1971.

Stead EA Jr: What we have learned about myocardial infarction from epidemiologic and dietary studies. Circulation 39 and 40 (suppl 4):85–90, 1969.

Stone NF, Levy RI, Fredrickson DS, Verter J: Coronary artery disease in 116 kindred with familial type II hyperlipoproteinemia. Circulation 49:476–488, 1974.

Strøm A, Jensen RA: Mortality from circulatory disorders in Norway, 1940–1945. Lancet 1:126–129, 1951.

Strong JP, McGill HC Jr: The pediatric aspects of atherosclerosis. J Atheroscler Res 9:251–265, 1969.

Strong WB, Rao PS, Steinbaugh M: Primary prevention of atherosclerosis: a challenge to the physician caring for children. South Med J 68:319–327, 1975.

Stuart KL, Schneckloth RE, Lewis LA, Moore FE, Corcoran AC: Diet, serum cholesterol, protein, blood haemoglobin, and glycosuria in a West Indian community (St. Kitts, W.I.). With observations on ischaemic heart disease. Br Med J 2:1283–1288, 1962.

Stulb SC, McDonough JR, Greenberg BG, Hames CG: The relationship of nutrient intake and exercise to serum cholesterol levels in white males in Evans County, Georgia. Am J Clin Nutr 238–242, 1965.

Sweeney MF, Etteldorf JN, Dobbins WT, Somervill B, Fischer R, Ferrell C: Dietary fat and concentrations of lipid in the serum during the first six to eight weeks of life. Pediatrics 27:765–771, 1961.

Syme SL, Marmot MG, Kagan A, Kato H, Rhoads G: Epidemiologic studies of coronary heart disease and stroke in Japanese men living in Japan, Hawaii and California: Introduction. Am J Epidemiol 102:477–480, 1975.

Tabaqchali S, Chait A, Harrison R, Lewis B: Experience with simplified scheme of treatment of hyperlipidemia. Br Med J 3:377–380, 1974.

Tamir I, Bojanower Y, Levtow O, Heldenberg D, Dickerman Z, Werbin B: Serum lipids and lipoproteins in children from families with early coronary heart disease. Arch Dis Child 47:808–810, 1972.

Taylor GO, Barber JB, Jackson MA, Resch JA, Williams AO: Lipid composition of cerebral vessels in American Negroes, Caucasians and Nigerian Africans: A comparative study. Stroke 6:298–300, 1975.

Taylor CB, Cox GE, Manalo-Estrella P, Southworth J: Atherosclerosis in rhesus monkeys. II. Arterial lesions associated with hypercholesterolemia induced by dietary fat and cholesterol. Arch Pathol 74:16–34, 1962.

Tejada C, Strong JP, Montenegro MR, Restrepo C, Solberg LA: Distribution of coronary and aortic atherosclerosis by geographic location, race, and sex. Lab Invest 18:509–526, 1968.

Thomas LH: Mortality from arteriosclerotic disease and consumption of hydrogenated oils and fats. Br J Prev Soc Med 29:82–90, 1975.

Toor M, Katchalsky A, Agmon J, Allalouf D: Atherosclerosis and related factors in immigrants to Israel. Circulation 22:265–279, 1960.

Trowell H: Ischemic heart disease and dietary fiber. Am J Clin Nutr 25:926–932, 1972.

Truett J, Cornfield J, Kannel W: A multivariate analysis of the risk of coronary heart disease in Framingham. J Chronic Dis 20:511–524, 1967.

Trulson MF, Clancy RE, Jessop WJE, Childers RW, Stare FJ: Comparisons of siblings in Boston and Ireland. J Am Diet Assoc 45:225–229, 1964.

Tsang RC, Fallat RW, Gueck CJ: Cholesterol at birth and age 1: comparison of normal and hypercholesterolemic neonates. Pediatrics 53:458–470, 1974.

Turpeinen O: Effect of cholesterol-lowering diet on mortality from coronary heart disease and other causes. Circulation 59:1–13, 1979.

Turpeinen O, Miettinen M, Karvonen MJ, Roine P, Pekkarinen M, Lehtosuo EJ, Alivirta P: Dietary prevention of coronary heart disease: Long-term experiment. I. Observations on male subjects. Am J Clin Nutr 21:255–276, 1968.

Tyroler HA, Heyden S, Bartel A, Cassel J, Cornoni JC, Hames CG, Kleinbaum D: Blood pressure and cholesterol as coronary heart disease risk factors. Arch Intern Med 128:907–914, 1971.

Vartiainen I: War/time and mortality in certain disease in Finland. Ann Med Intern Fenn 35:234–240, 1946.

Vesselinovitch D, Wissler RW, Fisher-Dzoga K, Hughes R, Dubien L: Regression of atherosclerosis in rabbits. Part 1. Treatment with low-fat diet, hyperoxia and hypolipidemic agents. Atherosclerosis 19:259–275, 1974.

Wagner WD, St Clair RW, Clarkson TB: Atherosclerosis regression in rhesus monkeys at plasma cholesterol levels achievable in man. Fed Proc 35:293, 1976.

Walker GR, Morse EH, Overley VA: The effect of animal protein and vegetable protein diets having the same fat content on the serum lipid levels of young women. J Nutr 72:317–321, 1960.

Walker WJ: Changing United States life-style and declining vascular mortality: Cause or coincidence? N Engl J Med 297:163–165, 1977.

Warner KE: The effects of the anti-smoking campaign on cigarette consumption. Am J Public Health 67:640–650, 1977.

Weidman WH, Elveback LR, Nelson RA, Hodgson PA, Ellefson RD: Nutrient intake and serum cholesterol in children. Pediatrics 61:354–359, 1978.

Weinstein MC, Fineberg HV: Cost-effectiveness analysis for medical practices: Appropriate laboratory utilization, in Benson ES, Rubin M (eds): Logic and Economics of Clinical Laboratory Use. New York: Elsevier North-Holland, 1978.

Weinstein MC, Stason WB: Hypertension: A Policy Perspective. Cambridge: Harvard University Press, 1976.

Weinstein MC, Stason WB: Foundations on cost-effectiveness analysis for health and medical practices. N Engl J Med 296:716–721, 1977.

Whyte HM: Potential effect on coronary-heart-diseae morbidity of lowering the blood-cholesterol. Lancet 1:906–910, 1975.

Whyte HM: The relative importance of the major risk factors in atherosclerotic and other diseases. Aust NZ J Med 6:387–393, 1976.

Whyte HM, Yee IL: Serum cholesterol levels of Australians and natives of New Guinea from birth to adulthood. Aust Ann Med 7:336–339, 1958.

Williams CL, Wynder EL: A blind spot in preventive medicine. JAMA 236:2196–2197, 1976.

Wilson JM, Jungner G: Principles of screenng for diseases. Public Health Papers No. 34, 1968.

Wilson WS, Hulley SB, Burrows MI, Nichaman MZ: Serial lipid and lipoprotein responses to the American Heart Association's fat-controlled diet. Am J Med 51:491–503, 1971.

Wissler RW, Hughes RH, Frazier LE, Getz GS, Turner DF: Aortic lesions and blood lipids in rhesus monkeys fed "table prepared" human diets. Circulation 32 (suppl 2):220–221, 1965 (abstract).

Wissler RW: Recent progress in studies of experimental primate atherosclerosis. Prog Biochem Parmacol 4:378–392, 1968.

Witte JJ: Recent advances in public health: Immunization. Am J Public Health 64:939–944, 1974.

Wood PDS, Stern MP, Silvers A, Reaven GM, von der Groeben J: Prevalence of plasma lipoprotein abnormalities in a free-living population of the Central Valley, California. Circulation 45:114–126, 1972.

Woodruff CW, Bailey MC, Davis JT, Rogers N, Coniglio JG: Serum lipids in breast-fed infants and in infants fed evaporated milk. Am J Clin Nutr 14:83–90, 1964.

World Health Organiztion. Mass health examinations. Public Health Paper No. 45, 1971.

Worth RM, Kato H, Rhoads GG, Kagan A, Syme SL: Epidemiologic studies of coronary heart disease and stroke in Japanese men living in Japan, Hawaii and California: Mortality. Am J Epidemiol 102:481–490, 1975.

Wright IS: Cardiovascular disease—unanswered questions. Problems that require intensive study and planning or basic or applied research. Circulation 47:A341–A357, 1973.

Younger RK, Scott WH Jr, Butts WH, Stephenson SE Jr: Rapid production of experimental hypercholesterolemia and atherosclerosis in the rhesus monkey: Comparison of five dietary regimens. J Surg Res 9:263–271, 1969.

Index